PROSTATE CANCER

Also by Professor Jane Plant

YOUR LIFE IN YOUR HANDS: UNDERSTAND,
PREVENT AND OVERCOME BREAST CANCER AND
OVARIAN CANCER

With Gill Tidey

THE PLANT PROGRAMME

UNDERSTANDING, PREVENTING AND OVERCOMING
OSTEOPOROSIS

EATING FOR BETTER HEALTH

PROSTATE CANCER

Understand, Prevent and Overcome

Professor Jane A. Plant

www.janeplant.com

This edition published in Great Britain in 2007 by
Virgin Books Ltd
Thames Wharf Studios
Rainville Road
London W6 9HA

First published in hardback in Great Britain in 2004
by Virgin Books Ltd

A catalogue record for this book is available from
the British Library.

ISBN 978 0 7535 1298 2

The paper used in this book is a natural, recyclable product
made from wood grown in sustainable forests.
The manufacturing process conforms to the regulations of the
country of origin.

Typeset by TW Typesetting, Plymouth, Devon
Printed in the UK by CPI Bookmarque, Croydon CR0 4TD

1 3 5 7 9 10 8 6 4 2

CONTENTS

AUTHOR'S NOTE

The diagnosis and treatment of medical conditions is a responsibility shared between you and your medical advisors. All diets should begin with a medical check-up to make certain that no special health problems exist and to confirm that there are no medical reasons why you should not undertake a change of diet.

ACKNOWLEDGEMENTS

I would like to thank my husband Peter Simpson for his support and practical help with the book and my children Emma and Tom for their help and encouragement. I would also like to thank Professor Jonathan Waxman from Imperial College for his help, especially with Chapter 1. I am most grateful to Henry Haslam for his assistance with the book and Rebecca McKinlay for her many helpful suggestions and references.

WELCOME

It is now 14 years since my breast-cancer secondaries disappeared following a fundamental change in my diet and lifestyle. My cancer had spread to the lymph nodes in my neck, in spite of radical mastectomy, three further operations, 35 radiotherapy treatments, irradiation of my ovaries to induce the menopause and several chemotherapy treatments. Despite all this treatment, my doctors had given me only months to live. I then recalled that people in rural China, where I had worked as a scientist, had a very low incidence of breast (and prostate) cancer. At that point I changed my diet and lifestyle, and to everyone's amazement, including, I have to admit, my own, the large cancerous lump in my neck disappeared within weeks.

Since that time I have not even had a scare, and my annual check-ups at Charing Cross Hospital have tended to focus more on my diet and lifestyle than on my cancer.

I have talked to senior doctors who have said that they personally have not met anyone who has survived such serious illness and had been very sceptical about my books until they had talked to me.

My experience, and that of many other women who had followed my diet and lifestyle, led me to write *Your Life in Your Hands*,[1] which was published in 2000, followed in 2001 by *The Plant Programme* and in 2005 by *Eating for Better Health*, written with Gill Tidey, cookbooks which complement the dietary advice in *Your Life in Your Hands*.[2]

In the first edition of *Your Life in Your Hands* I gave some information about prostate cancer because whenever and wherever I looked for information on breast cancer the same factors kept emerging as factors for prostate cancer too. I therefore included the data and information about prostate cancer in the book – and I included more in the second edition, published in September 2003. This book develops that work further and provides up-to-date science-based information specifically for prostate cancer sufferers.

I now help to run a website, www.cancersupportinterna tional.com, to provide information and support to cancer sufferers; this includes a forum for people to discuss their experiences of their illness, treatments, diet and lifestyle. From the many communications we receive from men and women who have complemented their conventional medical treatment with the Plant Programme dietary and lifestyle factors, I know that many people are now healthy and cancer-free. Indeed, when I attend functions these days I am always surprised by the number of men who come bounding up to me and the first thing they want to tell me is how good their test results are now that they follow my recommended diet and lifestyle!

Since the first edition of *Your Life in Your Hands* was published in 2000, more and more scientific evidence has appeared to support its findings and recommendations. It is perhaps worth noting that, despite the press seizing on one or two of the most sensational recommendations of the book – eliminating dairy produce and reducing exposure to hormone-disrupting and hormone-mimicking chemicals – there were seven food factors and five lifestyle factors to be addressed – there are now eight and eight, respectively, for prostate cancer.

Examples of new supporting evidence include the results of studies conducted by eminent researchers that show the link between prostate cancer and high dairy and calcium intake. There is also more and more evidence that the disease is associated with high circulating levels of a chemical messenger in the body called IGF-I and new evidence that this is linked to food factors identified in *Your Life in Your Hands*, especially high dietary intakes of dairy produce, as well as trans-fatty acids and refined carbohydrate and low dietary intakes of vegetables and fruit.

Also, there is further evidence of the importance of the correct balance of oils in the diet, as well as increasing evidence against consuming man-made vitamins and minerals, including mega-doses of vitamin C or calcium. Evidence of the association of carcinogenic chemicals such as those in pesticides and prostate cancer also continues to mount.

The reason all the recently published science has confirmed the findings and recommendations in my books and shown them to be so soundly based is not because I am clairvoyant or indeed particularly clever. It is simply because both books are based on research into the peer-reviewed scientific literature. Because of my scientific training, I am able to read information in publications written in the sort of scientific shorthand that all scientists tend to use to communicate with other specialists in their field, and translate it into simple straightforward English that makes it accessible to a wider readership. I am also able to recognise biased studies funded by vested interest groups such as the dairy or pharmaceutical industries. The extent to which medical practice is influenced by vested-interest groups is something that many others, including the *British Medical Journal* (*BMJ*), now take very seriously. The *BMJ* now requires that authors of any paper published by them should declare the funding sources of their study or other potential conflicts of interest. For this reason, many of the references in this book are from the *BMJ*. There is also concern about bias and misinformation in relation to our food. In *Save Yourself from Breast Cancer*,[3] Robert D Kradjian, head of the breast-surgery division at the Seton Medical Centre, Daly City, California, states the problem as follows:

The issue is clear. Much of our highly varied, desired, and profitable food supply has been found to be dangerous. The people who furnish this food and who are enriched by its sale do not want you to know this. They have generously contributed to scientists who have supported, and are willing to continue to support, their products. If those scientists suddenly have a change of heart, and seriously challenge the safety of that food, you may be certain that the bulk of the food-industry financial support will promptly disappear.

Whom are you going to believe? Those with no financial gain from the sale of food and with the backing of the world's scientific literature? Or are you going to follow those who have at times devised flawed studies and reaped millions of dollars in support of the industries that they fail to seriously criticise? You must decide, and your health will be substantially determined by your decision.

Happily, many medical professionals and scientists have been supportive of my work, and in 2005 I was given Life Fellowship of the Royal Society of Medicine. I am aware that many doctors are now recommending my books to their prostate-cancer and breast-cancer patients. Indeed, the recommendations have been found to be helpful to sufferers of many other types of cancer including colorectal cancer. Increasingly, I am invited to address medical societies and cancer support groups, with very positive feedback.

Perhaps it's worth mentioning that the diet will NOT cause osteoporosis. Quite the reverse. The book *Understanding, Preventing and Overcoming Osteoporosis*,[4] which I wrote with Gill Tidey, provides the scientific evidence that this disease, like breast cancer and prostate cancer, is strongly linked to the Western diet and has an extremely low incidence in countries such as China. The osteoporosis book contains many more delicious, healthy recipes which complement those in *The Plant Programme* and *Eating for Better Health*, and it is particularly helpful to those concerned about cancer spreading to their bones or who are taking medication that can cause bone thinning.

Prostate cancer is a serious illness: it is already the commonest type of male cancer in the USA, having increased by nearly 200 per cent between 1950 and 2001, and it is fast overtaking lung cancer as the number one cancer in men in most Western countries: in some countries death rates from it have trebled over the last thirty years. Conventional risk factors such as family history totally fail to account for the massive increase in the rates of prostate cancer.

Prostate cancer can cause incontinence and impotence, and some aspects and types of diagnosis and treatment can be unpleasant, with damaging short-term and long-term side effects. No man would want to go through all this unless it is essential.[5] This is definitely a disease for which prevention is better than cure, and one of the main messages of this book is . . . prevention

... prevention ... prevention. The book is packed with information to help to prevent prostate problems; and many men tell me that having followed the advice that it contains they no longer have to go to the loo several times a night so they sleep better, that their sex lives have improved and for those having regular PSA tests that the levels have fallen and they no longer have to worry about their results.

For a long time, the disease, unlike breast cancer, was surrounded by silence, but recently it has moved more into the public domain.[6] The fact that it is now talked about more openly has been helped by high-profile men such as former Mayor Giuliani of New York and the former Archbishop of Cape Town, Desmond Tutu, being prepared to admit publicly to having prostate cancer. Nevertheless, many men continue to bury their heads in the sand when, by making the simple dietary and lifestyle changes described in this book, they could cut their risk of ever suffering from the disease dramatically.

This new edition of the book also aims to bring you the most up-to-date scientific information on treatment. I look first at new developments in the conventional medical diagnosis and treatment of prostate cancer – though even screening and diagnosis are controversial, which is one of the reasons the disease is such a problem. Many men have only non-malignant but enlarged prostates; others have very slow-growing cancer, which could continue for ten or fifteen years before any treatment is really needed; while yet others have more aggressive disease.

I describe what cancer is in simple, unscary language and show that, instead of it involving some terrifying invasion of our bodies, it is simply our own cells behaving badly in conditions that encourage them to lose control.

I go on to describe some of the latest research findings into growth factors and hormone-disrupting and hormone-mimicking substances in our food, drink and environment, which I believe are responsible for the dramatic increase in prostate cancer throughout the West. I take forward the debate on chemopreventive substances in our diet and I provide simple, practical advice on how to reduce your risk of suffering from prostate cancer – advice that will also help to treat the disease in those already affected. I also look again at the politics of the problem, such as links between the pharmaceutical industry and medical clinicians, and the failure of the press to root out bias and flawed science funded by vested interest groups such as the dairy industry.

In each chapter I explain fully all the science and its implications and at the end of chapters 2 to 6 I summarise the main points 'in a nutshell' to help to make the arguments easier to follow. The scientific references on which the book is based are also included, should you or your doctor wish to follow them up.

Finally, I should like to reassure readers that I wrote this book in my own time, with no funding or influence from any vested-interest group, and that I have tried to ensure that the science on which it is based is, to the best of my knowledge, objective, authoritative and as free as possible from commercial, political or other such influences.

I hope very much that you can put the information in this new book on prostate cancer to the best possible use in your life.

Sincerely,

Professor Jane A Plant CBE, FRSM, FRSE, FRSA, FRGS, BSc (Geochemistry: Class 1), PhD, D Univ, DSc (Hon), DSc (Hon), FIMMM, CEng, FGS, CGeol, Freeman of the City of London

(I am not normally someone who uses titles. Everyone I know quickly calls me just 'Jane' and that is how I like to be addressed. However, I am a scientist and this book is based on what I believe to be sound science, so I include here my academic and professional qualifications and honours in order to reassure you, the reader, of my scientific credentials.)

1. PROBLEMS WITH THE PROSTATE?

In this chapter, I explain why, as a natural scientist, my approach to the problem of prostate cancer is different from that of many orthodox medical researchers. I then go on to examine the orthodox approach to prostate cancer. I review the conventional risk factors for the disease, the value and reliability of different diagnostic tests, the advantages and disadvantages of the various treatment options that are now available . . . and much, much more. I include brief case histories of three of the many men who are in touch with me about their disease after reading my first book, Your Life in Your Hands.¹ *By observing what has happened to all of them, I am convinced that the best outcome is achieved if the conventional medical treatments described in this chapter are combined with the dietary and lifestyle advice given later in the book.*

I t was my hope that my first book, *Your Life in Your Hands*, would serve two purposes. First, I wanted it to be directly useful to other people. I wanted to make the information I had access to as a scientist available to them as simple, straightforward advice, told in the context of my own story – a detective story which centred on my own breast cancer, the findings of which, I believe, saved my life. In this book I hope to do the same for men affected by prostate cancer, using my experience of helping many men to overcome their disease since *Your Life in Your Hands* was first published.

The straightforward advice and simple lifestyle suggestions described here will, I hope, be of practical benefit to men, in significantly reducing their risk of developing prostate cancer or other prostate disease. If you happen to be that one man in about 14 in the UK or one man in about 6 in the USA who has been diagnosed with prostate cancer, then you will also find much information here which will give you a better chance of survival and help you to cope with the rigorous treatment methods.

Secondly, it is vitally important that this book should take forward the debate within the scientific and medical communities – a debate that was ignited by *Your Life in Your Hands*. Science is, at heart, an adversarial process. This new book on prostate cancer backs up the evidence and hypotheses on the cause of the disease with the mounting evidence from the scientific literature on factors which promote it, especially the most dangerous form of the disease – metastatic prostate cancer. The inescapable conclusion is that the disease is almost entirely preventable and that relatively small augmentations to the orthodox medical therapies currently being used in clinics and hospitals would result in major improvements in patient survival. Providing prostate-cancer patients with sound dietary advice, as is common in cases of heart disease or diabetes, could greatly increase survival rates. Prostate cancer appears to be a particularly cruel disease, and I believe that so much suffering could be prevented, and so many lives could be saved, if the new evidence I have compiled in this book is acted on.

HOW ON EARTH CAN A NATURAL SCIENTIST CONTRIBUTE TO PREVENTING AND TREATING PROSTATE CANCER?

I am trained in a subject called geochemistry – a combination of geology and chemistry aimed at understanding the chemistry of the Earth. My speciality is in understanding the chemistry of the surface of the Earth, especially concentrations of chemicals where these occur either as natural concentrations in ore deposits or as a result of man's activity, for example, where there are landfill sites or contaminated land. When I studied this subject at university I had no idea how useful it would be in helping to deal with problems of human health (especially in developing countries), agricultural animals, and the environment generally.

I have frequently worked with biochemists, veterinarians, epidemiologists and medical geographers looking at the impact of chemicals in the environment on the health of humans, animals and crops. Early in my career, between 1975 and 1977, I served on a Royal Society committee concerned with geochemistry and health.[2] Since that time, I and my team of scientists at the British Geological Survey (BGS), often working in collaboration with Imperial College, London, where I am now a professor, became concerned with a wide range of human health problems related to the environment. Some of the methods we developed allow highly reproducible, high-resolution maps showing the distribution of chemicals over the Earth's surface to be prepared. We are then able to look on our computer screens at the distribution of, say, cadmium or lead (as potentially toxic chemical elements) or copper or cobalt (elements essential to animal and human health in trace amounts) in the same way people can look at the Earth's physiography – using remotely sensed photographs from space.[3] Almost from the beginning, and initially to our great surprise, these images, although intended for geologists, especially those exploring for metalliferous mineral deposits, created a lot of interest from veterinarians, who found them helpful in diagnosing environmental and nutritional animal diseases. For example, the veterinarians had an experimental farm to identify the levels of copper needed as a supplement in the diets of sheep and cattle in the north of Scotland. They could not understand why, when they gave the copper supplements developed on this farm to animals elsewhere, the animals quickly showed symptoms of copper poisoning. When they saw the maps we had produced, all became clear: their experimental farm contained soils with very high concentrations of another trace element, molybdenum, which blocks the uptake of copper, so the copper supplements they had developed contained far too much copper for general use. Seeing the natural variation in these two elements helped them to work out more appropriate doses of copper and other trace elements in relation to the natural variability of the soil. It was by working with veterinarians that I first began to learn of some of the amazing connections between geochemistry and biochemistry. I also learned, when I was ill, that veterinary was often better than medical literature in providing fundamental answers based on biochemistry. Eventually, I established a team that is regarded as one of the best in the world in tackling health problems related to the levels of trace elements in the environment: some elements such as arsenic and fluoride can occur at levels so high that they cause disease, such as cancer or severe bone deformity respectively, while others such as selenium, iodine, zinc and cobalt can occur at such low levels that they cause deficiency and ill health in man and animals. This is a particular problem in developing countries if the diet consists predominantly of locally grown crops and the underlying rocks are abnormally rich or depleted in particular chemical elements.

Very recent work that the BGS team has conducted includes studies of iodine deficiency and fluoride toxicity. The latter can lead to severe bone deformity and may be caused by the burning of poor-quality coals (in parts of China, for example) or by the presence of naturally high levels of fluoride in drinking water.[4]

What I learned as a result of this type of environmental detective work, time and time again, was that until you identified the fundamental cause of such problems, there was little or nothing that could be done to help the affected individuals. And until you've found the cause (whether it's of prostate cancer or any other disease) and effectively neutralised it, then you can never claim to have 'cured' the problem.

HOW SCIENCE SERVES US – AND WHY SOMETIMES IT DOESN'T

A good scientist will see things a little bit differently. As a science 'insider', I'd like to tell you something about the way that science works, which will help you to make sense of the approaches that scientists from different disciplines adopt when trying to treat diseases such as cancer. Also why any good scientist will want to probe, and know *why* something such as a disease has occurred.

I also want to look at why, despite vast expenditure, we have made so little progress against cancers such as those of the prostate.

There is a word to explain this situation, which also sums up what has happened to many branches of science in recent decades. This word, which is increasingly used pejoratively, is reductionism.

Let me quote from David Horrobin's article 'Not in the Genes', published in the *Guardian* on 12 February 2003, shortly before his death. Dr Horrobin was a prestigious medical researcher and author of more than 800 papers. In the *Guardian* article he states:

> Starting in the 1960s, molecular biologists and genome specialists took over biomedical science. Journals and grant-giving bodies came to be dominated by reductionists, who were scathing about the complexity of the whole organ, whole animal and especially whole human studies which were seen as too full of uncontrolled variability to be interpretable. Now we have an almost wholly reductionist biomedical community which repeatedly makes exaggerated claims about how it is going to revolutionise medical treatment, and which repeatedly fails to achieve anything.

For some time this reductionist approach dominated my own subject of earth sciences in the UK, and it is difficult to think of any memorable scientific breakthrough from that period. We have now returned to a systems-based approach, whereby all the Earth's complex interactions and feedbacks are taken into account to understand likely outcomes. We now grandly refer to our new approach as Earth Systems Science. In fact there is nothing new, except that the establishment now accept it again. As that great natural scientist James Lovelock explains in *Gaia: the practical science of planetary medicine*, published in 1991, 'To understand the physiology of the Earth as a whole system we need science, but it must grow from the top down as well as from the bottom up!' This was not the case in much of the earth sciences in the UK at the time.

Of course reductionist science is vital. It provides the pieces of the jigsaw, but too great a reliance on reductionism can lead to not being able to see the wood for the trees.

Reductionist science produces masses and masses of data. This is, in fact, a serious problem with science in general today: too many people are providing too much information, yet too few people have time to read and digest it. Sometimes scientists are repeating the same work without knowing about it. What happens to all the data this work generates? Well, it gets published in learned journals, helping to create scientists' reputations, and wins more funding for yet more research. But how much of this work is directly beneficial to cancer patients? Disappointingly little, I fear.

A better balance is needed, with more of the sort of science that involves analysing, synthesising or reviewing the work of others – putting the pieces of the jigsaw together. This is now highly unfashionable. It is thought not to be creative and not to provide the original cutting-edge ideas that 'bottom-up' science produces. Hence there are few prizes or distinctions for scientists carrying out such tasks and it is difficult for them to find sources of funding. Also, review papers are generally not welcomed by the prestigious research journals and they count for little on the CVs of individual scientists.

The implied aim of reductionist science in cancer research is to find the single 'magic bullet'. Modern medical research in general, and especially cancer research, is aimed at trying to find a pure form of a chemical compound which has a clearly defined chemical formula, can be administered in quantitative doses, and can be shown in statistically designed clinical studies to have a significant and reproducible effect on the outcome of the disease. This approach falls under the worthy-sounding title of 'evidence-based medicine' and is discussed further in Chapter 7.

But what if such a magic bullet doesn't exist?

What if our belief in magic bullets is just that – magical, illusory, not based in reality? In that case, no amount of scientific research and no amount of expenditure will ever find it. We will have wasted many fortunes, many decades and many lives for little or nothing.

In the meantime, we are left with surgery, radiotherapy and chemotherapy – albeit improved and refined – as the main front-line treatments against prostate cancer, as they have been since the 1950s, together with hormone-based methods. True, there have been small improvements in survival, but the reported incidence of prostate cancer continues to rise (*see* Chapter 3, p. 114). If I am feeling at my most cynical, I cannot help thinking how this must be the best of all possible worlds for those involved in 'the cancer industry'. This is discussed further in Chapter 7.

Too great an emphasis on a reductionist approach towards cancer research also, sooner or later, runs into the law of diminishing returns, whereby we have to spend more and more to achieve less and less. That's why all the cancer charities you know seem to have an inexhaustible appetite for money and why many of them are the best-funded charities in existence. In *Your Life in*

Your Hands, I complained that the only message we all seem to receive loud and clear is: 'Give us another billion or so, and give us another decade ... and then we may finally have a cure that works.' A few years ago, when I was listening to the BBC, I heard the then new Head of the Medical Research Council in the UK ask for a substantial increase in government funding to take forward [reductionist] medicine. In this way, he said, many chronic illnesses would be treatable in *twenty years time*!

Even if a cure were identified, would we be able to afford to prescribe it to cancer sufferers? The National Health Service in the UK is already in serious difficulty because of the cost of prescribing expensive new cancer drugs.

The high-technology approach to developing drugs for cancer is leading to many new drugs which are extremely expensive – which are then strongly marketed, often directly to patients via the World Wide Web or sometimes using patients to make emotional appeals through the media – although they may prolong life for only a few weeks or months and have unfortunate side effects. Hence there are increasingly highly charged emotional debates between individual patients and their families who, understandably, wish to have the latest treatment, and health authorities and organisations that find it difficult to justify the large aggregated bills for groups of patients for marginal benefit. Is this approach really helpful except in the very short term?

The modern era in cancer research really began in America more than thirty years ago when President Richard Nixon proclaimed 'war' on cancer in his State of the Union address in 1971. And, right from the beginning, it was dominated by reductionist scientific thinking, with its requirement for large-scale funding, extracted with the beguiling promise of a cure 'just round the corner'. 'Many people anticipated swift victory' recounts the news magazine *US News & World Report*, 'with the taming of the dread disease likened to a moon landing. Even as recently as 1984, the National Cancer Institute's director predicted that cancer deaths could be halved by the year 2000 in America.'

Such optimism was, of course, unjustified. Despite massive expenditure, the cancer death rate has continued to rise inexorably, and is now predicted by the World Health Organisation (WHO) to double worldwide by 2020.[5]

Certainly, there have been some success stories: for example, childhood cancers, particularly some leukaemias, can now be treated and cured effectively. But such bright spots are too few and far between. Moreover, what most people really want is primary prevention. As Jane Stephenson, Chair of the UK Breast Cancer Coalition, states 'For us it is not just gaining access to the best treatments available. It is about not getting cancer in the first place.'

So what, you may be wondering, is the alternative to relying so heavily on reductionist science? And is it any more effective in delivering tangible benefits to ordinary people?

Let me give you a couple of examples to explain how really significant medical breakthroughs have been made in the past with minimal resources but with great intellect and flair and a large measure of common sense. Most doctors would agree that the greatest contribution to all mankind in overcoming infectious diseases came not from the use of antibiotics but from improvements to public health: a clean water supply, improved sanitation, better nutrition and proper housing. These improvements came about as we gradually increased our understanding of why and how infectious diseases were transmitted. An early example of this type of work was carried out by Dr John Snow, who showed the value of studying the pattern of occurrence of disease. He made the famous dot map that showed the location of deaths from the epidemic of cholera which occurred in central London in September 1854. Deaths were marked by dots and, in addition, the area's eleven water pumps were located by crosses. Examining the scatter over the surface of the map, Snow observed that cholera occurred almost entirely among those who lived near (and drank from) the Broad Street water pump. He had the handle of the contaminated pump removed, ending the neighbourhood epidemic which had taken more than 500 lives. This 'scientific detective work' is called epidemiology – literally the study of epidemics – and it has been used successfully many times to identify the cause of disease and, through public-health medicine, to correct the things that society was doing wrong.

Professor Sir Richard Doll's epidemiological study of lung cancer in the 1950s was one of the most significant advances in understanding cancer in the twentieth century. Doll demonstrated beyond any shadow of a doubt the relationship between lung cancer and smoking tobacco. Lung cancer was shown not to be a curse visited on us by a wrathful God, nor to occur because of bad or faulty genes, but rather to be caused by something human beings were doing to themselves. For the first time we had a modern rationale and scientific understanding of the cause of a common type of cancer. Following Doll's work, we can now choose whether to smoke or not in the knowledge that by doing so we shall significantly increase our risk of getting lung cancer. Moreover, identifying the cause of lung cancer has led to people quitting the habit, approximately halving the death rate from the disease.[6] Since that time, rational explanations have been found for many other types of cancers. For example, mesothelioma – a type of chest-wall cancer – is now known to be caused by exposure to asbestos dust, skin cancer to be caused by exposure to ultraviolet light or arsenic poisoning, and cervical cancer is known to be caused by infection by the sexually transmitted human papilloma (wart) virus. In all of these cases the risk of cancer ever developing can be minimised by lifestyle changes as individuals or as a society.

Many doctors tend to see non-communicable diseases like prostate cancer as simply an inevitable result of ageing. For example, a recent article in the *British Medical Journal* (*BMJ*) spoke of '. . . the growing burden of non-communicable disease – in both developed and developing countries – as a consequence of population ageing. Cardiovascular disease, cancer, neuropsychiatric conditions, and injury are fast becoming the leading causes of disability and premature death in most regions.'[7] There is no mention in the article of the influence of 'Western diet and lifestyle' or other possible underlying causes of non-communicable diseases. According to this line of reasoning, age is a primary cause of cancer. I, for one, think this is far too simplistic.

Before we proceed, let me tell you a little more about the scientific method and the way I was trained to approach problems. This involves five stages:

1. **Gather existing information.** Previous facts and theories are reviewed as objectively and impartially, but as critically, as possible.
2. **Produce new information.** This is collected by experiment or observations, without emotional involvement. In some cases

new ideas are produced by analysis and synthesis of information produced by other scientists. To be a good scientist you must be prepared to admit you are wrong: arriving at the truth is what is important, not personal prestige. If you raise a question, even if you arrive at the wrong answer, you will be respected if you work with honesty and openness. At the beginning of my science career, I learned a saying that has always stayed with me and guided my work: 'the person who asks the questions solves the problem'.

3. **Evaluate.** The new results are evaluated in relation to existing theories, and new insights or ideas are identified.

4. **A new hypothesis is proposed.** Speculation must be identified as such and clearly separated from facts.

5. **Test the hypothesis.** If the hypothesis works, submit it for further testing and validation until you have a new theory. If it doesn't work, begin again.

The characteristic values to which scientists have traditionally aspired are:[8]

- Honest experimentation
- Meticulous respect for evidence
- Candid admission of mistakes or error
- Pursuit of truth
- Moral and intellectual independence of all political authority and economic power
- Openness to the public scrutiny of research by one's peers. (You will see that throughout the book I use the term 'peer reviewed' to indicate science published after it has been critically reviewed by other scientists. This type of information is distinguished from newspaper reports and other sources of information.)

This logical and ethical framework has been successfully used by scientists (whether they realised it or not) for centuries. It is how I and my team have successfully solved many human health problems related to environmental factors, and it is precisely how I approached the challenge of my own breast cancer and also prostate cancer.

There is a wealth of research – some of which goes back many decades – on the factors involved in prostate cancer. As you read the chapters that follow, I am sure you will be just as astonished as I was initially to learn how much has been discovered already but has not reached the public. While it is true that some of the risk factors for prostate cancer – such as increasing age or a family history of prostate cancer – are completely outside our control, there are many other risk factors which we can control – easily. These 'controllable' risk factors readily translate into simple changes that all men can make in their day-to-day lives to help prevent or treat the disease.

My message is: even advanced cancer can be overcome.

I know, because I've done it – and I have helped many, many prostate-cancer (and breast-cancer) sufferers to do the same.

RISK FACTORS

A risk factor is something that increases your chance of getting cancer. Different cancers have different risk factors. For example, smoking is a risk factor for cancers of the lung, mouth, larynx, bladder, kidney and some other organs.

But having a risk factor, or even several, does not mean that you will automatically develop cancer. Some men who have one or more prostate-cancer risk factors never develop the disease, while many men with prostate cancer have no known risk factors.

According to the University of Michigan website, the following are the key known risk factors for prostate cancer in the USA:

- **Age.** Prostate cancer is found mainly in men over age 55. The average age of patients at the time of diagnosis is 70. In the UK, the average age at diagnosis of prostate cancer is 72.[9]
- **Family history of prostate cancer.** A man's risk for developing prostate cancer is higher if his father or brother has had the disease.
- **Race.** This disease is much more common in African American men than in white men. It is less common in Asian, African and native American men.

Scientists have studied (see below) whether benign prostatic hyperplasia (BPH), obesity, lack of exercise, smoking,[10] radiation exposure, or a sexually transmitted virus might increase the risk for prostate cancer. At the present time, there is little hard validated evidence that these factors contribute to an increased risk.

In the UK, the following risk factors for prostate cancers have been suggested:

Factor	Variable
Demographic	Increasing age
	Place of residence
Genetic	Family history of prostate cancer
	Family history of breast cancer
	Race – black
Dietary	High fat consumption
	Low green-vegetable consumption
Occupational	Cadmium exposure
	Radiation exposure
	Farming

Source: Factsheet 20.3 1994 (Cancer of the Prostate) of the Cancer Research Campaign, adapted from Dearnaley, DP, 1994. Cancer of the prostate. *BMJ*, 308, 780–784.

These are fairly standard risk factors, and smoking and sedentary lifestyle are also included on the websites of some charities.

One authority, Professor Jonathan Waxman of Imperial College, London, a distinguished oncologist specialising in prostate treatment,[11] indicates that the Chinese diet is protective, and he attributes this to the consumption of yellow beans (even though I have worked in China, I am not sure what these are: perhaps he is referring to soya beans).

I am impressed that dietary and lifestyle factors are mentioned in the factsheet above, by many other prostate cancer charities and by Professor Waxman; I have yet to see such factors included in discussions of breast cancer Indeed as soon as dietary and lifestyle factors are mentioned in relation to breast cancer, somebody from a breast cancer charity can almost be guaranteed to try to undermine the findings, however eminent the researcher or however sound the research (see further in Chapter 7). Do these people not understand that multifactorial diseases can be prevented and treated by eliminating controllable risk factors? (See further in Chapter 3.)

Why me?

One of the first questions that I think everyone asks when they are diagnosed with cancer is 'Why me? Why has this awful thing happened to me?' Eventually, I believe I found the answer to this question for breast-cancer and prostate-cancer sufferers, and it is very disquieting, because it brings home the high risk that people living a Western lifestyle are taking – a risk that increases more and more each year, despite the fact that, like me, most of the sufferers I know thought they were living a healthy lifestyle.

Prostate cancer rates have increased dramatically since the 1970s, more than doubling in the USA between 1973 and 2000.[12] Throughout the West, prostate cancer is now one of the most commonly occurring cancers affecting men. In the UK, for example, it is the commonest cancer in men, with a lifetime risk of being diagnosed of 1 in 14; it is rare under the age of 50.[13] In the US, it is the most commonly diagnosed cancer among men, with a lifetime risk of 1 in 6; one man there loses his life to the disease every 20 minutes.[14]

No man living a Western lifestyle should be surprised, therefore, to be one of those affected. The odds are high. However, what struck me very forcibly when I first became aware of these figures was the contrast between the comparatively high risk Western men and women run of contracting prostate or breast cancer, compared with the much lower risk of people living in the East (see Chapter 3). This was the first suspicion that there might be a cause for such cancers, just as there is a specific cause for the high risk of lung cancer that smokers run. In the following chapters, I will tell you what I think that is: but first, let us look at how to equip yourself to fight against the disease.

HOLDING YOUR GROUND

The typical route through cancer treatment is surgery, radiotherapy and chemotherapy, although new treatments such as photodynamic therapy (PDT) and high-intensity focused ultrasound (HIFU) have become available to treat prostate cancer. Many people use the analogy of cancer treatment as a battle between the disease and the treatments – with the patient as the battlefield. Although this analogy is unpopular with cancer charities or doctors, one of the things you must realise from the outset is the heavy toll that surgery, anaesthesia, radiotherapy and chemotherapy will take on your body. Many people have to take breaks or give up treatments, especially chemotherapy courses, because they become too ill – for example, if their blood cell counts fall to too low a level. To cope with treatment you need to ensure you are equipped physically, emotionally and practically. When I was being treated for breast cancer, I found that dietary and other methods to keep my body as well nourished as possible helped me cope physically (*see* Chapter 5 and *The Plant Programme*[15]). Using my scientific knowledge, I developed other coping strategies to ensure that radioactive substances (used for diagnosis) or chemotherapeutic substances (used for treatment) were removed from my body as soon as possible after they had done their job. I outline these coping strategies in a tips section at the end of this chapter. I have found that other cancer sufferers find such tips very helpful. One of the first and most crucial things you have to do is to understand how to work with your doctor.

A GOOD DOCTOR-PATIENT RELATIONSHIP

Cancer patients often feel as if the disease is their 'fault' – either a genetic defect, something to do with 'blocked emotions' (research shows that there's no such thing as a 'cancer personality' – see Chapter 6) or the result of some other personal failing. This isn't true. Additionally, conventional cancer therapy can 'process' patients to the extent that they no longer understand what is really being done to them. A cancer patient is a vulnerable person and the relentless procedures may induce a feeling of loss of control, but it is vitally important to retain control and develop a constructive working partnership with all your medical team. Let me show you how to work with your doctors and set out to recover your health.

When trying to understand cancer treatments, it is important to understand the different roles of research scientists and clinical doctors. Scientists generally are trying to answer the question 'why?' Doctors are professional human biologists who have taken an oath – now modified from the Hippocratic oath – which requires that they follow a strict code of ethical and professional behaviour. They tend to use only orthodox procedures established by clinical trials, usually based on pure chemical substances or standardised technical procedures validated by controlled, statistically based experiments using cell cultures, laboratory animals and, finally, patients. The growing threat of litigation against medical practitioners is making it more and more difficult for them to depart from orthodox medicine – though some alternative medicine is gaining acceptance by a profession that is necessarily conservative. Our GP treated my daughter Emma's repetitive strain injury with acupuncture rather than pills, for example. She said she felt a bit achy the following evening but was fine the next morning and has had no recurrences after five years.

Like most groups of professionals, doctors range in their ability from excellent to poor. My experience with medical doctors encompasses both, and is probably typical. I was fortunate, in some ways, because right from the beginning, I was not in awe of them as many patients are. Even before I embarked on a career in science, I had developed something of a questioning approach towards medical custom and convention.

Your relationship with your doctor, be it your GP or cancer specialist, is crucial to how well you manage the disease. Although it is only natural to be anxious and afraid (and believe me, I was terrified), try to show your doctors that you will work with them to recover your health and that you wish to be fully involved in decisions.

How can you quickly tell whether your doctor is going to be a good bet? Here's a quick-and-easy ready reckoner I use: it makes no claim to be scientific, but it will help you focus your mind on the most important issues.

A CHECK-UP FOR YOUR DOCTOR

Possesses lots of common sense and explains things clearly and effectively	Treats you arrogantly or impatiently and falls back on confusing jargon if questioned
Follows his or her chosen vocation because s/he obviously cares about people	Authoritarian – gets a kick out of telling you what to do, gets angry when you ask questions or suggest what is wrong with you

Demonstrates s/he is up to date in their knowledge	Indicates s/he is ignorant of subjects that they should understand. Dismisses information, even from the peer-reviewed scientific literature
Technically skilful e.g. knows how to carry out a thorough physical examination	Fails to give thorough examination or to come up with a meaningful diagnosis
Prepared to discuss your health with you on a partnership basis and to recommend dietary, lifestyle or other factors you can change yourself	Uninterested in underlying cause and displays a clear preference for empirical (suck it and see) methods to suppress symptoms; reaches for the prescription pad or computer keyboard almost before you have started your second sentence

Interestingly, a systematic review of the literature on patients' priorities for general-practice care, conducted as part of a project by a European task force,[16] raises similar points. The most highly rated aspect of care was 'humaneness', followed by competence and accuracy. Provision of information and opportunities for participation also featured highly in most studies of patient satisfaction. It was noted that patients increasingly expect to participate in decisions about their care, but these aspirations are rarely met. Most patients want to be able to trust the health professionals they consult, but this did not mean they want to be deceived about the nature of their illness or the risks and potential harms of medical treatment. The authors suggest that in order to avoid putting greater burdens on doctors' time, they should: provide information and educational packs, and help patients to think through their preferences with training to manage their condition by nurses, counsellors, information officers or fellow patients.[17] The success of the approach centres on having access to and understanding information.

In an article in the *BMJ*, the Chief Medical Officer of the Department of Health, Sir Liam Donaldson, wrote 'The patient as expert and partner in care is an idea whose time has come and has the potential to create a new generation of patients who are empowered to take action to improve their health in an unprecedented way.'[18]

Of course, this is the whole principle behind this book and my previous books, *Your Life in Your Hands*, *The Plant Programme*, *Understanding, Preventing and Overcoming Osteoporosis* and *Eating for Better Health*[19] and I am aware that these books, or references to them, are increasingly included in patient packs provided by good GPs and hospitals.

Another factor of particular relevance in prostate cancer, with a possible bearing on the relationship between patient and health professional, is gender. Initial statistics suggest that men are significantly less likely to visit their GP than women, and anecdotal evidence suggests that they are more likely to present with their disease at a more advanced stage. The reasons for this are not known. According to some doctors, many men are reluctant to accept personal vulnerability, and this may affect their judgement. It may also mean that they prefer not to see their own GP, or even attend their own practice, about 'embarrassing problems'.[20] On the other hand, many patients would prefer to see the same doctor all the time. While some general practices regard this as the preferred procedure, this is by no means always the case. If you have cancer and insist that you need this kind of support and your practice refuses, you might wish to consider changing your practice. Discussing a diagnosis of prostate cancer with elderly men (aged 65 or more) may require considerable care, since it has been reported that serious physical illness, including cancer, is associated with increased risk of suicide, especially in men.[21] Patients in emotional distress who find it difficult to talk to friends and family may find it helpful to talk to the Samaritans, a charity devoted to providing a free 24-hour telephone counselling service.

According to the Director of the Patients Association,[22] there are some key things that patients want from their doctor:

- **Eye contact.** Apparently some doctors continue to look at their computer screen while greeting their patients.
- **Partnership.** Patients want to be people who doctors do things with, not people who doctors do things to. They want to be consulted about their condition and treatment [including more information about the possible side effects of any drug they are prescribed[23]].
- **Communication.** Communication from doctor to patient and vice versa is the key to a successful consultation. In many cases

patients are scared and don't understand (or can't take in) what the doctor is saying. With the shock that follows a diagnosis of cancer, the doctor's description of the illness may have been inaccurately heard or misrepresented. It may even be remembered variably, with the patient repeating their description of events in different ways, depending on who they are talking to. For these reasons it is important that patients who may receive a diagnosis of cancer are accompanied by a friend or companion who can sit in and, if possible, make written notes of the conversation.[24] [I would add that I sometimes accompany people and observe just how confused people are about what the doctor really said to them. Often partners are equally distressed and confused.]

- **Time.** Patients want to spend more time with their doctor.
- **Appointments.** Patients want to see their doctor within a reasonable time.

It is also considered important, in the case of prostate cancer, to understand fully the patient's main goal, which may be survival, or postponing or relieving symptoms, or minimising the side effects of treatment such as incontinence or impotence.[25]

Medical professionals are now being advised to:[26]

- Build the doctor-patient relationship
- Develop a shared understanding of the situation
- Agree a way forward

On the other hand, patients should realise that many doctors will find it difficult to tell them of a diagnosis of prostate cancer and to discuss aspects of the disease that are important but uncomfortable to discuss, such as incontinence and other possible side effects. People who have had such cancer describe how sexual difficulties were ducked and how they struggled to maintain their previous persona.[27]

A frequent problem that patients encounter is the use by the medical profession of language which seems calculated to be obscure. Before a medical student can become a doctor, they must be initiated into a language which, it has been estimated, contains 10,000 new words – words which, to most of us, seem just as dead as the Greek or Latin from which they originated.[28] Why, for example, is a foot clinic described as podiatry? Why should itching be called 'pruritis' or a runny nose 'rhinorrhea'? – though it is easy to see why the term idiopathic hypercalcuria is used to describe the condition of too much calcium in the urine, of unknown origin. These are extreme examples, it is true, but they make a useful point.

With the increasing bureaucratisation of the NHS, even English is being turned into gobbledegook. Describing the aims of the new Commission for Patient and Public Involvement in Health, the chief executive is quoted in the *BMJ* as saying 'We would want to have highly effective knowledge databases that people could draw on so that they could have constructive, meaningful debate that moves the agenda forward in a constructive way. What we're talking about are intelligent, informed, democratised challenges that provide better outcomes for everyone'. The new body's aims are therefore described in anything but lucid terms.[29]

Always insist on fully understanding what your doctor or other health professional is saying to you, and if they start to use new and alarming-sounding words, ask them to explain precisely what they are trying to tell you in simpler language. Clarify any details by asking them to draw you a diagram, for instance. Then you will be in a much stronger position to evaluate, influence and, if necessary, query your diagnosis and treatment. Once my doctors realised I was a scientist, they tolerated my questions and tried hard to answer and reassure me. But even then I felt I didn't know enough. It wasn't that they were holding anything back. It's just that their approach seemed so different from mine.

THE PROVINCE OF THE PROSTATE

As with breast cancer,[30] there remains great controversy among health professionals about the value of screening and early detection for prostate cancer.

The common-sense thing to do is to learn about your own body – to become body aware. It always amazes me how little men know or understand about the prostate gland until it causes trouble. We should all learn the basics of our anatomy and how our body feels normally and examine ourselves regularly to find out when things are wrong – especially when they are seriously wrong. Although self-examination is out of the question in the

Spine

Bladder

Pubic bone

Prostate

Penis

Urethra

Testis

Scrotum

Rectum

Figure 1.1 Male urino-genital tract, showing position of the prostate gland.

case of prostate cancer, there are several symptoms to be aware of, as discussed below. Let us first learn a little more about the prostate gland.

Looking at the simplified drawing of male reproductive organs and urinary tract (Figure 1.1), you will see that the prostate gland is situated between the pubic bone and the rectum, and surrounds the urethra, the tube through which urine passes from the bladder to the penis. The tubes of the reproductive system through which the sperm pass meet the urethra in the prostate. The prostate gland provides the fluid in which sperm are carried and it contracts at orgasm to propel the sperm out of the penis. Hence it is connected with the whole urinary and male reproductive system, so that prostate disease and its treatment can damage urinary and sexual function.[31] Interestingly, the embryonic tissue that gives rise to the prostate gland in males develops into a womb in females.

In a young boy, the gland is the size of a pea, growing at puberty to the shape and size of a walnut. At the same time growth within the prostate leads to the development of microscopic glands which produce the prostatic secretion called prostate-specific antigen (PSA). This fluid, which is rich in sugar and enzymes, is important in sexual activity. The PSA, which drains through tiny prostatic ducts, provides the fluid in which sperm are carried. The PSA nourishes the sperm, keeping them alive until fertilisation can occur. PSA also clears residual matter left in the prostatic ducts after orgasm.[32] The level of PSA normally present in the bloodstream reflects the activity and health of the prostate gland. This can be measured in a PSA test (see pp. 26–33). The development and growth of the prostate at puberty is influenced by the pituitary gland, the master gland of the body, which sits in the centre of the brain, produces growth hormone and another important hormone called prolactin, and orchestrates thyroid hormone production – all of which are important in the development and growth of the prostate gland.[33]

Certainly in the West, however, the prostate seems to grow again in men in their late forties, and herein lies the problem.[34] Prostate growth increases with age, and enlargement of the gland in older men can cause significant difficulties with urination, including as a result of obstruction of the neck of the bladder by an enlarged prostate.[35]

PROSTATE CONDITIONS[36]

Let us now look at diseases of the prostate generally.

Benign prostatic hypertrophy (BPH)

Benign enlargement of the prostate, otherwise known as benign prostatic hypertrophy (BPH) is the commonest cause of prostate problems and is considered a condition of ageing. Treatments to limit its size include surgery such as transurethral prostatectomy (TURP), in which a tube is inserted through the penis along the urethra to remove physical obstruction. Alternatively, drug treatments can be used to reduce the size of the prostate. Because prostate enlargement can be a slow process that takes many years, medical treatment is generally less effective than surgery and often takes a considerable time to improve symptoms; it is usually reserved for patients who are unfit for surgery. A TURP will lead to an improvement in nearly all patients. Drug treatments are hormonal and include the LHRH agonists and finasteride (see p. 59). Herbal medicines can also help (see p. 70).

More than half of the men in the United States between the ages of 60 and 70 and as many as 90 per cent between the ages of 70 and 90 have symptoms of BPH. For some men, the symptoms may be severe enough to require treatment.[37] The symptoms of BPH and cancer are very much the same and are principally the symptoms of enlargement of the gland.[38]

According to Wilt, treatment options for BPH depend on how men, in discussion with their doctor, balance the bother of lower-urinary-tract symptoms with the relative effectiveness and likely adverse effects of various types of treatments.[39] For men with mild to moderate urinary symptoms, management by GPs is appropriate. Alpha-blocking drugs are the preferred pharmacological treatment for improving symptoms and urine flow, regardless of the extent of prostate enlargement, although they are associated with side effects such as dizziness and headache. Combining these drugs with another drug, finasteride (which inhibits the activity of an enzyme that converts the androgen testosterone into its active form dihydrotestosterone (DHT) (see p. 58), provides no greater improvement in symptoms than alpha blockers alone. Alpha blockers have not been clearly shown to prevent complications from BPH or the need for surgery in the long term.

A study to compare two drugs, doxazosin and finasteride, alone and in combination, for the treatment of symptoms of BPH showed results for finasteride that were not significantly different from the placebo. Doxazosin was effective in improving urinary symptoms and urinary flow rate, and was more effective than finasteride alone or a placebo. The addition of finasteride did not provide further benefit to that achieved with doxazosin alone.[40]

Another study showed that a drug called tamsulosin was more effective than finasteride for short-term treatment of BPH, with a better safety profile.[41]

Men with severe symptoms (see below) should be referred to a urologist. If the conditions are due to BPH, surgery is thought to result in a lower incidence of complications, including the need for blood transfusions and hospital stays. Another systematic review compared surgery with laser treatment for BPH and showed that the former led to greater improvement in urinary symptoms than either contact or non-contact laser therapies. However, men treated with lasers had fewer complications (although many trials did not report adverse events). There were no differences between the groups in the incidence of sexual problems or incontinence.[42]

In another study, comparing TURP, non-contact laser therapy and watchful waiting, Brookes and colleagues[43] found that older men needing treatment for urinary symptoms and wanting to retain or improve sexual function should consider standard surgery rather than non-contact laser therapy.

Prostatitis

Prostatitis is an inflammation of the prostate gland and can be caused by infection or sometimes sexual activity. Symptoms include significant pain, usually with a temperature and frequency of urination. Treatment with antibiotics, in some cases intravenously, may be required. Prostatitis can be a recurring problem for some men, requiring repeated courses of antibiotics.

Prostate cancer

Prostate cancer can vary from a relatively harmless condition to a serious illness, and its frequency increases with age. A small amount of prostate cancer is commonly found in older men who have died from other causes, with up to 80 per cent in 80 year olds. According to Waxman, little spots of cancer occur in 70 per cent of 70 year olds, 60 per cent of 60 year olds and 50 per cent of 50 year olds, but their relationship with the development of aggressive cancer is unknown.

A non-aggressive type of prostate cancer is known as prostatic intra-epithelial neoplasia, or PIN. Some doctors regard PIN as being a precursor of aggressive cancer, likely to lead to the development of an invasive tumour, although most remain unconvinced that PIN is related to overt prostate cancer. If you are diagnosed with PIN, you should be reassured that it is unlikely to progress to invasive cancer, but you will be advised to have an annual check-up including PSA testing (*see* p 26).

Difficulties with urination caused by prostate cancer can be due to the physical enlargement of the gland or to the invasion of the prostatic urethral valves by cancer so that they are unable to open and shut normally. In serious cases, it becomes impossible to pass urine; this causes considerable pain, because of the pressure on the bladder, and requires catheterisation to remove the obstruction.

SYMPTOMS OF PROSTATE CANCER

Remember that although any of the symptoms listed below can indicate cancer, they are more likely to be caused by a non-cancerous disease. In any case, if you find any of the symptoms described, see your doctor as soon as possible. Even if you are reassured that nothing is wrong, monitor changes and return to the doctor and press for a referral if you think there is a problem, certainly if any of your symptoms become worse.

Such symptoms include:[44]

- difficulty or pain when passing urine
- the need to pass urine more often
- broken sleep due to the need to pass urine
- waiting for long periods before urine flows
- dribbling during urination
- incomplete emptying of bladder, which may lead to urinary infection accompanied by pain in the penis and a high temperature

These symptoms are the same as those for BPH. Prostate cancer may additionally cause:

- blood in the urine and/or semen

This and associated symptoms can be caused by other factors such as bacterial infection.[45]

Other symptoms of advanced prostate cancer may include:

- swollen lymph nodes in the groin area
- impotence (difficulty having an erection) and reduced quantities of ejaculate

- pain in the pelvis, spine, hips, or ribs

These symptoms, too, may be due to other diseases (for example, pain in the spine, pelvis or hips frequently reflects arthritis, especially in older men) and do not necessarily mean that a man has prostate cancer.[46]

A TESTING TIME

The time taken to diagnose prostate cancer in the UK is longer than for any other tumour type, for a range of reasons, one of the most significant being the non-specific nature of the symptoms of the disease.[47] Urinary frequency, for example, the commonest symptom of prostate cancer, can also reflect BPH, and hence affects almost all older men. Typically, the symptoms will have developed gradually over many years and may be ignored until the problem becomes critical. For the same reasons, GP referrals of their patients to hospitals may fail to indicate any need for urgency.

Another problem is that even if the tumour is cancerous, to date there is no way of telling how aggressive the growth will be. The problem is that some small yet rapidly growing cancers have not been spotted in time. Others with enlarged and malignant prostates may have had slow growth for ten years or more, with no spread to other tissues.[48]

In America, the American Cancer Society (ACS) recommends that a PSA test and a digital rectal examination (DRE) should be offered annually beginning at age 50 to men who have a life expectancy of at least 10 years. Men at high risk (*see* p. 11) should be tested beginning at age 45. Some men, apparently, ask their doctor to make the testing decision on their behalf, and they should be tested.[49] A clinical policy of not offering testing, or discouraging testing in men who request early prostate cancer detection tests, is considered inappropriate in the US. It is recommended, however, that if health-care professionals offer men the option of PSA and/or DRE tests they should, prior to testing, discuss the potential benefits, side effects, and uncertainties regarding early detection and treatment to help them make an informed decision.[50] In the UK, advice is more equivocal, but if you are concerned go to see your GP.

On visiting your GP to discuss symptoms, give the fullest, clearest information possible. They should listen to an account of your symptoms, assess your general physical condition, check for bladder enlargement, perform a DRE and blood tests for blood count, kidney function and PSA levels (*see* below). During the DRE, you will be asked to lie on your side and adopt a foetal position, drawing your legs up to your stomach. The doctor will insert lubricating jelly on a gloved finger to determine the size and shape of the prostate, which is likely to be much bigger with BPH and become knobbly if cancer is present.[51] Be reassured that even abnormal findings on DRE, such as nodularity or induration of the prostate, leads to a diagnosis of prostate cancer as a result of biopsy in only 15 to 25 per cent of cases. This compares with prostate cancer prevalence of less than 5 per cent among men of similar age without abnormal DRE. Although neither accurate nor sensitive for prostate cancer detection, abnormal DRE is associated with a 5-fold increased risk of cancer present at time of screening.[52]

PSA TEST

As discussed earlier, PSA is produced by the normal prostate and secreted in the seminal fluid in large quantities. Prostate cancer changes the cellular barriers that normally keep PSA within the ductal system of the prostate, and thereby alters blood serum levels. The result of the PSA test is reported in ng/ml (nanograms per millilitre – very tiny amounts).

Doctors have had a hard time establishing an absolute cut-off level at which more testing is needed. Most (but not all) doctors agree PSA levels below 4 are normal, and levels over 10 indicate that a prostate biopsy (in which tissue is removed and examined under a microscope) is needed. But a grey zone exists for levels between 4 and 10. About one in four men whose PSA is in this range have prostate cancer and in such cases some doctors recommend that a biopsy should be performed immediately. But the biopsy can be uncomfortable and carries a risk of infection and bleeding, so other doctors suggest repeating the PSA test at a later date or using other tests.[53]

In the US,[54] many doctors now recommend a biopsy when PSA levels are higher than 4, but there is controversy about the exact cut-off point that separates 'normal' from 'abnormal' PSA levels and some doctors use 3.0 or 2.5 as the upper limits of normal.

PSA levels can be used, together with clinical examination results and the tumour's Gleason score from biopsy samples (*see* p. 36), to decide which additional tests are needed. The PSA test is also used to monitor the effectiveness of treatments and indicate evidence of recurrence.[55]

Since the first use of the PSA blood test in the 1980s, doctors have been able to detect many more cases of prostate cancer at an earlier stage and, unlike mammography for detection of breast cancer, which involves irradiation, the PSA test has no effect on the body, but the test is not perfect, and several important questions have yet to be answered. For example, it is not yet known if screening with the PSA test will save lives or prolong patients' survival. Prostate cancer is thought to be more curable if detected at an early stage. But some doctors argue that the test may be detecting some cancers that would never cause symptoms in a normal lifetime because they are so slow growing.[56]

This is important, because some treatment for prostate cancer can have lasting adverse side effects, and patients with abnormal PSA, particularly those who have no other symptoms, should weigh their options carefully before proceeding with radical forms of treatment. Certainly, a biopsy must be performed before proceeding with treatment, but even this carries a risk of infection since it is generally carried out through the rectum, which is full of bacteria.

Let us look further at some of the pros and cons of the PSA test to help you and your doctor decide what is best for you.

The pros of the PSA test

According to a recent article in *The Times* by Dr Thomas Stuttaford,[57] evidence in the US, and in most of the developed world, where most doctors recommend regular testing with the PSA blood test, strongly suggests that this policy is paying off. The PSA reading for those with a prostate-gland-confined cancer is vital. The chances of long-term survival fall dramatically if the PSA is over ten [not in my experience of communicating with prostate-cancer sufferers who follow my diet and regime]. It is therefore important to have regular testing so that any cancer can be detected while the PSA is still low. In the US, doctors consider the PSA to be fundamental. In the UK, research has shown that if the PSA is over ten only 34 per cent of the patients treated do not have evidence of a spreading tumour after five years.

A qualitative study by Chapple and colleagues[58] shows that the reasons why men with prostate cancer advocate screening include beliefs about the benefit of early diagnosis and the need to have responsibility. Policy makers, politicians, and doctors, the authors say, need to understand why people want wider access to PSA testing.

Herxheimer and Ziebland also found that men with prostate cancer felt strongly that healthy men should be offered PSA testing, despite the false positives (indications of cancer that turn out to be false) and the fact that earlier diagnosis has not been shown to lead to more effective treatment. They believed that early diagnosis would reduce mortality, improve quality of life and save the NHS money. They argued that testing should be available because (1) symptoms can be ambiguous, (2) screening is seen as responsible behaviour and would encourage men to look after their health, and (3) there is equivalent screening for women's cancers.[59] A related finding was that many men for whom 'watchful waiting' (see p. 46) would have been an appropriate option would not contemplate it, and indeed few of those who might have chosen it remembered any mention of it[60] in discussion with their doctor.

In Europe, unlike the US, a system of screening men for prostate cancer once in every four years is considered sufficiently effective in catching nearly all tumours in time. Researchers on the ongoing European Randomised Study of Screening for Prostate Cancer studied more than 17,000 men and reported that 'very few, if any, aggressive prostate cancers escape screening'[61] at this interval.

It has also been pointed out by an individual patient that had he not had a PSA test his prognosis might have been worse than others who presented with bone metastases and high PSA values. He points out that during his decision-making process he came across a paper on dilemmas in treating early prostate cancer.[62] It was easy, he said, to work out that there just aren't enough experienced urologists (able to carry out this tricky operation successfully) to carry out the number of radical prostatectomies that early detection by PSA screening would require. A sample of

244 urologists had a mean of 14.1 years experience, and 130 of them managed 100 patients or more with prostate cancer. Expertise in performing radical prostatectomy was restricted to comparatively few – 98 reported having ever performed the procedure and only 12 (14 per cent) that they performed 20 or more operations yearly. He also suspects that the United Kingdom is far short of the number of three-dimensional conformal radiotherapy machines (*see* p. 51) needed to offer that treatment option.[63]

The cons of the PSA test

Opponents of PSA testing claim that the use of this test is responsible for the observed increase in incidence of the disease. It is also claimed that PSA screening causes over-diagnosis in about 29 per cent of white men and 44 per cent of black men in the USA who would otherwise have died of another cause, without their prostate cancer being detected in their lifetime.[64] One recent study compared data on prostate-cancer mortality in the Seattle – Puget Sound area of the USA, where screening and aggressive treatment were adopted early, with Connecticut, where adoption of these procedures was slower. In 1987–1990, men aged 65 to 79 in Seattle were five times as likely to undergo PSA testing, twice as likely to undergo biopsy, and rates of radical prostatectomy and radiotherapy were also substantially higher. Nevertheless, through eleven years of follow-up, prostate-cancer mortality was similar in the two areas.[65]

A high PSA test result suggests that cancer may be present – it can also reflect inflammation of the prostate, urinary retention, prostatic infection, BPH, and prostatic manipulation. According to some authors, neither DRE nor PSA tests are accurate or adequately sensitive for prostate-cancer screening.[66]

In one research study, factors found in the blood from high dairy consumption and some medications increased PSA levels, as did vigorous exercise (though it has been suggested that bike riding does not influence PSA levels[67]). Moreover, it has been stated that the test does not seem able to distinguish between malignant and non-malignant prostate tumours, and one US report concluded that as many as two thirds of those testing positive probably do not have cancer.[68]

Physicians have speculated that PSA screening may be responsible for the reduction in prostate-cancer mortality observed in the late 1990s, but the results of a recent survey suggest that, for the study population, PSA screening cannot explain the decline in prostate-cancer mortality.[69]

Another study reported that only 15 to 25 per cent of cases with PSA greater than 4.0 were found to have prostate cancer on biopsy.[70]

An editorial in the *Journal of the National Cancer Institute* commenting on the PSA controversy under the title, 'The More We Know, the Less We Understand', stated, 'Only one man in four with a PSA level greater than 4.0 is found to have prostate cancer on biopsy ... and about one-third of prostate cancers are detected in men with a normal PSA level'[71] (the problems of false positives and false negatives respectively).

In a review article in the *BMJ* entitled 'The PSA storm', Yamey and Wilkes describe how questioning cancer screening can be a risky business in America.[72] They conclude that they angered a group of urologists who are protagonists of the PSA test by challenging its 'wishful thinking'. They also suggest that they 'stepped on the toes of a very wealthy and powerful pro-screening lobby that stands to make money from encouraging men to get tested. Even some of the patient support groups in this lobby have a conflict of interest, since they rely on support from pharmaceutical companies.' 'With the widespread belief in America that every man should know his PSA, a belief driven by politics and not evidence,' Yamey and Wilkes fear that 'sceptical voices like theirs will always be drowned out.'

Improved methods of testing

Efforts are under way to improve the reliability of the PSA test. Scientists have discovered variations in a gene that controls levels of PSA in men – a finding that could make PSA screenings for prostate cancer more accurate.[73]

One new study shows that genetic variations can directly influence levels of PSA that can be detected in a man's bloodstream. It is estimated that 29 million men may have the genes that produce levels of PSA about 30 per cent higher than average. PSA levels are generally higher in African American men.[74] It is too early to know whether men with higher levels are at higher risk for cancer. It is also too soon to know whether men with lower-than-normal PSA levels are at risk of having their cancer remain undiagnosed.

If the results of the study are confirmed, it is suggested that $12 billion a year could be saved in unnecessary biopsies. Testing for the newly discovered gene variants is quick and inexpensive and could become a part of the PSA screening regimen.[75]

In another study, scientists have reported that measuring a precursor form of PSA called proPSA improves the accuracy of testing. By measuring the proportion of proPSA relative to PSA they were able to identify the men with aggressive cancer earlier, and they believe that this method could also reduce the number of unnecessary biopsies.[76]

Some PSA circulates unbound to other substances in the blood and is called the per cent free PSA. PSA results between 4 and 10 combined with a low per cent free PSA means that a prostate cancer is more likely to be present. The laboratory doing the testing will provide this information to your doctor. Another refinement uses the PSA velocity (which is the increase in PSA level over time), which is calculated from the results obtained from three specimens over at least an 18-month period. A PSA velocity over 0.75 per year is considered high and suggests the need for a biopsy. Certainly I like to have plots of the PSA results against time for the men I advise. One can quickly see if the rates of increase in PSA test results are increasing or decreasing.

Other, less common, methods of using PSA results include PSA density, to adjust for men who have large prostate glands, and age-specific PSA levels. Doctors are looking at whether the latter may be a more accurate indicator of the presence of cancer, because levels increase naturally with age, but neither of these methods has been validated.[77]

The PSA test – some suggestions

In summary, according to the ACS,[78] there are many uncertainties regarding the early detection and treatment of prostate cancer. Cancers found by PSA testing and/or DRE are, on average, smaller and have spread less than cancers discovered because of the symptoms they cause, but prostate cancer is unlike many other cancers in that it often grows very slowly.

For men with cancer that has not spread beyond the prostate, the 5-year relative survival rate is almost 100 per cent, whether or not they are treated. On the other hand, before early detection tests were widely used, most men with prostate cancer were diagnosed with advanced disease, and most died within a few years of the diagnosis.

Although early diagnosis and treatment of prostate cancer can help some men to live longer, it may not affect the life span of other men. For a man who has poor health or other serious medical illnesses and is not likely to live more than 10 years, there may be no benefit in an early diagnosis of prostate cancer, and it may do more harm than good, by affecting their quality of life.

Certainly, I think the suggestion that a high PSA test result should be repeated at least once before an invasive biopsy is performed[79] is sound advice. The lead author of the study is quoted as saying, 'Even if the repeat test shows an elevated level, prostate cancer will only be discovered in about one quarter of men who undergo biopsy . . . A single elevated PSA level does not automatically warrant a prostate biopsy'. Yet another study found that the PSA test may fluctuate from year to year. In some cases, levels that were abnormally high returned to normal on their own – with important implications for the need for immediate biopsy.[80]

There are certain measures you can take to make your PSA test as accurate as possible. Because ejaculation can cause a temporary increase in blood PSA levels, abstinence from sexual activity is recommended for two days before the test is performed. Also, urinary tract infections, BPH and inflammation of the prostate can all elevate PSA levels. On the other hand, several medicines (including finasteride and some anti-androgens) and herbal preparations (such as PC-SPES, a herbal mixture that contains saw palmetto, see page 71) can lower PSA levels **so that early prostate cancer is undetected.**[81] Ask your doctor for advice on the length of time you should stay off such drugs and preparations before having your PSA test.

I now have considerable experience of working with men who have had a diagnosis of prostate cancer. I would advise all men over 45 to have regular PSA tests and to ask for such a test if they have any of the symptoms of prostate cancer listed above for more than a couple of weeks. If you are at risk because of a family history of prostate cancer, for example, cut your avoidable risk factors by following the dietary and lifestyle advice in Chapters 5 and 6. I have known people's PSA levels fall dramatically when they simply follow this advice.

REFERRAL

If, after taking your symptoms and test results into account, your GP finds significant evidence of prostate disease, you will be referred to a consultant urologist, or to an oncologist if a diagnosis of cancer is suspected. Most patients will be found to have BPH and their care will remain with the urologist.[82] Those with suspected cancer will generally be referred to an oncologist specialising in prostate cancer, and will normally have the same examination, tests and case histories that their GPs carried out repeated at the hospital.

If you are referred to a hospital consultant, my general advice to all UK patients is to obtain treatment for serious illnesses such as cancer at NHS centres of excellence. I am aware of several people whose cancer remained undiagnosed by their private hospitals or physicians, and by the time they attended NHS clinics their cancer was very far advanced. A recent study has shown that patients in for-profit hospitals in the US are more likely to die than those in non-profit hospitals.[83]

Most good hospitals treating prostate cancer now have a specialist unit with a team that includes oncologists, radiotherapists and chemotherapists. I still hear from men who have been treated, some of them privately and expensively, by general surgeons using an approach which can only be described as in the best tradition of 'muddling through', with no attempt to assess the nature and scale of the problem at the outset. Being treated by a specialist team is essential. Ensure that your GP knows your views and refuse to be fobbed off with anything less than treatment at a specialist centre of excellence. Your life, quite literally, may depend on it. In the case of surgery, for example, ensure that you are treated by a surgeon who carries out at least thirty such operations a year, and ask about his or her success rates compared with the national average. Also ask about survival rates generally at the centre at which you are being treated. (Asking for such information is particularly important for men having prostate operations because this operation is quite complicated.) Such statistics need to be treated with caution, however, because some doctors will treat patients whom others regard as incurable. I remember asking senior doctors at Charing Cross at what point did they give up – was it when patients had less than a 50:50 chance of survival? I found their reply very moving. They said that, providing the patient wanted to survive, they would never give up.

BIOPSY

A *core-needle biopsy* is the main method used to diagnose prostate cancer accurately. The doctor will commonly use TRUS (*see* p. 38) for guidance.[84] Biopsies are performed using fine, spring-loaded needles inserted into the prostate through the wall of the rectum. Six to ten core biopsies may be taken, from different places in the prostate. A local anaesthetic is normally used. Some patients find the procedure painless, others report some discomfort, while some experience severe pain. The biopsy procedure can leave some patients in pain for quite a time. It results in infection (since the needle passes through the rectum) in 1 to 2 per cent of patients in the UK, and it may even lead to incontinence and impotence for a time. The specimens taken should be examined by a pathologist experienced in staging and grading prostate cancer (*see* below).[85] Some blood in the urine or in bowel movements can be common for 2–3 days following the biopsy. Blood in the semen may last for up to 2–3 weeks.[86]

Lymph-node biopsy may also be performed to find out if cancer has spread from the prostate to nearby lymph nodes, and it is only done in, for example, men with a high Gleason score or young men with a high PSA level. A specially trained radiologist may take a sample of cells from lymph nodes using a technique called *fine-needle aspiration* (FNA), using a computed tomography (CT) scan image to guide insertion of the long, thin needle used to take a small sample from the lymph node.[87] If cancer cells are found in the lymph node biopsy specimens, treatment options other than surgery are likely to be used.

STAGING AND GRADING

The **stage** of a prostate cancer indicates how far it has spread within the gland, neighbouring tissues and other organs. It is an important factor in selecting treatment options and considered to be highly significant in predicting outcome. The TNM System of the American Joint Committee on Cancer (AJCC) is the most commonly used system in the US and is the basis for the WHO system. It describes the extent of primary tumour (T), the presence or absence of spread to nearby lymph nodes (N), and the presence or absence of spread (metastasis) to distant organs (M). The stages described here are generalised from the 1992 version of the AJCC staging manual. Ensure that your doctor is using the 1992 version before trying to apply it to the guidelines below – but note that it predates the widespread use of the PSA test.[88]

T stages There are two types of T classifications for prostate cancer: the clinical stage, based on DRE, needle biopsy and TRUS findings, which is used in making treatment decisions; and the pathological stage, following surgery, which is based on full investigation of the entire prostate, the seminal vesicles (two small sacs next to the prostate that store semen) and, in some cases, nearby lymph nodes, and is therefore more accurate in prognosis. There are four T stages. T1 refers to a cancer that is not felt during a DRE, although cancer cells are found in a prostate biopsy or prostatectomy specimen. T2 means that the doctor can feel the prostate cancer by DRE and that the cancer is thought to be confined to the prostate gland. T3 cancers have spread beyond the outer rim of the gland and have reached the surrounding tissue and/or the seminal vesicles, but do not involve any other organs. T4 cancers have spread to tissues next to the prostate.

N stages N0 means that the cancer has not spread to any lymph nodes. N1 indicates spread to one lymph node in the pelvis, but its size is less than 2 cm in diameter. N2 means that the cancer has spread to one lymph node, and is between 2 and 5 cm in diameter; or that it is in more than one node, but none are larger than 2 cm. N3 means that there is at least one lymph node larger than 5 cm. Nx means that tests to detect lymph-node spread have not been done.

M stages M0 means that the cancer has not metastasised beyond the nearby nodes. M1 means that metastases are present in distant (outside the pelvis) lymph nodes, in bones, or in other distant organs such as liver, lungs or brain. Mx means that tests to find distant spread have not been done.

GLEASON RATING[89]

One system used to assess the severity of prostate tumours, known as the Gleason rating system, can be used by doctors when discussing treatment options with their patients.

Gleason scores are determined by examining prostate biopsy samples, or by examining the entire prostate after surgical removal. Since biopsy samples represent only a small portion of the entire prostate, they may not be representative of the gland as a whole. The Gleason score as determined from the biopsy specimen, however, has been shown to be one of the best methods of predicting how prostate cancer will progress. An accurate Gleason score can help one decide on the best treatment options.[90]

The Gleason score indicates the aggressiveness of the tumour, according to how well it is differentiated (cells that are completely differentiated are good, healthy cells). Gleason Patterns 1 and 2 are well differentiated; Pattern 3 is moderately differentiated; and Patterns 4 and 5 are poorly differentiated. Perfectly differentiated prostate cells are happy to go about their business in the prostate making PSA and ejaculatory fluid. They look and act like the mature prostate cells they are. They interact with other perfectly differentiated prostate cells to create the tiny tubular structures that the prostate requires to deliver its product to the urethra. Once they become malignant, however, they become less differentiated and start behaving badly. The tubules they make with other malignant cells are distorted and arranged haphazardly, and they may eventually form solid clumps and even go off on their own to make new colonies elsewhere in the body. See further in Chapter 2.

The Gleason score, which should always be calculated by a pathologist with considerable experience in examining samples of prostate tissue, is written as the sum of the two most prominent Gleason patterns. So a Gleason score of $2+3=5$ has a dominant well-differentiated pattern (i.e. pattern 2) and a less dominant moderately differentiated pattern (pattern 3). A score of $4+3=7$ means that a poorly differentiated component (pattern 4) is dominant. If 95 per cent or more of the tumour is composed of one pattern, the corresponding number is counted twice; thus, a wholly moderately differentiated tumour would be scored $3+3=6$. Ask to see your score, and check that it adds up: e.g. $2+3=5$, not some other number. Mistakes can happen!

Ensure that you thoroughly understand the difference between the Gleason pattern and the Gleason score, before discussing such information with your doctor, and remember that other terms such as 'Gleason grade' or 'Gleason degree' are meaningless.

Among untreated patients with clinically localised prostate cancer, those with a low Gleason score (5 or less) have a very small risk (4 to 7 per cent) of dying of their cancer within 15 years, even if their cancer is never treated. Men with cancers with a Gleason score 6 have a 15 to 30 per cent risk of cancer death if untreated for 15 years. Those with cancers with a Gleason score 7 have a 50 per cent risk of cancer death if untreated for 15 years. Those with poorly differentiated tumours (Gleason scores 8 to 10) have an 87 per cent risk of dying from the disease within 15 years if untreated[91] (but remember that these are just statistical risks, and all my experience of communicating with prostate cancer sufferers indicates you can greatly improve your odds).

OTHER SCREENING TECHNIQUES, INCLUDING SCANNING

Blood tests

A **full blood count** (FBC) determines whether the patient's blood has the correct number of various types of blood cells. Abnormal test results may suggest spread of cancer to the bone marrow, where blood cells form, but doctors repeat this test regularly in patients being treated with chemotherapy because the drugs used affect the bone marrow temporarily. Spread of prostate cancer to the bones or liver can be detected by other blood tests. Some of the drugs used in hormone therapy can interfere with liver function and are also identified by blood tests.[92]

Researchers in the United States have developed a simple blood test that can be used to identify which patients with prostate cancer need the most aggressive treatment even among those whose tumours seem to be at the same stage of development. The research is published in the journal *Cancer*,[93] and the authors include Donald Gleason, who developed the Gleason system of rating prostate cancers (*see* p. 36). The new test involves measuring the level of an enzyme (cathepsin beta) involved in the progression of cancer cells and the level of natural inhibitors of the enzyme (called stefins). The researchers found that more aggressive types of prostate cancer showed a higher ratio of the cathepsin beta to stefin A than less aggressive types.[94]

Scanning

Several types of imaging may be used to look for cancer within the prostate as well as cancer that has spread, but all have imperfections:[95]

Transrectal ultrasound (TRUS)   uses sound waves to create a computer image of the prostate on a video screen, but if there is the possibility of prostate cancer a biopsy is the only way it can be diagnosed definitively.[96] In addition to providing information about the configuration of the prostate, the ultrasound probe gives an idea of the shape of the structures around the gland. It can also establish if there are changes in the capsule of the prostate suggesting that it may have been breeched.[97]

If the specialists feel that the cancer may have spread, they may also suggest a CT (or CAT) scan, an MRI scan or a bone scan, which provides additional information of the extent of the cancer. Remember, though, that a CT scan and a bone scan use ionising radiation (*see* p. 45).[98] Also, abnormalities detected by bone scans can include arthritis and other degenerative bone diseases and simple bruises (e.g. to the ribs).[99] The choice between MRI and CT scans depends on the physician's preference and the availability of scanners.

Radionuclide bone scan   The bone scan involves injection with a radioactive substance called technetium in a phosphate compound designed to 'stick' to the bones. The radioactivity of the technetium decays quickly and the total amount of radioactivity is low compared with the much higher doses used in radiation therapy, and generally does not cause side effects. The radioactive substance is attracted to diseased bone cells throughout the skeleton and can therefore be seen on the bone scan image. These areas may suggest that metastatic cancer is present, but arthritis or other bone diseases can give the same pattern.[100] If required to have such a scan, do follow the instructions carefully so that the procedure does not have to be repeated and you minimise your exposure to any unnecessary ionising radiation.

After the test, drink several glasses of a well-known cola which contains phosphoric acid to try to encourage your body to exchange the radioactive phosphates for the non-radioactive phosphate compounds in the cola as soon as possible. (Otherwise I never drink such products.)

Computed tomography (CT) A CT (or CAT) scan uses a rotating X-ray beam to create a series of pictures of the body from many angles. A computer combines the information from these pictures, producing a detailed cross-sectional image. The CT scan may reveal abnormally enlarged pelvic lymph nodes, which could be a sign of a spreading cancer (or a sign that the immune system is fighting an infection). The CT scan can also detect cancer that has spread to other internal organs, such as the liver, and is frequently performed prior to treatment, especially if there is evidence of lymph-node involvement.[101]

Magnetic resonance imaging (MRI) MRI is like a CT scan except that magnetic fields are used instead of X-rays to create detailed cross-sectional pictures of selected areas of your body. These pictures can identify cancer that has spread from the prostate, and, as with the CT scan, may be performed if there is evidence of lymph-node involvement.[102]

Some new techniques

A new advanced technique of **high-resolution magnetic resonance computerised imaging** is being developed, which uses magnetic nanoparticles to seek out lymph nodes.[103]

This method should help doctors to distinguish more accurately between normal nodes and those affected by cancer. The studies reported found detectable metastases, confirmed by pathological examination, and also showed that some lymph nodes, which might otherwise have been removed, contained no cancer. Forty-five of the 63 malignant nodes were so small they would not have been identified as malignant by conventional imaging techniques.[104]

ProstaScint scan This is still a relatively new type of test, which, like the bone scan, uses low-level radioactive material to find cancer that has spread. In this test, the radioactive material is attached to a monoclonal antibody, a type of antibody engineered in the laboratory to recognise and stick to a particular marker on cancer cells. The disadvantage of this method is that it often suggests spread when there is none.[105]

Sentinel lymphadenectomy is a new method of identifying spread of cancer into the lymph nodes. The sentinel node is defined as the first node to receive drainage from a tumour and is identified by injecting a special substance around the primary tumour and noting its spread via lymphatic channels. This method has been reported to have a 95 per cent success rate in identifying cancer spread to lymph nodes.[106] It is replacing removal and pathological examination of lymph nodes and is suitable for many, but not all, patients. This method may reduce the incidence of lymphoedema (build-up of fluid due to disruption of normal lymph drainage following surgical removal of the lymph node).

Positron Emission Tomography (PET) is a relatively new method of detecting cancer spread. It is based on radioactive labelling of glucose, which is taken up more readily by cancer cells than normal cells, or sometimes radioactive labelling of ammonia or water. Again, it depends upon computer images of radioactive emissions from high-energy short-lived particles from radioactive isotopes such as fluorine-18. At the time I wrote the first edition of this book, the technique was being used mainly for the early detection of lung and brain cancer. It is now more widely available and is used to detect spread of several types of cancer including prostate cancer. The main advantage of PET is that it identifies centres of unusual metabolism, whereas most other methods can only identify the presence of lesions which may or may not be active cancer.

DIAGNOSIS AND PROGNOSIS IN LOCALISED PROSTATE CANCER

According to Dr Stuttaford, research has now shown convincingly that in the great majority of cases there are four factors that are fundamental in assessing risk in those patients in whom the tumour hasn't already spread beyond the prostate gland (cancers that have metastasised form a different group).[107]

1. The PSA reading
2. The Gleason score

3. The age of the patient
4. The extent of tumour spread within the prostate.

There are now tables taking these factors into account, which estimate the average survival time. Medicine isn't an exact science. Some patients do better than the average, others worse.[108]

I think he should add a fifth point: the extent to which men are keeping closely to my diet and lifestyle recommendations. These are the men bounding up to me or emailing me to tell me how low their PSA test results are – in some cases having fallen from above 100 to below 1. At a conference dinner recently a girlfriend commented ruefully on how I always appeared to be surrounded by men. 'Don't worry', I said. 'They just want to tell me how well they or their wives are doing now they are following my programme.'

WHAT NEXT?

In the UK, it is common that all tests and scans will have been carried out before treatment options are considered, although this may not always be the case. I think that it is essential that you have the fullest possible information before making any decisions about your treatment options with your doctors. For example, having radical surgery to remove the prostate is usually not worthwhile if the cancer has already spread beyond the prostate gland.

Generally, you will be seen by a consultant oncologist or urologist to be given your diagnosis and the results of all the tests and scans.

In cases of cancer I think it important that doctors are compassionate but honest and that this is preferable to giving false reassurances.

The mainstays of prostate-cancer treatment continue to be surgery; radiotherapy (the use of radioactive rays – usually high-energy X-rays – to destroy cancer cells); chemotherapy (the use of chemicals to disrupt the physiology and biochemistry of the cancer cells); or hormone treatment to prevent the androgen hormones, especially testosterone, from reaching the receptor cells in the cancer or prostate tissue cells generally. Recently, new methods of treatment such as High Intensity Focused Ultrasound

(HIFU) and photodynamic therapy (PDT) have become available. The problem with some of these treatments (mainly radiotherapy and chemotherapy) is that they can give rise to side effects so harmful that they compromise the benefits of the treatment (in some extreme cases causing other different types of cancer such as leukaemia). Also, they can, for reasons which are not understood, fail in a significant proportion of cases. Hence doctors can only quote survival statistics to their patients. They cannot offer any assurance of a cure to an individual. Remember that your body is as unique as your personality and your fingerprints. Although understanding your cancer's stage and learning about your treatment options can help to predict what health problems you may face, no one can say precisely how you will respond to cancer or its treatment.[109]

It is important for patients to understand that medical procedures can often be the subject of far more controversy within the medical profession than the public usually realises. Different specialists may have very different views about the best treatment options.

Professor Waxman points out that the efficacy of a particular course of treatment is arrived at from an analysis of the results of different clinical trials, but the relative advantages of different types of treatment for prostate cancer have often not been clinically proven. In other words, there is, as yet, no proof that there is one certain and 'correct' way to manage the disease. As a result, opinions sometimes differ as to which might be the best course of treatment for the individual patient.[110]

Moreover, it has been argued that any figures comparing different outcomes and side effects are of questionable validity because there is a significant bias in the selection of patients for trials. All of this can cause understandable anxiety in some patients.[111]

Before agreeing to any invasive procedure, it would be wise to ask these questions (some of which are taken from a prostate-cancer website[112]):

- Is my cancer only in the prostate or has it spread?
- Will I need additional tests? What are the purposes of the tests?
- What are my treatment options? How long does treatment last?
- What is the overall success rate for the procedure? (and how is 'success' defined?)

- What other therapies are available, and how do they compare?
- What is the likely outcome in my own situation?
- What is the individual success rate of the specialist/surgeon involved?
- How does this compare with other specialists in the same field?
- What are the side effects (both common and rare) and their chance of occuring?
- Will the treatment cause serious bone thinning, and hence osteoporosis?
- What are the chances that I will have problems in urinating?
- What are the chances of my becoming sexually impotent following treatment?
- What are the chances of chronic colitis and diarrhoea?
- What is the quality of my life going to be after the procedure?
- What are the chances of my cancer coming back?
- What are the new and promising drugs and treatment for prostate cancer management?
- Is there anything else I should know?

A good doctor will take the time to answer these questions for you.

One issue you should also discuss with your doctors before undertaking any treatment is methods to prevent blood clots developing. Many oncologists underestimate the risk of these blood clots, although many cancer patients are vulnerable to the condition. Most oncologists included in a recent survey reported that they were not using preventive methods routinely in chemotherapy, hormone therapy, or radiotherapy.[113] The authors of the report say that national guidelines are needed for this.

While I think it wise that you should tell your oncologist and other health professionals if you are following the dietary and lifestyle factors I recommend, if you wish to do so, do not be put off if they are not convinced. Try to persuade them to read the book and show them the lists of references from the peer-reviewed science it is based on. Many doctors have been persuaded of the value of my approach by their patients, some of whom are doctors or other health professionals themselves, thereby helping other sufferers. If you cannot persuade them, then do not worry. Make your own decision, bearing in mind that all my recommendations are based on sound science and dietary principles based on thousands of years' experience (*see* p. 173). Above all, my regime fits with Hippocrates view that it can do no harm.

THE HALF-TIME SCORE

Some questions to ask yourself at this stage. Have you:

- found the strength to admit to yourself that you have a prostate problem?
- sought medical advice as soon as possible and obtained information to calm your fears and reassure yourself as much as possible?
- ensured that your GP has sent you to a specialist hospital, not to a general surgeon, and that you have confidence in the team who will be treating you?
- involved your friends and family who are prepared to help (*see* further in Chapter 6)?
- attended for all the tests and followed instructions closely?
- listened to people with a positive supportive approach?
- tried to remove old wives' tales and irrational fears from your mind and developed a more rational, less frightening concept of prostate cancer based on scientific understanding (*see* Chapter 2)?

Or have you:

- panicked and scared yourself by thinking of all the awful things that could happen?
- listened to people with scary stories?
- gone alone to be given the diagnosis or the results of tests and become confused and frightened?
- been influenced by too many different doctors? (Take the advice of the consultant in charge of your case. They will have treated the most cases and will have the greatest real experience of prostate cancer, as distinct from simply theoretical knowledge.)

In the section which follows, I shall explain the reasoning and rationale for current cancer therapy.

TREATMENT OPTIONS

If you are diagnosed with prostate cancer and have had all of the tests, the next step is to decide with your oncologist which is the most appropriate course of treatment for you. Modern doctors will try to involve you in such discussions. This does not mean they do not know their facts and have their own views. It simply means that they wish you to engage with them and work together to decide on treatment options to defeat your prostate cancer.[114]

The result of early screening, particularly in Europe and the US, means that more and more men are receiving early diagnosis of prostate cancer, and more and more patients are therefore faced with the dilemma of deciding on treatment options.[115]

Also do try to bear in mind that today a diagnosis of cancer no longer equates to a death sentence: a significant proportion of patients are completely cured, whilst a further proportion may have their symptoms eased for a significant time. Survival is a probability, not a slim possibility.[116] In the US more than 90 per cent of all prostate cancers are now discovered in the early stages, and the five-year survival rate for these patients is almost 100 per cent. Over the past twenty years the five-year survival rate for all prostate-cancer patients there has increased from 67 per cent to nearly 100 per cent, with ten-year survival at 93 per cent and fifteen-year survival at 77 per cent of patients. In England, the five-year survival rate has increased from only 31 per cent before 1975 to 71 per cent in 2000–2001 – but it is only 60 per cent in Scotland.[117]

If you need treatment, the specialists will generally recommend some combination of surgery, radiotherapy and hormone treatment, and they may recommend chemotherapy if the cancer is found to have spread.[118]

Let us look first at some of the treatment options for localised prostate cancer (confined to the prostate gland).

- observation, with treatment at a later date if necessary ('watchful waiting')
- radiotherapy: external-beam radiotherapy; or brachytherapy (internal radiotherapy, which involves the insertion of small needles carrying radioactive pellets)
- surgery

- high-intensity focused ultrasound (HIFU) treatment
- photodynamic therapy (PDT)

WATCHFUL WAITING

A good strategy for some patients with prostate cancer may be watchful waiting.The cancer is regularly and carefully observed and monitored, but there is no immediate active treatment. This approach may be recommended if the cancer is not causing any symptoms, especially if it is very small and confined to one area of the prostate, if it is expected to grow very slowly, or if the patient is elderly or frail or has other serious health problems. Because prostate cancer often grows very slowly, many older men with the disease never need any treatment. Some men may decide that the side effects of treatment outweigh the benefits. Watchful waiting does not mean that more aggressive therapy cannot be used if the cancer begins to grow more quickly or causes symptoms.[119]

The following are Professor Waxman's criteria for patient selection for the watchful waiting option for patients with localised prostate cancer:

- good histology (low Gleason score)
- minimal infiltration
- lack of symptoms
- older men
- patient preference

One recent study[120] showed that men with prostate cancer who decided not to have surgery and instead opted only for treatment of their symptoms did as well as men who had surgery, at least in the first six or seven years after diagnosis. Men having surgery had only half the risk of dying from prostate cancer, but this was balanced by an increased risk of death from other causes. The researchers suggested that reasons might include a variety of complications such as blood clots following surgery.

SURGERY

Surgeons treating prostate cancer generally prefer to go through the abdomen, often removing the entire prostate, the seminal vesicles and the pelvic lymph nodes. This route allows the surgeon to see how far the disease has spread. This is major surgery, and as patients tend to be older it is risky, with the chances of complications increasing with age. After surgery, there is a 70 per cent risk of impotence and a 5 per cent risk of incontinence.[121]

Surgery for prostate cancer requires enormous skill – a skill that develops with practice. Radical prostatectomy has been refined over the last 20 years, so that damage to nerves controlling sexual function can be limited. These will now not be removed, unless they are affected by the cancer. The name of the operation has been changed to reflect these advances: it is now called a radical nerve-sparing prostatectomy.[122]

Admission to hospital is usually on the day before the operation. Prior to surgery, an anaesthetist will examine you, reviewing your overall medical state – in particular the state of your heart and lungs – to determine your fitness to undergo the procedure.

Try to talk to both your surgeon and your anaesthetist well ahead of the operation (standard practice at all good hospitals). It is also standard practice at good hospitals for the surgeon to mark the area to be incised with a black felt-tip pen while you are fully awake. Although this is disturbing, just think how much more distressing it would be to come round from anaesthesia and find the wrong bit had been removed. If necessary, insist that this is carried out before you are given your 'pre-med' or tranquilliser.

There have also been reports of problems related to blood transfusion, mostly because the wrong type of blood has been used. If you may need a blood transfusion and you are likely to be unconscious at the time of the transfusion, make sure that you know your own blood group and insist that the health professional checks that the blood is the correct one for you before allowing them to begin the transfusion or operation.[123]

Several hours before the operation you will be given a pre-med injection to help you to relax. After the injection your throat may feel very dry and you will become sleepy. You will then be given a suppository to cause the bowel to empty, making surgery easier and reducing the risks of side effects such as infection. You will also be fitted with thigh-length support stockings to prevent blood clots forming in your leg veins. Patients are usually given an injection of Heparin, a drug that prevents blood clots forming (which happens more commonly in people undergoing operations). Antibiotics may also be given. Before the operation you will be wheeled into an anteroom and given an injection by an anaesthetist which will make you unconscious within seconds. Following removal of the prostate, the bladder neck must be reconstructed, which requires great skill because scarring can cause many of the side effects of such operations. A catheter is placed through the reconstructed bladder neck to drain urine before the abdomen is repaired. You are likely to spend two or three hours under observation in a recovery room before being sent back to the hospital ward.[124]

On waking back on the ward, you will find that you have a drip in your arm, a catheter in your penis and plastic tubes draining blood and serum from the surgical wounds in your abdomen. In most cases the drains are removed after five days and the catheter after one to two weeks. In a few cases problems due to scarring around the surgical join of the bladder and urethra cause complete inability to urinate, and this may require further minor surgery.

After the operation, it can take a minimum of three months to recover. Take it easy, gradually returning to a regular pattern of exercise.

Another type of operation, radical perineal prostatectomy, involves removing the prostate through an incision between the scrotum and anus. Nerve-sparing operations are more difficult by this approach, and lymph nodes cannot be removed.[125] Robotic surgery guided by scans is being developed for prostatectomy operations to try to improve their precision and reduce the side effects such as incontinence and impotence.

The following are Professor Waxman's criteria for patient selection for radical surgery:

- age less than 70 years
- poorly differentiated tumours (high Gleason score)
- PSA less than 12–15
- sexual potency not an issue
- no pre-existing radiation (not absolute)
- informed consent
- patient desire
- patients without heart conditions or other serious illnesses

There was a report in the *Lancet* about the possible spread of prostate cancer during surgical operations. Although it was considered that the jury was still out, the article noted that even a solid tumour such as prostate cancer may already have shed some cancer cells into the blood or lymph system, and that surgery could potentially worsen the situation. There is no doubt that anaesthesia damages the immune system, and in China they frequently use acupuncture rather than anaesthesia for such operations for this reason.[126] Giving men radiation therapy after removal of their cancerous prostate gland has been found to lower the chance of recurrence by about 8 per cent.[127]

RADIOTHERAPY

Radiotherapy owes its origins to the first separation of the naturally occurring radioactive isotope radium-226 from a type of uranium ore known as pitchblende, by Marie Curie, who was a student of Henri Bequerel, the person who first discovered radioactivity.

Radiotherapy now relies on irradiating cancer with powerful X-rays (invisible but very powerful electromagnetic waves of energy) delivered using an externally applied beam, or in some cases by implanting radioactive sources which emit gamma rays (even higher energy rays). The machines most commonly used deliver powerful X-rays created by a machine called a linear accelerator. The exact method by which radiation destroys cancer cells is not known, but it is thought either to inflict genetic damage sufficient to kill cells directly, or to induce the cells to commit suicide by the process doctors call apoptosis. It relies on the fact that healthy tissues can repair the damage from radiation exposure more readily than cancer cells.

One of the main benefits of radiation therapy is that it can preserve the anatomical structure around the cancer so it is less mutilating and disfiguring than surgery. Radiation can also destroy microscopic extensions of cancers that surgery can miss and is a safer option for older, frailer patients. Nevertheless, it sometimes fails to eradicate all the cancer cells in tumours and, like surgery, it is primarily a local treatment. It does not help in cases of metastastic cancer, except to relieve symptoms. Whole-body radiation exposure sufficient to kill all dispersed cancer cells would destroy tissues vital to life.

Many people are afraid of radioactivity, and rightly so. It is used a great deal in diagnostic medicine, including X-rays and bone scans, and in radiotherapy. It is worth remembering that in the UK, about 14 per cent of the average dose of ionising radiation to a UK citizen is from medical diagnostic procedures and treatment, compared with less than 1 per cent from industrial activity plus fallout from nuclear weapons; the remainder (about 85 per cent) comes from natural sources, including rocks, soils, buildings and food.[128]

In an investigation of hospital doctors' knowledge of radiation exposure,[129] it was found that few had any knowledge about the level of radiation that their patients were likely to be exposed to during investigations, although they had all taken the radiation protection course. This lack of awareness is particularly unfortunate considering the number of cancer patients who receive repeat investigations and treatments. This is unlikely to be a problem with radiotherapists, however, who, in my experience, are very knowledgeable about this subject.

There are two types of radiotherapy used to treat prostate cancer: external radiotherapy, which requires six weeks of treatment and kills all fast-reproducing cells in its line of fire, and brachytherapy, which involves implanting radioactive pellets into the prostate; this one-to-two-day treatment is more localised. It is growing in support in the US, but the UK still has relatively few centres. No long-term side effects of brachytherapy have yet been noted.[130]

External-beam radiotherapy

Radiotherapy involves sophisticated machinery and highly trained medical professionals. The first step in such treatment is planning. This involves determining precisely how to deliver the radiation to the area of the prostate to be treated and calculating the dose to be used, based on all the information obtained, especially from scanning. Planning should now routinely involve the use of computer imagery.[131]

Planning is a complex and highly skilled process, normally carried out by physicists to determine how to maximise the effects of radiation on malignant tissue, while causing as little damage as possible to normal tissue.

A newer form of external-beam radiotherapy, known as *Three-dimensional conformal radiation therapy* (3D-CRT), uses computers to map the cancer precisely and appears likely to increase the success rate and reduce the side effects of radiotherapy. Short-term results suggest that by aiming the radiation more accurately it is possible to reduce damage to tissues near the prostate and increase the radiation dose to the cancer.[132]

Recently intensity-modulated radiotherapy (IMRT) treatment for prostate cancer has been introduced. This is a refinement of conformal external-beam therapy, but employs a non-uniform beam to create greater conformity between the distribution of the radioactive dose and that of the cancerous tissue.[133]

Prior to radiotherapy, you will be taken to the radiotherapy treatment centre to ensure that the plan is accurate. Be prepared for a room that looks like something from a science-fiction film. During this stage, one or more tiny permanent tattoo marks will be made on your skin, to determine the positions of the radiotherapy delivery during the treatment process. I can still see the one above the top of my breastbone, but no one else seems to notice unless I point it out to them! The commonest treatment plans involve daily treatment as an outpatient, apart from weekends, for a period of six weeks, and many people continue to work daily (as I did during my treatment). It is entirely normal to be worried about radiotherapy, especially if there is a long wait for treatment, but once it begins most people adjust quickly.

Normally when you arrive for treatment you will be asked to wait in a waiting area with other patients.[134] Ensure that you talk only to patients with positive attitudes to calm any nerves. Always end conversations abruptly – rudely, if necessary – at the merest suggestion of a horror story.

When it is your turn for treatment you will be taken into the radiotherapy treatment room by a radiographer, who will position you and the radiotherapy machine correctly, using laser beams and your tattoo or tattoos. The staff will then leave the room to reduce their exposure to radiation, but they will continue to observe you using a video camera. You should keep as still as possible throughout treatment. The radiotherapy treatment takes only a few moments, and you will be allowed to leave the hospital almost immediately afterwards. In most centres the time taken from arrival to completion of treatment is about 30 to 45 minutes.[135]

The following are Professor Waxman's criteria for patient selection for external-beam radiotherapy for patients with localised prostate cancer:

- patient preference
- well-differentiated cancer
- small-volume tumours
- sexual potency not an issue
- age over 70 years
- any pre-existing history of colitis is a contra-indication to treatment, as colitis can be made worse

Brachytherapy (internal radiation therapy)

Brachytherapy sounds very modern, but it is a method that has been around for decades. The procedure is relatively quick, requires short anaesthesia, and, after a few hours, you will usually be allowed to go home.[136]

The planning and administration of treatment is similar in many respects to external-beam radiotherapy, although it is initially more complex and involves an ultrasound probe being inserted into the rectum to take many measurements to assess the dimensions and configuration of the prostate and its relationship to other structures, such as the urethra. Up to 40 needles may be used to insert radioactive pellets (each about the size of a grain of rice) of particular isotopes, such as iodine-125. These will keep their radioactivity long enough to treat the tumour, but the radioactivity will then gradually die away. A urinary catheter is frequently inserted into the prostate while the procedure is being carried out.[137]

Needles containing more radioactive material, high-dose rate (HDR) brachytherapy, are generally used for less than a day, and in combination with low-dose external-beam radiation. For about a week following insertion of the needles, patients may experience some pain and may have discoloration of their urine.[138] The treatment is more expensive than external beam radiotherapy and is not available under the NHS in all parts of the UK.

The following are Professor Waxman's criteria for patient selection for brachytherapy for patients with localised prostate cancer:

- younger men
- all tumour grades
- tumour stage less than T2
- PSA less than 10

These highly selected patients would also be likely to have a very good prospect for cure by standard radiotherapy or surgery, or indeed a very low chance of progression of their tumour without any invasive treatment.

Effects of radiotherapy on the skin

Initially, the treatment has little or no effect, but gradually the skin looks and feels as if it has been very badly sunburned. Indeed it is wise to be careful about ever sunbathing after having radiotherapy. Wash the burned area only with plain water using a low-power shower and never use soap or shower gels on the affected area. There are many different recommendations, for treating the soreness caused by radiotherapy, including Aloe vera cream, but even herbal remedies contain preservatives which can aggravate symptoms. It is best to buy an Aloe vera plant and use a segment of a fresh leaf to rub on the affected area. Aloe vera has been used for centuries by desert Arabs against sunburn.

Some foods contain chemicals similar to those used in antiradiation pills given to astronauts (more about this later).

Radiotherapy and chemotherapy have different side effects. In my own case, apart from the burn in the immediate irradiated area, I had no other problems after radiotherapy. I know of no one treated by radiotherapy for prostate cancer who has lost his hair or felt nauseated (although irradiation of the head or digestive tract for other types of cancer can cause such symptoms). Throughout the radiotherapy you will be given blood tests to ensure that you can continue with the treatment. Also ask about the regularity with which the equipment is serviced and checked. This is very important, because poorly maintained radiotherapy equipment can be extremely dangerous. At the end of the treatment you should be given a thorough physical check-up, and this should be repeated after six weeks.

SOME OTHER SIDE EFFECTS OF RADIOTHERAPY AND SURGERY

Incontinence[139]

Incontinence is the inability to control the urine stream, resulting in leakage or dribbling of urine. There are three types: stress, overflow and urge incontinence.

- Stress incontinence, which is the commonest type after prostate surgery, occurs when coughing, laughing, sneezing, or exercising and is usually caused by problems with the muscle valve, or sphincter, that keeps urine in the bladder. Prostate cancer treatments may damage the valve or the nerves that keep it working.
- Overflow incontinence is associated with a dribbling stream of urine with little force, usually due to blockage or narrowing of the bladder outlet, by cancer or scar tissue.
- Men with urge incontinence often have a sudden need to pass urine, because the bladder is over-sensitive to stretching caused by urine build-up.

Depending on your situation, there are several ways to improve this condition, including surgery, medicine, and exercises, so do not be afraid to ask your doctor for help. They will have dealt with this problem many times before.

Cystitis (inflamed or sore bladder)

Cranberry juice is often recommended for cystitis but it is useless where there is no infection and the problem simply reflects irritation. A patent medical cure known as Mist Pot Cit, which contains potassium citrate, should be avoided because it can increase the risk of heart problems.[140] It is best to drink lots of boiled, filtered (but certainly not fizzy) water.

Impotence[141]

Impotence, the inability to achieve an erection of the penis, can occur because of damage as a result of radiation therapy or radical prostatectomy. It is considered less likely after brachytherapy. Several solutions are available.

- Prostheses (penile implants) can restore the ability to have erections.
- Mechanical pumps, placed around the entire penis before intercourse.
- Certain drugs, such as sildenafil (Viagra), prostageandin E (administered as a urethral suppository (MUSE)), or injection of prostaglandin directly into the penis.[142] According to the orthodox doctors, the earlier that Viagra, or more modern alternatives, are tried, the more likely they are to work – and the later, the less likely.[143]

Do discuss such problems with your doctor and with your sexual partner.

Rectal damage and diarrhoea

Both external beam and brachytherapy can damage bowel and rectal tissue (proctitis), causing diarrhoea and colitis, and burning pain and diarrhoea, respectively. The doctors can treat this with drugs, but the symptoms should stop soon after the completion of treatment – though in some patients the radiation causes permanent scarring, leading to longer-term diarrhoea and sometimes rectal bleeding. In severe cases, surgery is required. Steroid enemas may be offered, but see my comments on steroid use in cancer treatment (*see* p. 60–61).[144]

DEALING WITH PAIN

Do not hesitate to discuss pain with your doctors. Enduring unnecessary pain has no benefit, and pain medication does not interfere with cancer treatments. In fact getting effective pain relief can help some patients to be more active and may indirectly help them to live longer.[145]

I was lucky to have suffered very little pain after surgery. If I had suffered severe pain I would have tried acupuncture rather than chemical painkillers such as morphine. Acupuncture is said to have originated in China over 4,000 years ago, when it was realised that it often enabled arrow-wounded soldiers to make surprising recoveries from long-standing illnesses.

Acupuncture for pain relief is one of the most widely accepted of all complementary medical disciplines. Indeed, the British

Medical Association published a report on 'Alternative Therapy' in 1986, in which it accepted that there is a scientific basis for claims that acupuncture is effective as an analgesic (pain-reliever),[146] and it is now widely available on the NHS. Some veterinary surgeons routinely use it for chronic pain relief for animals.[147] Overall, evidence from randomised controlled trials supports the use of acupuncture in pain conditions including post-operative pain. Such trials also provide evidence of an effect on nausea, so acupuncture is a potentially valuable method of contributing to relieving some of the effects of cancer and cancer treatments – with the additional advantage that it does not add to the chemical burden of the body or cause other side effects.[148]

Acupuncture needles are extremely fine and do not hurt in the same way as, say, an injection; patients may even be unaware that a needle has been inserted. Many patients say they find acupuncture relaxing and sedating, though the method does not work well on everybody. If you use acupuncture it is essential to use only a fully qualified member of the British Acupuncture Council (or equivalent).

Variations include acupressure, where pressure is applied using studs on elasticated bands to the points traditionally used for acupuncture, and electroacupuncture (EAP), which uses an electrical pulse instead of inserting a needle in the acupuncture point. Lasers are sometimes used now instead of needles. Transcutaneous nerve stimulation or TENS does not use acupuncture points but stimulates nerves which block pain messages and it can be used at home. Hypnosis is another option for pain relief which is also thought to work by increasing endorphin production in the brain.

I refused, and continue to refuse as far as possible, to take medication prescribed by doctors or available over the counter from pharmacists. Steroids are sometimes given to suppress various types of discomfort associated with cancer or its treatment, but since they depress immune function, I have always refused them. I also try to minimise my use of antibiotics and I cannot remember when I last used painkillers. None of these types of drugs is known to cause cancer, but I just do not like taking man-made chemicals if I can avoid doing so.

HORMONE OR DRUG TREATMENT*

This method is often used, as prostate cancer is frequently hormonally driven. All hormonal treatments aim to negate the effects of androgens (more specifically testosterone) on prostate tissue, which they do in a variety of ways. It is given to patients with localised cancers, or if the cancer is advanced and spreading to other tissues. Some types may be prescribed indefinitely. Injections may be given to block testosterone production, or tablets to neutralise the hormone; an operation may be recommended to remove the testes; or oestrogen tablets may be recommended to balance the testosterone. Lowering testosterone levels can make prostate cancers shrink or grow more slowly, but the therapy alone does not cure the cancer. Moreover, some prostate cancers are androgen-independent and some become androgen-independent after a few years of treatment. All forms of hormone treatment can have such side effects as: impotence, loss of sex drive, hot flushes, breast swelling and osteoporosis.[149] Adjuvant hormonal therapy refers to treatment used in addition and prior to the start of surgery or radiotherapy, and it is claimed that it improves outcomes, especially for aggressive prostate cancers.

Orchiectomy This is the medical name for surgical removal of the testes (castration). It is a relatively quick operation carried out under general or spinal anaesthetic. Some medical practitioners argue in favour of this treatment on the basis that it can be forgotten relatively quickly(!!) Another argument of advocates of orchiectomy is that it is cost-effective – i.e. cheap – although this is disputed. It continues to be used if patients prefer this treatment having been fully informed about all of the options available.[150]

Oestrogen therapy Oestrogens have been used to treat prostate cancer for more than 60 years. The main drug used is diethylstilboestrol (DES), a synthetic version of a female hormone, oestrogen, generally taken in tablet form up to three times a day. This works by blocking the release of LHRH (*see* Chapter 2, p. 98), leading to the shutting off of testosterone production. Research has shown an increase in deaths from cardiovascular

---

* The interaction of hormones with prostate tissue is described more fully in Chapter 2 and only abbreviations are used here, for example LHRH is used for luteinising hormone-releasing hormone.

disease from this treatment, dating back to the mid-1960s.[151] Other symptoms include gastrointestinal problems and mood changes, and all patients suffer from swelling of the breasts, which can be very tender and profoundly enlarged. Waxman concludes that this treatment would now seem to be unnecessary, since there are so many alternative treatments for prostate cancer. The argument for treatment with oestrogens in the UK is again that they are cheap! I am aware that men find swollen breasts distressing and embarrassing, and it is possible for them to have their enlarged breasts reduced by cosmetic surgery.

Anti-androgens work by blocking the binding of testosterone and DHT to androgen receptors in prostate tissue. The first drug of this type, Flutamide, was introduced for prostate-cancer treatment in the 1970s. Side effects can include severe depression, diarrhoea and in rare cases liver damage which is sometimes fatal.

In the late 1980s, another drug of this type called Bicalutamide was introduced for prostate-cancer treatment and is without major known side effects other than nipple tenderness, which may require radiotherapy! Approximately 40–60 per cent of all patients treated with this drug alone retain sexual potency.

Cyproterone acetate may cause fluid retention, strokes and heart attacks, and is so toxic to the liver that it can be used only for a very short period of time.

Gonadotrophin-releasing hormone (GnRH) agonists treatments began in the early 1980s. They work by causing a decrease in LH and FSH levels produced by the pituitary. Subcutaneous implants requiring three-monthly replacement have been developed – a method regarded by Waxman as a humane and effective treatment of prostate cancer. Side effects include hot flushes (treated with yet more drugs) and, less commonly, anaemia and osteoporosis (on average about 2 per cent bone loss for every year of treatment). Any osteoporosis is treated with drugs called bisphosphonates (*see* below).

Other hormone drugs Megestrol acetate is sometimes used if first-line hormone treatments lose effectiveness. Ketoconazole, initially used for treating fungal infections and later found to also work as an antiandrogen, is another drug used for second-line hormone therapy.[152]

Other methods include combinations, for example of LHRH agonists with anti-androgens. Intermittent hormonal therapy may also be used in an attempt to allow the return of sexual potency, but the efficacy of this for treating prostate cancer remains unproven. Drugs that can prevent the adrenal glands from making androgens are sometimes used with other methods of hormone treatment for total androgen blockade, but once again doctors do not know whether this is more effective than treatments with single drugs.

Other drugs called bisphosphonates, previously used principally for treating osteoporosis, may also prolong the life of patients whose prostate cancer has spread to the bone. There has been debate for some years as to whether bisphosphonates have an anti-carcinogenic effect on malignant tumour cells, or whether they merely alter the bone so that the tumour doesn't spread as easily or grow so fast.[153] A systematic review of the role of bisphosphonates on damage to the skeleton (e.g. fracture, nerve-root compression and reduced mobility) in patients affected by metastatic cancer also found that bisphosphonates reduced these problems and extended the time to their onset.[154]

As with most prostate-cancer treatments, opinions as to the best methods are divided.[155] Working with people at risk of prostate cancer spreading to their bones, I have found that they find my book on osteoporosis,[156] which contains lots of advice on protecting bones, extremely helpful.

One recent report suggested that 'hormone drugs attack a man in every department where he feels he is a man' – impotence, mood, lack of energy, inability to work. Patients may not be warned about these possible effects, and by the time they have had the treatment it is too late.[157] I have to say that I know many men on these types of treatment who appear to be coping very well. Sometimes it is a matter of changing treatment methods until the best one for the patient is found.

CHEMOTHERAPY

The first chemotherapeutic drugs were developed during the 1940s and were a spin-off of the work carried out by the Nazis to develop methods of chemical warfare. Unfortunately, solid tumours such as prostate cancer are only rarely curable with chemotherapy alone.[158]

Chemotherapy involves the administration of anti-cancer drugs that travel throughout the whole body via the blood-circulation system. Hence it is a systemic anti-cancer treatment. Many chemical compounds are currently in use, and new ones are constantly being screened and tested.

Chemotherapeutic drugs act by preventing cells from multiplying by interfering with their ability to replicate their DNA. In at least some cases, anti-cancer drugs (like radiotherapy) are thought to induce suicide or apoptosis of cancer cells. Unfortunately, while the chemotherapeutic agents are in the body they attack all cells undergoing cell division (mitosis). This is why they particularly affect tissues which have a fast turnover of cells such as the lining of the digestive tract, hair follicles and bone marrow. This is the reason for the common side effects of the treatment, which include nausea and vomiting, loss of hair, mouth sores, anaemia and increased risk of infection.

Damage to the rapidly replicating cells of the bone marrow can be particularly problematic because, as well as causing anaemia, it can damage the immune system. This reduces the ability to fight infections and can increase the potential for internal bleeding because too few red and white blood cells and platelets (the cells responsible for clotting) are produced.

One recent study[159] claims that doctors should be wary of starting their patients on newly approved drugs because of the high rate of adverse side effects which can be undetected until late in the post-marketing surveillance period. New anti-cancer drugs reaching the European market between 1995 and 2000 offered few or no substantial advantages over existing preparations, yet cost several times – in one case 350 times – as much.[160] Four of the drugs considered were chemotherapeutic agents for advanced metastatic breast cancer.

I find the following statement, from the ACS's website, particularly interesting, since some of the prostate sufferers I have communicated with have been in remission following treatment with chemotherapy and keeping to my diet and lifestyle. The website states that chemotherapy is an option for patients whose prostate cancer has spread beyond the prostate gland and for whom hormone therapy has failed. It is not expected to destroy all of the cancer cells, but it can slow tumour growth and reduce pain.[161] Chemotherapy, combined with my diet, and lifestyle, saved my life when I had been given at best a few months to live. I refused to take steroids, however, because they suppress the body's immune system. Steroids are designed to relieve symptoms, and I understand why they are prescribed in cases of advanced cancer. My doctors insisted, but fortunately they were administered as pills which I hid under my tongue and then spat out. This was my decision, and you should discuss their use thoroughly with your doctor and agree what to do.

Chemotherapy drugs used in treating prostate cancer that has returned or continued to grow and spread after treatment with hormone therapy include doxorubicin, estramustine, etoposide, mitoxantrone, vinblastine, paclitaxel, and docetaxel, and many new ones are being developed. Two or more drugs are often given together to reduce the likelihood of the cancer cells becoming resistant to chemotherapy. Small-cell carcinoma is a rare type of prostate cancer that is more likely to respond to chemotherapy than to hormone therapy. Cisplatin and etoposide are the drugs recommended for treating such cancers.[162]

Do maintain an active interest in what is going on. Some years ago, I accompanied a friend for her chemotherapy treatment and she was almost accidentally given chemotherapy of twice the strength it should have been – and this had not been picked up by the doctor prescribing it, the computer system, the pharmacy or the senior nurse in charge of the ward. Had I not helped her collect her drugs and read the labels she could have had serious liver or kidney failure.

Some tips for coping with chemotherapy

If you are worried about losing your hair, treat yourself to a really good wig from a reputable company. A simple tip that many people facing chemotherapy find helpful is to involve your normal hairdresser, who can help you to choose a wig of the right colour and texture and trim it so that it looks almost identical to your normal hairstyle.

Ensure that you are given good anti-sickness pills such as those that actually block the receptors in the brain that tell you to feel sick. Also some people develop horrendous haemorrhoids as a result of constipation caused by their anti-sickness pills. These can be dealt with easily by eating Linusit, which is organically-grown linseed (also called flax seed) and is widely available in health-food shops and has other benefits in combating cancer (*see* Chapter 5).

Additional advice from the National Cancer Institute (NCI) of America[163] includes telling your doctor about any side effects of the treatment, asking before you take any other medicine or supplement, including ones recommended by complementary or alternative health practitioners, and talking about your feelings (to counsellor, friends or family). Some further tips for eating if your appetite is badly affected by your treatment include:[164]

- Eat frequent, small meals or snacks whenever you want, perhaps four to six times a day, rather than three regular meals.
- Keep snacks (such as seeds, nuts, and fresh and dried fruits) within easy reach, so you can eat something when you feel like it.
- If you do not want to eat solid foods, try to drink soup, juice and herbal or green tea.
- When possible, take a walk before meals to stimulate your appetite.
- Eat with friends or family members, or, when eating alone, listen to the radio or watch TV.

You can vary your diet by trying the new foods and recipes from this book and from *The Plant Programme* and *Eating for Better Health*. One of the commonest observations of patients following the diet recommended in this and my previous books when undergoing chemotherapy is how well they are able to withstand treatment, and this is often noted by their health-care professionals.

NEW TREATMENTS

A recent NIH Workshop on Selective Receptor Modulators (SRMS) focused on their potential use for treating hormonal-dependent cancers, including those of the prostate. Some SRMS, such as finasteride, are already being used for the clinical treatment of BPH and prostate cancer.[165]

A cancer treatment that encourages cancer cells to commit suicide by using biocatalysts that single out diseased cells is being developed by scientists at Exeter University.[166]

The US FDA and the UK National Institute for Clinical Excellence (NICE) have approved a new drug, Gleevec, for patients with a rare but life-threatening form of leukaemia, and is being tested on prostate cancer.[167]

Other new drugs with mechanisms of action that are not fully understood include Genasense, which is designed to work against a protein called Bcl-2 which allows cancer cells to ignore signals to commit suicide. When given to patients over several days before standard chemotherapy, Genasense is thought to help the other drugs kill the cancer cells. Bcl-2 over-expression plays a role in many types of cancer, including that of the prostate.[168]

Another drug that could prove a success story is Kahalalide F, which is based on a protein produced by tiny Hawaiian sea snails. The drug has proved effective in tests on patients with prostate cancer. Molecules harvested from sea urchins, clams, algae, snails and sea cucumbers found off the coast of Venezuela are also under investigation as potential cancer cures. Laboratory tests showed that minute quantities of substances they produce can kill 50 per cent of cancer cells. One researcher is quoted as saying, 'Some outstanding growth inhibition was observed, suggesting that these organisms could be very promising sources of novel compounds.'[169]

Two of the most important new treatments for prostate cancer are high-intensity focused ultrasound (HIFU) and photodynamic therapy (PDT).

HIGH INTENSITY FOCUSED ULTRASOUND (HIFU) (ABLATHERM)

Ultrasound treatment can work at depth in the body without harming healthy tissue, unlike lasers or radiotherapy; and unlike some types of radiotherapy, the effects cease as soon as treatment ends. Ultrasound has been used for scanning, including during pregnancy, for a long time. HIFU works by concentrating an ultrasonic beam on the prostate cancer, destroying it by applying controlled heat almost instantaneously.

During treatment, a probe which generates the focused ultrasound beam is inserted into the rectum (where the prostate gland is most accessible) through the anus. The probe then moves under computer control according to an image of the prostate cancer prepared from scans.

The technique is claimed to improve the precision of treatment, improve outcomes and have fewer and less serious side effects than conventional treatments. The first use of HIFU on humans was in 1993. Since then tens of thousands of patients have been treated with it at more than 120 centres throughout the world. In the UK, the main centres are the Guy's and St Thomas's NHS foundation trust and the Royal Marsden NHS foundation trust. There are several published studies of clinical trials of the technique. Like PDT, the technique can be used on patients on whom other treatments have failed. One advantage of the method is that it can be regarded as simply an extension of diagnostic ultrasound scanning. Although available in many European countries, Canada and Australia, HIFU is not yet approved in the USA, where the results of further clinical trials are awaited.

The main criteria for patient selection for HIFU include

• tumour contained within prostate with no evidence of spread.

PHOTODYNAMIC THERAPY (PDT)

Photodynamic therapy uses laser or other light sources combined with a drug that is activated by light, called a photosensitising agent, to destroy cancer cells. The types of drugs used are ones that are preferentially taken up by cancer cells rather than normal cells and which, when they are activated by light, destroy cells. Clearly it is essential that the light reaches the cancer cells. Hence PDT was used initially to treat skin cancers or those on or near the lining of internal organs, such as cancers of the lining of the mouth or the lining of the bladder which could be easily reached using lasers or light probes. Fibre-optic cables are now being used to treat solid tumours such as prostate cancer. If the cancer is confined to the prostate, the aim will generally be to cure the cancer but for advanced metastatic cancer the aim of PDT is usually to reduce symptoms by shrinking the tumours. PDT treatment can be given to patients in hospital, although it is more frequently used to treat patients as outpatients.

The first stage of treatment involves an injection of the drug, or it may be given as a drink or in tablets. The second stage involves shining light directly on to the cancer. This may involve a laser or non-laser light delivered through flexible tubes to ensure that it is taken as close as possible to the cancer. The interval between the two stages of treatment allows the drug to accumulate in cancer cells; its length depends on the type of drug used, and can vary from about 90 minutes to four days. Healing causes much less scarring than surgery. The time taken to heal depends on how deeply the light has penetrated, and it can take several weeks.

Clinical trial results for PDT treatment of prostate cancer are becoming available. In a report in the *Journal of Urology*, Dr Timothy Nathan and colleagues of University College Medical School, London, reported that a form of PDT benefits prostate cancer patients whose disease has recurred after radiation treatment. They found that PDT destroyed localised areas of cancer with safe healing and without the cumulative toxicity associated with ionising radiation. Fourteen patients with rising PSA scores and known recurrences of prostate cancer after radiotherapy were given PDT using an experimental chlorophyll drug followed by red-light treatment administered using fibre-optic cables inserted into the prostate gland through needles.

PSA scores decreased in nine patients and to below the limit of detection in two of them. Five patients had no viable tumour tissue when needle biopsies were performed, and CT and MRI scans showed tissue breakdown of cancer involving up to 91 per cent of the prostate after treatment. However, four men developed incontinence and of seven men who had been able to have sexual intercourse following radiotherapy four suffered long-term impotence. The researchers concluded that 'The results suggested that this kind of PDT merits further investigation.'

Side effects

Side effects of PDT include incontinence and impotence, which are described above. Other side effects can include skin damage and eye damage, if suitable precautions are not taken, and other, usually minor, temporary discomforts.

Sunburn and eye damage As with all kinds of treatment, the side effects of PDT vary from person to person. They also reflect the type of photosensitising drug used and the time between giving the drug and applying the light treatment. Although the drugs used are mostly taken up by cancer cells, they can make normal skin cells, including those of the eyes, highly sensitive to light. People undergoing PDT are advised to protect themselves not only from sunlight but also from bright indoor lighting for a period of time, which can be up to weeks depending on the drug used. Patients may be advised to wear shady hats, and to be well covered, wearing gloves and dark glasses if they go outdoors. Sunscreens do not help. It is possible to become severely sunburnt even on a dull winter day or through glass if the sun is strong. Indoors, low-level lighting, maximum 60 W bulb, is advised. Opticians' appointments should be avoided and you should avoid any bright light being shone in your eyes. Your doctor or nurse should advise you on a schedule to expose yourself gradually to normal light when it is safe to do so.

Pain   Treatment with PDT can cause pain in the tumour area, which can be treated with painkillers.

Swelling   This can occur with some drugs. It is usually very temporary and can be treated with steroid drugs to reduce inflammation if necessary.

Other side effects can include constipation, which can be treated with a high-fibre diet such as the Plant Programme, or nausea, which can be treated with acupuncture and ginger tea.

Further research

Clinical trials are in hand to maximise the effectiveness and minimise the side effects of PDT. Research is being carried out into different photosensitising agents, which may be green (based on chlorophyll) or red (derived from blood), and on laser versus non-laser light delivered by fibre optics. Your doctor can advise you whether PDT is an appropriate treatment in your situation.

A word of warning and some advice

Because PDT treatment is, in principle, relatively simple, carries little risk to those operating the equipment and is enormously profitable, some private clinics are offering it to patients with advanced prostate cancer. Unfortunately, they may not be using it in a way that will help to treat the cancer. For example, some patients I have talked to have simply been placed in a whole-body red light field after being given the photosensitising drug. This is Cytoluminescent therapy (CLT), not PDT. It is difficult to understand how the light can reach the tumour in this situation, and I can find no evidence of successful outcomes for people with deep solid tumours such as those of the prostate. When these patients come to see me, it is usually because their PSA levels have risen, in some cases quite dramatically, after being treated in this way. Some of the patients had been doing very well, previously, with their NHS treatment combined with my regime. I have become concerned that the drug that is preferentially absorbed by the cancer if not activated by light may actually stimulate the cancer. I emphasise that I have no evidence for this – it is just my instinct as a scientist. My advice is always to discuss treatment with your doctor, to confirm the drugs that are to be used and the way the light will be administered.

TREATMENTS OF RECURRENT PROSTATE CANCER

Unfortunately, for some patients, prostate cancer can and does come back. Having repeated occurrences of cancer can be very distressing. I remember feeling suicidal the fifth time my cancer returned, and thinking that whatever I did to fight my cancer there was no escape. But try to remember that it is possible to recover from even advanced cancer. I did it, and I am aware of many men who have had recurrences of prostate cancer and are now in remission – some of them have been in remission for years.

Recurrence frequently requires chemotherapy and, in advanced cases, radiotherapy or radioisotope treatment to control pain.

The use of chemotherapy agents depends on many factors, including the type and stage of prostate cancer, the medical history of the patient and, in some patients, their state of mind. The oncologist prescribing treatment will consider all of these factors and many others – including their own experience of clinical successes and failures – and I would always follow their recommendations as to which chemotherapeutic agents to use. The drugs in use in the past were highly toxic and more suited to treating younger men who could withstand their toxicity and side effects. Improved chemotherapy agents are available, including Mitozantrone (often given with steroids to limit its side effects – but *see* p. 60). The side effects of this drug are reported to be minimal, with a very few cases of nausea, vomiting or infection, and no hair loss. The treatment does not improve life expectancy significantly but benefits the patient's well-being.[170]

Systemic radiation therapy, involving radioactive isotopes such as strontium-89, is used to treat bone pain caused by metastatic prostate cancer. This is usually more successful than external-beam radiation, but in the UK its high cost is an issue in treatment under the NHS, where half-body (upper or lower half) radiotherapy is more commonly used. This treatment can have significant side effects, including anaemia, sickness and infection.[171]

I believe that prostate cancer has the same root cause as breast cancer, however, and I have survived for fourteen years cancer-free after five occurrences of breast cancer.

SUMMARY OF TIPS FOR COPING WITH ANTI-CANCER TREATMENT

General

1. Insist that you are treated at a hospital with a specialist prostate cancer team, which includes a urologist – not just a general surgeon – a radiotherapist and a chemotherapist and ideally a doctor trained in HIFU.
2. Try to take a partner or discreet friend when you go for consultations with your doctors. Ensure that they are equipped with a notebook and pen to take notes to minimise confusion and additional stress.
3. If you know you are panicking or feeling emotional, ask your doctors for more time before making irrevocable choices about treatment options. Ensure that you are as calm as possible when you make important decisions or choices and try to involve your partner in your decisions.

Diagnosis

4. Listen and read instructions carefully and follow them closely to minimise the need for repeat tests and thus to minimise your exposure to radioactivity and other impacts of diagnostic procedures.
5. If you have a bone scan, drink cola containing phosphoric acid afterwards, to try to flush the radioactive agent used for testing from your body as soon as possible. (This agent is usually attached to a phosphate compound so it will attach to your bones during testing.)

Surgery

6. Before surgery, while you are awake and fully conscious, ensure that the area to be operated on is clearly marked with a felt-tip pen by the surgeon who will be operating on you, and that your blood type has been recorded correctly.

Radiotherapy

7. Wash the affected area with water only, using a low-power shower. Do not use soap. Use olive oil or the leaves of Aloe vera plants on the skin but no creams – even herbal ones – that could contain irritating preservatives.
8. Eat seaweed, an organic egg a day and lots of garlic to give your body cysteine-like chemicals to repair DNA – as used by astronauts (*see* Chapter 5).

Chemotherapy

9. Buy a wig with guidance from your normal hairdresser and have him/her style it to your usual hairdo. Drink juices to minimise or prevent the hair loss associated with some types of chemotherapy (*see* Chapter 5).
10. Drink only filtered water that has been boiled to kill organisms that can cause sickness and diarrhoea in immunosuppressed patients (*see* Chapter 5).

Photodynamic therapy

11. Follow advice to prevent skin burn and eye damage by dressing appropriately and avoiding strong light, even indoors.

COMPLEMENTARY AND ALTERNATIVE TREATMENTS

The international market for complementary and alternative medicine was worth an estimated $21.2 billion in the United States in 1997, more than half of which was paid directly by patients, and £450 million in Britain in 1998, with 90 per cent purchased privately.[172]

Complementary medicine is marginalised in many healthcare systems, but calls for an integrated approach, using both conventional and complementary therapies, are growing louder. Basic courses in various complementary therapies are now available in many medical schools in Britain and the United States, albeit on an optional basis.

Complementary therapies are often seen by patients as more 'natural' and having fewer side effects than conventional treatments. The enthusiasm for them shows people's desire to help themselves, as well as their frustration with the limitations of conventional medicine. The holistic and patient-centred approach of many complementary therapists appeals, as does the sense of empowerment gained from their philosophies of care. One of its great benefits is that users appreciate the greater amount of time devoted to the consultation.[173] Here I shall look only at herbal therapies. Some other complementary therapies, including hypnosis, will be considered in Chapter 6.

Herbal therapies

Natural substances have been used in Chinese medicine and Indian Ayurvedic medicine for about 3,500 years, and, as the WHO has pointed out, most of the people on Earth still rely on herbal treatments. Until the nineteenth century, drugs in western Europe, too, came mainly from plants – and botanic gardens were established so that Renaissance medical students could be trained to recognise medicinal plants.

The potential benefits of herbal medicines have been reviewed in an article by Ernst,[174] who suggests that a potential benefit could lie in their high acceptance by patients, their efficacy, their relative safety and their relatively low cost. He nevertheless points out how few clinical trials have been carried, in view of the very large number – several thousand – of different plants being used for medicinal purposes worldwide. He attributes the relative paucity of such trials to the small size of the sector compared with that of pharmaceuticals. He also points out, however, that records of adverse effects associated with herbal medicine from 55 countries are tiny compared with the adverse effects associated with conventional drugs held on the WHO monitoring centre database for the period 1968–1997.

It is worth remembering that the pharmaceutical industry sources several of its chemotherapeutic drugs from plants, including Pacific yew pine needles, Japanese marine algae and the periwinkle plant.[175]

Aspirin, which originally was a herbal medicine and one of the first to be commonly accepted by orthodox medicine, has been found to reduce the incidence of several types of cancer.[176] This is attributed to its content of salicylic acid.[177] I can find no specific studies of its use against prostate cancer, however. Remember to keep aspirin-based products – and indeed all medicines – away from children.[178]

In herbal medicine, Saw Palmetto has been used as a treatment for BPH. It may well be that Saw Palmetto might be of use in cancer prevention and the reduction of prostate hypertrophy, but again it has yet to be subjected to randomised clinical trials. If you plan to take Saw Palmetto, have your doctor monitor the concentration of dihydrotestosterone (DHT; a substance which is known to stimulate growth of the prostate) in your blood before you start and after you have taken the preparation, to see if the treatment is helping to reduce DHT levels, and adjust the dose up or down.[179]

Astralagus, a traditional Chinese herbal medicine used for two thousand years or so for the treatment of cancer, has recently been studied extensively in the West. There are reports that cancer patients receiving Astralagus have twice the survival rate of those receiving placebos. Some herbalists in the West routinely provide chemotherapy and radiotherapy patients with Astralagus, and apart from boosting the immune system (which is damaged by such treatments) it is also claimed to stop the spread of cancer cells. The EU is apparently planning to ban it on the pretext that, although it is a herb, it has not been on sale or in use in Europe for 30 years or more.[180] What a waste of time! Such products are easily available over the internet.

Several prostate-cancer books variously recommend that sufferers of enlarged prostates take: Saw Palmetto oil (about 350 mg); Panax ginseng (about 3 to 5 mg); or Pygeum bark (about 100 mg).[181]

PC-SPES, yet another herbal formula, contains *Chrysanthemum morifolium*, *Gandoderma lucidium*, *Glycyrrhiza glabra*, *Isatis indigotica*, *Panax pseudoginseng*, *Robdosia rubesceus*, *Scutellaria baicalensis* and *Serenoa repens*. The mixture has been shown to lower PSA in patients with prostate cancer and to inhibit the growth of prostate cancer cells *in vitro*.[182] These results are encouraging but require confirmation in clinical trials.[183] PC-SPES contains plant equivalents of DES (*see* below) and has the same drawbacks.[184]

One of the most authoritative reference books on herbal medicine[185] recommends the following treatments for prostatitis and BPH, some of which might be helpful with the symptoms of prostate cancer:

Teas: Horsetail, Pulsatilla, Goldenrod.
Tablets or capsules: Echinacea, Pulsatilla.
Formula: Black Willow, Saw Palmetto, hydrangea, poke root, Thuja.

An extract of stinging nettles is also claimed to help against prostate cancer.

If you are going to use any of these treatments, inform your doctor and ideally ensure that your herbal treatment is supervised by a suitably qualified doctor, for example from the British Society for Integrated Medicine. Also check that they have an MBChB or equivalent basic medical qualification. I am wary of some herbalists and herbs which can come from unreputable sources. A few years ago, an importer in California brought in a Chinese herb mix, which he named PC-SPES. Word-of-mouth reports said that it relieved pain and symptoms of those with prostate cancer, especially advanced cancer. Researchers recently found, however, that apart from the eight natural herbal ingredients, the mix also contained DES (the synthetic oestrogen used in hormone treatment), indomethacin (an anti-inflammatory drug) and warfarin (an anticoagulant). Apparently, pre-1999, the Chinese had been adding the three compounds to the formula before shipment, and latterly just the warfarin. Doctors had been using PC-SPES with great success but noticed side effects like breast enlargement (typical of taking DES). When some people had blood clots and bleeding problems, investigations started. One wonders why they can't ask the Chinese to provide pure PC-SPES and test whether it works without the addition of Western drugs. In Europe, there is a herbal product called Protasol with many of the same ingredients but no trial results to date.[186]

Eye of newt and toe of frog?

For many other treatments, there is little evidence that they improve outcomes and in some cases such as shark-fin extract their production can involve cruelty. As a scientist I fail to follow the logic that goes something like this: sharks don't suffer much from cancer; they are cartlilagenous fish; therefore, if we eat their cartilage it will help treat cancer. I suspect that the real reason sharks don't get cancer is similar to the reason that gorillas in the wild do not get much cancer – because they eat the food they have evolved to eat in environments relatively free from man-made chemicals.

I am also concerned about the use of pancreatic enzymes from young livestock to treat cancer. This dates back to the theory that malignant cancers are false placentas, as first proposed by Scottish embryologist John Beard in 1902. The placenta stops growing on day 56 of human pregnancies at the same time the pancreas starts to function in the foetus. He surmised that the same substances that stopped the growth of the placenta would stop cancer cells growing. He extracted juices from young animals and injected them into cancers and reported that they shrank in animals and humans, but his findings were never duplicated. It has recently been suggested that this is because other experimenters used enzymes that had lost their effectiveness. The ideas are being re-examined by Dr Gonzalez in the US according to the theory that cancer reflects the pancreas's inability to produce trypsin, in the same way that diabetes reflects its failure to produce insulin. The enzymes concerned in the enzyme theory of cancer, trypsin and its precursor chymtrypsin, still cannot be synthesised and must be extracted from young livestock. I understand that these enzymes digest protein in the intestines, but I fail to see how such large molecules could enter the bloodstream and tissues and kill cancer cells. I would prefer to eat pineapple, which contains the protein-digesting substance bromelain, on which the first biological washing powders were based, or papaya, which contains the protein-digesting enzyme papain. I am also concerned that pancreatic enzyme might contain growth factors, although I can find no analysis of it, and that some of it is in a lactose (milk sugar) base.

I also have serious concerns about the use of high concentrations of vitamin C. This treatment derives from the findings of

Linus Pauling winner of the Nobel prize for chemistry, when he developed prostate cancer. He learned that male gorillas in the wild did not suffer from the disease and wisely looked at their diet. Being a chemist, it seems he was looking for the chemical that was protecting the gorillas and calculated that they were having more than 10 times as much vitamin C as there is in a typical Western diet – but he missed the main point that the gorillas were living on a vegan diet packed with fresh fruit and vegetables (see Chapter 6, lifestyle factor 1, or www.cancersupportinternational.com for further evidence against taking man-made vitamins, minerals and extracts). Likewise, apricot kernels which contain vitamin B17, laetrile, were recommended by those studying the Hunza people in Asia who suffer little cancer or other degenerative disease. Again, the answer is most likely to be their vegan diet. Professor Colin Campbell, perhaps the world's greatest ever nutritional scientist describes laetrile as 'a prime example of a health scam' and records that animal studies have repeatedly shown that it had no effect on tumours.[187] Personally, I can see no sense in the use of coffee enemas or colonic irrigation. If the diet is good, elimination of faeces will remove toxins naturally.

Personally, I prefer to use conventional medical treatment combined with the Plant Programme diet and lifestyle, which is natural and healthy and involves no animal suffering. One of the things that occurs to me is that pharmaceutical companies are always quick to move treatments from alternative to mainstream medicine where they can profit by doing so. For example they have developed several natural plant alkaloids from yew that are used as powerful chemotherapy agents. There are only two reasons that they have not done so for the therapies described in this section, all of which are amenable to double-blind randomised clinical trials: either they cannot make a profit from them, and they would damage sales of other more profitable anti-cancer treatments – or the treatments do not work.

There are many alternative and complementary treatments, from acupuncture to reiki and reflexology, which can help cancer patients a great deal. Moreover, the best alternative and complementary therapists will give you that most precious thing, their time. Just talking to people like Jan de Vries is, I am sure, healing. If they do not help to comfort and support you in this way find a different therapist!

PREVENTION ACCORDING TO CONVENTION[188]

The drug *finasteride* was studied in the Prostate Cancer Prevention Trial, which involved thousands of men across the US for seven years, until 2004.

Scientists are also looking at ways to prevent recurrence among men who have been treated for prostate cancer. These approaches involve the use of drugs such as finasteride, flutamide, and LHRH agonists. Some studies have shown that hormonal therapy after radiation therapy or after radical prostatectomy can benefit certain men whose cancer has spread to nearby tissues.

The NCI-supported Prostate, Lung, Colorectal, and Ovarian Cancer Screening Trial is designed to show whether certain detection tests can reduce the number of deaths from these cancers. This trial is looking at the usefulness of prostate-cancer screening by performing a digital rectal exam and checking the PSA level in the blood in men ages 55 to 74. The results of this trial may change the way men are screened for prostate cancer.

Also, researchers are (at last!) investigating whether diets that are low in fat and high in soy, fruits, vegetables, and other plant foods might prevent a recurrence. The early results show considerable success (*see* Chapter 5).

THREE STORIES

Let me look briefly at what has happened to three close colleagues and friends who were diagnosed with prostate cancer shortly before *Your Life in Your Hands* was published and who followed my advice and are now alive and well. They are relatively free of symptoms, apart from one who is on a hormone-related treatment, and their initially very high PSA results have fallen to very low values – in one case below detection limit.

Take the case of Alec (a combination of a number of case studies of several people merged together), an engineer who I have worked with for many years. I remember on one occasion when we were driving somewhere together to work being surprised when he stopped the car at a motorway service centre and I saw his food choices – a meat-and-cheese burger, fries, peas and milky tea – but I said nothing at the time.

I still remember the day when I was told grimly by another male colleague that Alec wanted to speak to me – but he would not say what this was about. Anyway, almost immediately I returned to my office. Alec telephoned me and asked if there was anyone else in the room. Having been reassured that I was alone and had closed the door to my secretary's office he began to tell me about his problem. He had just been diagnosed with advanced prostate cancer and had been given a fairly poor prognosis. He sounded depressed and anxious. My first reaction was to say that I would do everything I could to help and to try to reassure him as much as I could by pointing to my own survival against the odds. He was so sure that he would soon die that he gave up many of the positions he held on the committees of learned societies and other organisations, despite my advice not to do so – and he still regrets this. Anyway, he went on my diet and followed it to the letter. He is still so evangelical about it that many of our mutual friends complain to me about how he nags at them if they do not follow my line – and of course this is all my fault (although I always refuse to behave like the food police). In discussions with his doctor (and I always refuse to be involved in orthodox medical choices, because I am not qualified to give such advice), Alec opted for external beam radiotherapy, combined with my diet and lifestyle. He takes no ongoing medication. He now looks a picture of health and spends hours of enjoyment playing golf with his friends or taking his grandchildren out – but no longer for burgers, chips and milkshakes!

Then there is Paul, a professor who lives a whirlwind lifestyle travelling around the world. His prostate cancer was detected by a very high PSA score (around 70) when his university first offered free health screening. He chose to have brachytherapy and went to a hospital in America for treatment. He also follows my diet and lifestyle closely and is on no other drug treatment. When I last saw him he told me delightedly that his latest PSA result had been less than 1.

Finally, a former senior executive from a leading UK company who loved his French cheeses and red wine. Again, he was found to have prostate cancer, with a PSA test result of about 15. He has followed my diet since he was first shown it in the *Daily Mail*. He chose to have radical surgery and continues to have hormone therapy of a type that has caused his breasts to develop – though he is always very smartly dressed and his breasts are not apparent.

The three examples I have chosen are all aged between about 46 and 75 years. I cannot tell you whether any of them have had other side effects. I am not medically trained and feel that I cannot question men – especially old and dear friends – about their sexual potency or their ability to urinate! All I know is that all three, and many, many other friends and colleagues who I am in contact with look well and healthy and tell me how well they are doing, frequently against the odds (with initially bad prognoses or recurrences of prostate cancer).

CONCLUSION

If you have read this far, you will have realised that, where prostate cancer is concerned, prevention is far, far better than cure. Shyness is a big problem. If a woman finds a lump in her breast she doesn't hesitate to go to the doctor, but men feel that talking about the prostate is embarrassing and so tend to avoid a visit to the doctor until it may be too late. Under-funding is perceived as another result of this shyness (but *see* Chapter 7). Men should be shouting about prostate cancer as much as women do about breast cancer. Although the UK government has increased funding for prostate-cancer research, it still falls short of that devoted to breast-cancer research from the government and via breast-cancer charities. The biggest UK prostate-cancer charity was founded only in 1996. The increased budget is, however, starting to work. Already new treatments like cryosurgery (freezing the prostate to kill cancer cells) or building viruses that attack the cancer cells and leave the healthy ones alone, are being developed. Unless new and successful treatments are developed, the poor diagnostic techniques, the horrid nature of some current treatments with their unpleasant side effects and the lack of an understanding of the real cause combine to make having no treatment a real option.[189]

Meanwhile, the word is **PREVENT**. And in the following chapters I shall try to help you to do just that; prevent you ever suffering from the disease or of having a recurrence if you are already a sufferer.

A FINAL QUOTE

The biomedical community needs to recognise and advocate approaches to prevent cancer with the same enthusiasm that it currently directs towards treating it.

Peter Greenwald
Division of Cancer Prevention, National Cancer Institute
National Institutes of Health, Bethesda, Maryland, USA[190]

2. CELLS BEHAVING BADLY

In this chapter I explain what cancer is in a way I wish I had been told when I was first diagnosed with the disease. The material is drawn from medical textbooks and recently published scientific papers, including papers about the latest stem-cell theory of cancer, but it is explained in unscary, everyday language. The evidence shows that, with a few exceptions, prostate cancer is not caused by inherited faulty genes but by environmental factors that translate into avoidable risks.

The chapter also deals with the roles of two groups of powerful biochemicals – hormones and growth factors – which act as chemical messengers in the body. They do this by docking with specific receptors within cells or on cell membranes to initiate processes in the cell such as growth, differentiation and proliferation. Growth factors and hormones are important in regulating these processes in normal cells, but an increase in their activity and expression can promote cancer and help it to proliferate.

W hen I first told my mother of my illness, she said: 'But we've never had anything like *that* in our family!'

At first, I was startled by her reaction. Then I remembered that people used to look upon cancer as something almost shameful: a family secret to be concealed at all costs, as mental illness often is to this day. Instead of saying someone had died of cancer, obituaries often euphemistically said the person had died 'after a long illness'. Perhaps the reason for this was fear, an emotion that the word cancer still invokes in most people to this day. The word cancer, in fact, comes from the Greek word 'karkinos', literally meaning 'crab', a word that was first used to describe the disease by Hippocrates. The name is particularly unfortunate, conjuring up, as it does, visions of a creature that won't let go. We shall learn here that this image is totally wrong and that cancer cells are just some of our normal cells that have started to behave badly.

I think that a lot of the fear of cancer stems from a basic lack of understanding of what it is. When people have a modern, rational understanding, they can cope with the disease more effectively.

As a scientist confronted with my own cancer, I had to find out as much as possible about what I was dealing with. I found that getting to grips with the most up-to-date facts enabled me to clear my mind of unhelpful old wives' tales, and having a modern understanding of cancer and its treatment helped me to feel less frightened. On one level, cancer is very easy to understand: it is a certain way in which some cells in the body begin to behave badly. What is 'bad' or odd or unusual about the behaviour of cancerous cells? Well, normally, parts of your body do not start to grow out of control, do not attack or consume other parts of your body and do not take off and start up a new colony elsewhere in your body. But cancer cells *do* act in these ways.

In order to understand why cancer is so hard to treat and cure, we need to look at it in a bit more detail and to acquire some basic information. If you're tempted to skip this short chapter, let me beg you not to – this isn't *Mastermind* and you're not going to be tested on it afterwards! Knowledge is power: if you understand the basic science of cancer, you're in a powerful position to protect yourself, to get involved in your treatment if you ever become a patient, and to play a role in the public debate about this increasingly important threat to men's health.

WHEN BAD THINGS HAPPEN TO GOOD CELLS

As you probably know, your body is made up of millions and millions of cells living in complex interrelationships with each other. Normally, your cells do not grow out of control, they do not invade each other's territory, and cells from, say, the lining of your intestines or parts of your prostate gland do not take off and start growing in other organs such as your bones or liver, a process called metastasis. But, as indicated above, it is the property of cancer cells to do precisely these three things that makes them so dangerous.

Even when cancer cells are removed from the human body and grown in a laboratory culture, they behave very differently from normal cells. For example, normal cells are fussy about the nutrients they consume, but cancer cells are not. Also, normal cells reproduce only until they just touch each other, and then they stop (a phenomenon known as contact inhibition). By contrast, cancer cells keep on propagating and will pile up in mounds because they produce a substance called telomerase which stops them from counting how many times they have reproduced themselves. Also, whereas normal cells make their energy in special organelles called mitichondria, cancer cells make their energy throughout the cell by an anaerobic process called glycolysis that is very inefficient. One researcher has suggested that cancer cells switch to glycolysis as a source of energy because in the middle of tumours they do not receive enough oxygen for their mitochondria to work properly – so they are switched off.

Telomerase is an enzyme that regulates the length of chromosomes in higher organisms, known as telomeres. In most human cells, the activity of telomerase is suppressed, and telomeres shorten progressively with each cell division. By contrast, 80–90 per cent of human cancers have been found to have active telomerase, resulting in continued cell proliferation.[1]

So *why* do cancer cells start behaving badly? Why do they grow out of control and eventually, if unchecked, start migrating across the body, establishing secondary tumours in a process called metastasis? To understand why, you need first to be aware of the simple fact that your body must make new cells when necessary – and in some tissues 'necessary' is, in fact, almost constantly. As your body wears out, new cells are created to replace older, dead or damaged ones. This process is called cell division or, more technically, mitosis.

When cells reach a certain critical size and metabolic state, they divide and create new daughter cells. The daughter cell inherits an *exact* replica of the heredity information (an exact replica of the types of genes in an exact sequence) of the parent cell. Not all cells divide at the same rate. For example, liver cells in the adult do not normally divide, but they can be stimulated to do so if part of the liver is removed surgically. On the other hand, the stem cells in human bone marrow are a good example of cells that divide rapidly and almost constantly. The average red blood cell lives only about 120 days. There are about 2.5 trillion of them in an adult body. To maintain this number, about 2.5 million new red blood cells must be produced every second. In total, about 2 trillion cell divisions occur in an adult human every 24 hours; that's about 25 million a second!

We also know now that many of our tissues other than bone marrow contain stem cells that help regeneration if tissue is damaged. For example, the hippocampus in the brain, which is responsible for memory, can shrink in people under chronic stress or suffering from severe depression, but it can regenerate when things improve because it contains a large number of stem cells. Unlike normal cells, these cells have the ability to renew themselves and to change into many other cell types. (It is these properties in embryonic stem cells that are under study by scientists all around the world as a means of trying to regenerate damaged tissue: for example, spinal nervous tissue in people paralysed as a result of a serious accident.)

Normally, the cells in your body reproduce only when instructed or allowed to do so by the cells around them, according to a complex and highly evolved system, which maintains the size and shape of your body throughout your life. Hence your ears and eyes, feet and legs stay in proportion to the rest of your body.

Now you can begin to imagine what would happen if this process goes wrong. If something happens to increase the rate at which one group of cells reproduce, the result will be an ever-increasing number of cells that have no beneficial function to the body, yet are absorbing nutrition at an increasing rate. And that's what a tumour is. If the cells remain in their place of origin and do not directly invade surrounding tissues, the tumour is said to be benign (or non-cancerous). If the cells invade neighbouring tissue and cause distant secondary growths (metastases), the tumour is known as malignant.

THE WRONG KNITTING PATTERN

How can this process go wrong? Well, it's all a matter of control. Cell division, mitosis, happens according to a well-established cycle. First, the cells increase in size and make new proteins before a resting phase; then they make two exact copies of the cell chromosomes. (Chromosomes are the strings of DNA that contain our gene sequence and they carry all the instructions about how to make us: blue eyes, curly hair, and so on.) Next, the chromosomes line up and finally they divide into two. The whole process is designed to make new cells that are exact copies of the ones they are replacing. This sequence of events is controlled by the cell's genes.

We know now as a result of the Human Genome Project to document all human genes that each cell in the human body, whether a normal cell or a stem cell, contains about twenty six thousand genes, which provide detailed instructions that determine not only the colour of our eyes or hair, but also instructions about cell division, growth and death. Genes can be thought of as knitting patterns or computer programs which, in the case of cancer cells, have somehow had a few mistakes introduced. Just think how a sweater would turn out if it was made from a pattern with a mistake in it. It's the same idea.

Most cells, no matter what their shape or function, have an outer surface – the cell membrane – inside which is a thick fluid called cytoplasm. Then, with the exception of red blood cells, all cells have a 'control centre', called a cell nucleus. In the cell nucleus are the chromosomes, made of strands of a special substance called DNA that contains our genes. The genes specify how to make particular proteins that carry out their work. When a gene is activated it causes such proteins to be made. Mutations (mistakes in genes) can cause the wrong amounts or types of the protein to be produced thus sending the wrong message. Then, when the cell begins its cycle of mitosis, there are errors – just like the misshapen sweater made from the misprinted knitting pattern.

All cells, including prostate cells, have receptors for chemical messengers such as hormones and growth factors and other chemical messengers that control our immune system called cytokines. Receptors are special parts of the cell designed to allow chemical messengers such as particular hormones or growth factors to dock and deliver their messages. In the case of growth factors, for example, one end of each receptor protrudes into the fluid between the cells, while the other end projects into the cell's cytoplasm, and in this way creates a conduit along which the message starts to be transmitted. So, for example, when a growth factor docks on to an appropriate receptor its message is passed directly into the cytoplasm. There it begins the relay of a message that is carried from one protein to the next until it reaches the cell nucleus, just like the baton in a relay race. This relay occurs along what is sometimes called a pathway. Once in the cell nucleus, the message activates genes to initiate their instructions – in this case, for the cell to begin its growth cycle. But cells can receive other messages as well.

NEW THEORIES FROM OLD

Until recently, most scientists thought that the cells in a cancer were descended from a common ancestral cell, which, until that point, had been a fairly normal cell in the prostate gland (for example) and which at some point in time – probably years before any tumour was detected – initiated a programme of inappropriate reproduction. Recently other scientists have suggested that tumours arise from more specialised cells called cancer stem cells, which have the properties of normal stem cells, particularly the ability to self-renew and differentiate into multiple cell types. They suggest that a distinct sub-population of these cells persists in tumours; and that it is these that cause the cancer to recur and metastasise.[2] Analysis of the cellular origins of cancers of different organs supports this theory because it indicates that the most likely ancestral cell of all the tumours studied was, in each case, a stem cell required for normal tissue renewal. Opponents of the theory do not deny the existence of cancer stem cells. Rather they suggest that most cells in a tumour have stem-cell properties. The theory explains the genetic instability of cancer cells – that is to say, they can quickly become resistant to many types of treatment.

As long ago as the mid-19th century, pathologists noted the similarity between embryonic tissue and cancer and suggested that tumours arise from embryo-like cells. The idea that adult tissues contain embryonic remnants that generally lie dormant but that could be activated to become cancer was formalised in 1874 as the embryonic rest theory of cancer. The idea that cancers arise from tissue stem cells in adults is simply a modern version of a theory first proposed more than 130 years ago!

The cancer-stem-cell theory has particular importance when we consider the role of growth factors in promoting cancer, because the fate of normal stem cells (i.e. what type of cells they will finally turn into: for example, prostate cells or skin cells) depends on cellular signals, especially those from growth factors. It now seems likely that growth factors control what happens to all stem cells, including cancer stem cells. Indeed, cell-signalling pathways are now thought to be the same in embryonic cells and cancer cells.[3]

DAMAGED GENES

So what can go wrong to cause cancer? Most scientists agree that it involves damage to the genes that control cell growth and differentiation.

There are basically three types of genes in cells that can go wrong to produce cancer: those that say 'grow', called proto-oncogenes by doctors and researchers; those that say 'don't grow', called tumour suppressor genes; and those that say 'fix it', instructing the cell to repair damage or, in extreme situations, self-destruct, called apoptotic genes.[4]

In cancer, one or more of the 'knitting patterns' for the 'grow', 'don't grow' and 'fix it' genes crucial to cell mitosis accumulates a series of mistakes resulting in the ancestral cancer or cancer stem cell. Normally, the body has a complex 'quality control' system to ensure that such errors are detected and eliminated – to the extent of causing damaged cells to self-destruct (the cell's ability to commit suicide, a process called 'apoptosis'). But somehow, the initiated cancer cell avoids the body's quality control safeguards and begins to grow out of control. Normal DNA repair mechanisms don't work and, for some reason, the body's immune system does not recognise the cancer cells as abnormal, and so fails to kill them off. Even the 'final solution' of apoptosis fails to work. You can see from this sequence of events that cancer is actually the result of a series of failures, starting from mistakes in the cell's genes – the knitting patterns.

These mistakes in the genes are called mutations, and most cancers possess mutations in one or more of the three main gene categories. The progression of cancers from an individual damaged cell to a cluster of damaged cells, then to non-aggressive cancer and finally to highly aggressive cancer is generally considered to result from the continued accumulation of mutations. Cells from advanced cancer typically have many genetic changes and chromosome rearrangements, although these are considered to be the result rather than the cause of malignancy. The number of mutations required for the development of cancer varies with the type of cancer.

THE GROW GENES

The first genes that can go wrong are the grow genes, the genes that produce normal growth proteins in our cells, which relay signals to the nucleus (the control centre of the cell), stimulating growth in response to proteins and other substances in the intercellular fluid. The signalling process involves a series of steps which begin at receptors on the cell membrane (or within the cell,

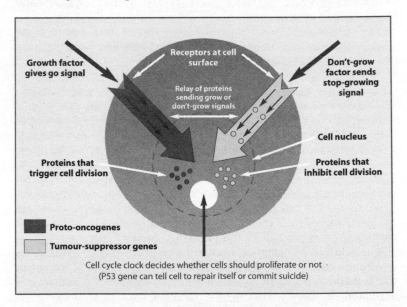

Figure 2.1 'Grow' and 'don't-grow' signalling in normal cells.

in the case of steroid hormones), then involve a host of intermediary proteins in the cell cytoplasm and end with the activation of factors in the cell nucleus which help to move it through its cycle of growth and replication (Figure 2.1). The abnormal degree of proliferation in cancer-cell populations generally results from over-activity in one or more of these steps.[5] Interestingly, one of the diagrams in Woolf's *Pathology, Basic and Systemic*, a book for medical students, illustrating how cancer cells behave, shows a marked increase in growth factors in the intercellular fluid followed by an increase in growth-factor receptors and in signal transmission, followed by an increased response to their signalling, leading to cancer. The role of growth factors, especially insulin-like growth factor-I (IGF-I) in promoting cancer has been investigated for many years, but recently, as discussed in Chapter 4, the quality and quantity of evidence of its role in promoting prostate cancer has increased greatly.[6] Many other growth factors are implicated in the development of other types of cancer. For example, epidermal growth factor (EGF) is implicated in HER2-receptor-positive breast cancers and in some types of lung cancer.

The activation of a normal grow or proto-oncogene to become a cancer-causing oncogene can occur in several ways: by altering DNA at a particular point on the chromosome, by rearranging chromosomes, or by increasing the numbers of normal proto-oncogenes in a cell.[7] There are several such genes which, when damaged, become oncogenes involved in prostate cancer. One of them, ERBB2, codes for an epidermal-growth-factor-like protein; this oncogene is also involved in ovarian and other cancers. Others include: FGF3, which codes for fibroblast growth factor; MYC, which codes for a factor involved in activating growth-promotion in the cell nucleus and is also involved in ovarian and colon cancer; and ROS1, which codes for insulin-receptor-like proteins on the cell membrane. The location of proto-oncogenes at particular sites on particular chromosomes is now well documented as a result of the Human Genome Project.

The relay of information between a receptor and a cell nucleus is sometimes called a pathway. When growth factors – present in the fluid between cells – attach to cell receptors, a pathway is activated or 'fired'. That is, the relay of the 'grow' message is begun. In cancerous cells, the relaying proteins maintain their activity when they should have stopped, or 'switched off'. In the case of prostate cancer, the proto-oncogenes with the mistakes – those that keep telling the cell to 'fire' when it should have 'switched off' – are thought to be those that control how the receptors for growth factors behave.

Pharmaceutical companies are currently working on drugs intended to 'shut down' growth-factor receptors that have gone wrong. Shut-down methods have been shown to work in cultures of cancer cells, but they have not yet been shown to work in the human body. Research is in progress to formulate a substance that will increase the activity of IGF-binding protein 3[8] in prostate-cancer patients, either directly or by stimulating its production in the body.

THE DON'T GROW GENES

The second class of genes which can go wrong to produce cancer are called tumour-suppressor genes. In normal cells, these genes encode for a sequence of proteins to restrict cell growth, including by cell-to-cell signalling via the fluid between cells – the intercellular fluid. So if a cell is growing out of control, these genes can make a set of proteins to send a different relay of signals to the nucleus. This time it is to say 'don't grow'.

It is the inheritance of mutated forms of the BRCA-1 gene and the BRCA-2 gene (both tumour-suppressor genes) that is thought to cause an estimated 5–10 per cent of all inherited or familial breast-cancer cases. There is also evidence that these same genes are involved in inherited prostate cancer. For example, work by a team at Cambridge University, UK, has shown that men who carry the mutated BRCA-2 gene are four to five times more likely to get prostate cancer.[9]

In recent years, much more has become known about the behaviour of the BRCA genes. More than 2,000 papers have been published in peer-reviewed journals on the BRCA1 gene alone. From this work, scientists have learned that this gene, in its normal, unmutated form, helps to guard DNA against damage from free radicals, radiation and chemicals. The BRCA1 protein seems to act like a plumber, fixing breaks in the genome as they occur. The BRCA1 protein physically binds to damaged DNA and then recruits other molecules to assemble the equivalent of a DNA repair kit. Scientists have further demonstrated that the absence of the BRCA1 protein does not directly cause cancer but makes cells more susceptible to changes that can lead to cancer.[10] It has been suggested that the BRCA1 protein works via the intercellular fluid, from where it interacts with surrounding cells to keep them cancer-free.[11]

ALL IN THE FAMILY?

Within affected families, the BRCA-1 or BRCA-2 gene can be passed directly from generation to generation, through either the male or the female line. However, not everyone who carries the mutated genes goes on to develop cancer. Furthermore, just because a close relative has had prostate cancer it does not mean that there is genetic cancer in your family.

Several studies have looked into the family history of patients with prostate cancer. One study carried out in Canada and published in 1995 showed that, out of a sample of over 7,000 men with prostate cancer, only 159 had a positive family history, unlike the situation for many other cancers. These results indicate that for most patients inheritance has little to do with the development of their prostate cancer.[12] It has been suggested that true hereditary prostate cancer occurs in a very small number of men and tends to develop at a very early age (less than 55 years old).[13]

Some researchers have suggested that faults in the BRCA genes are involved in types of prostate cancer other than familial, so presumably the genes can be damaged during an individual's lifetime. Unlike some other cancer genes, which produce proteins that are more unreachable because they are located deep in the pathway within the cell near the cell nucleus, the proteins that the BRCA genes encode for are secreted into the fluid between cells. In healthy cells, these proteins are thought to be the method by which the prostate protects itself against unruly cell division and, hence, cancer.

It may be important for people to know if they have inherited the mutated forms of the tumour-suppressor genes involved in predisposing them to prostate cancer. If you wish to find out whether or not you have inherited faulty genes, you will need to consult an appropriate medical specialist. However, I believe that since the inherited mutated genes implicated in prostate cancer are tumour-suppressor genes, they are simply failing to 'close the door after the horse has bolted'. I believe that changing certain aspects of your diet and lifestyle could help to reduce your individual risk by reducing your exposure to growth factors, as discussed under proto-oncogenes, above, and hormone and hormone-mimicking substances.

THE FIX IT GENES

The third group of genes involved in cancer are those controlling the replication and repair of DNA – the 'fix it' genes. These instruct the cell to repair faulty DNA or commit suicide. An example of this type of gene, which is defective in many human cancers, is the p53 gene.

The p53 gene, although often grouped with tumour-suppressor genes, actually operates within the cell nucleus, by inducing repair or apoptosis. Damage to the p53 gene, which can produce a protein capable of halting the whole cell cycle and hence cell division until DNA damage is repaired or cell-suicide is triggered, continues to be regarded as a key factor in human cancers. More than half of all human cancers have mutations in the p53 gene and hence no functioning p53 (messenger) protein. It has been suggested that a virus called SV40, which knocks out the p53 gene, was a contaminant in polio vaccines administered in the US and possibly other countries between 1955 and 1963.[14]

Injecting tumours with viruses containing high concentrations of the p53 gene is already in use in China, but in the West the risks have yet to be fully evaluated.

WHERE IN THE CELL?

In several types of cancer the genes that have gone wrong encode for proteins deep within the cell. In the case of prostate cancer, recent research is hopeful and suggests that the problems are related to proteins responsible for transmitting messages to stimulate or slow down growth, between the cells and intercellular fluid, rather than deep in the cell as in the case of some other types of cancer. This suggests that changes in body chemistry such as those achieved through changes in diet or lifestyle can help to prevent and treat the disease. This is discussed further in Chapters 4, 5 and 6.

ALL IN THE GENES?

One of the first things patients do when they receive a diagnosis of cancer is to look to their lives to try to establish what it is that has caused their illness. They often ask themselves, 'Is it me, or is it something I've done?'[15] In other words, 'Have I got cancer because of my genes or because of my particular lifestyle?'

According to Professor Waxman, all the evidence seems to point to predominantly environmental causes for prostate cancer. I agree with him completely.

Following the Human Genome Project, we have all been encouraged to believe that we are simply a bag of genes in a hermetically sealed bag and that developing a disease is the result of a faulty gene switching in.

Because there is a clear, obvious and unambiguous genetic component in the causation of cancer, many scientists and lay people seem to take for granted that cancer is, by definition, a genetic disease. Let me explain the way this reasoning runs:

1. Cancer results from genetic errors
2. Cancer is therefore a genetic disease
3. There's nothing you can do about your genes, so there's nothing you can do about your risk of getting cancer
4. The cure for cancer will therefore be a genetic one: spend a few more billion on researching 'gene therapy' and we'll one day find the answer.

This is faulty logic and it is unscientific. Unfortunately, many people who ought to know better seem to believe this mistaken line of reasoning. I do not.

Even the term 'proto-oncogenes' which literally means 'first cancer genes' (it is quite a mouthful!) implies that we have genes in our body whose only purpose is to lurk in hiding just waiting for their opportunity to malfunction and cause cancer. In fact, these genes are *essential* for the growth cycle of normal cells. Only *mutated* or *damaged* forms of these genes lead to cancer. But you wouldn't think so from the name.

As I wrote in *Your Life in Your Hands*, the simplistic genetic model totally fails to take account of our interface with our environment – such as exposure to toxic chemicals like those in tobacco smoke, which are known to trigger lung cancer. I do not believe that most of those suffering from tobacco- or asbestos-induced lung cancer would be affected if they had not been exposed to cancer-causing agents (now referred to as epigenetic factors). Neither do I believe that most men have genes that will lead them to suffer from prostate cancer without being exposed to something that promotes it. As we shall see, damage to the DNA, the material that makes up our genes, is critical to the initiation of cancer,[16] and both this damage and the promotion and progression of prostate cancer are critically linked to factors in our lifestyle and environment. There are various repair mechanisms, and it is only when damage persists that cancer becomes established as a disease.

RESEARCH FOR CURES AND NEW TREATMENTS

So why has all the research, including that arising from the much-vaunted Human Genome Project, not led to readily available cures? Probably because all the 'new' methods face the same problems and must overcome many of the same obstacles faced by standard chemotherapy: for any method to be effective, it must find, penetrate and then change or destroy cancer cells without irreparably damaging normal, healthy cells.

One of the main results of all the recent scientific research activity has been to show that there are only minimal differences between cancer cells and normal cells.[17] Indeed, the very latest research suggests that cancer cells are just our own somewhat damaged embryonic stem cells,[18] and only a minute fraction of the tens of thousands of genes in individual cancer cells are damaged. Hence it is extremely difficult to devise treatments against cancer that will not damage normal tissue as much as cancerous tissue. Some new drug treatments being proposed depend on fundamental differences between cancer cells and normal cells, for example the fact that all cancer cells make their energy by an inefficient process called glycolysis throughout the cell rather than in distinct organelles called mitochondria, A new drug called dichloroacetate (DCA) is being tried out as a means of re-activating the mitochondria in cancer cells so that they cause the cancer cells to die. The treatment has been shown to attack cancer cells in culture and to shrink cancers in experimental rats but no clinical trials have been performed on humans. Unfortunately, cancer treatments may work well in cultures of cancer cells or sometimes in laboratory animals. In the human body, however, not only must the anti-cancer agent, whether chemical or biological, find the cancer, but it must also find a way to penetrate tumours sufficiently to be effective *without* causing such serious side effects that it cannot be used on human patients. Solid tumours, such as those of the prostate, typically, have many barriers to drug delivery; not much blood flows within them, and some agents do not easily diffuse out of the blood vessels into the cancer itself.[19] Also, there are the problems of toxicity, side effects and the emergence of drug resistance in the tumour cells and immune resistance to foreign proteins in the body generally. Moreover, cancer cells are highly genetically unstable and can mutate or change so rapidly that they can readily evade recognition by immunology-based treatments and/or rapidly become resistant to many different methods of treatment, including those based on chemicals or gene therapy. Finally, as discussed in Chapter 1, the cost of researching the 'new' methods of treatment is extremely high in the West, and any drugs developed are likely to be so expensive that they may not be widely available for prostate-cancer patients – even if they could be made to work in human beings with active cancer.

Many new methods of cancer treatment are being developed. They include methods based on gene therapy to correct defective genes (in the past these failed to deliver genes to a high-enough proportion of cells in cancers and in some cases were claimed to be directly responsible for patient deaths. New gene therapies that use high concentrations of the p53 gene are becoming available. These carry the gene in a virus and are injected directly into solid tumours, often accompanied by chemotherapy. The side effects from the gene therapy are claimed to be minimal. These treatments have been tried in America to treat advanced breast cancer and in China to treat several different types of cancer including cancer of the lung and naso-pharyngeal cancer with, it is claimed, a high degree of success. The drug used in China, marketed as Gendicine, was developed by Chinese scientists and is much less expensive than many of the latest drug treatments available in the West. Unfortunately, not all cancers have defective p53 genes, and even in those that do the treatment may fail. Moreover, research suggests that inactivation of the p53 gene is rare in primary prostate cancer and is unimportant in metastatic prostate cancer.

Other new cancer treatments are based on molecular medicine aimed at correcting the proteins produced by faulty genes; methods to induce apoptosis in cancer cells; methods of blocking the formation of small blood vessels to choke off the blood supply that cancers need in order to grow (angiogenesis inhibitors); and methods to prevent cancer cells metastasising. New immunological methods designed to stimulate the body's own immune system into recognising and destroying cancer cells are also under development. These include drugs based on monoclonal antibodies manufactured to bind to specific proteins, called antigens, which are present on all cells. The monoclonal antibodies are created to target a particular antigen or antigens carried on specific cancer cells. Such methods generally increase time to disease progression by only a few months, however – hardly a triumph compared with my survival of fourteen years due to a simple, low-tech, low-cost approach based on science and common sense!

Recent work[20] provides a scientific basis for the success of my approach. The authors of this research point out that, while much recent attention has focused on the Human Genome Project, the genes that have been identified as causing cancer so far account for only a small proportion of major cancers. The rapid increase in the incidence of the cancers that accompany economic development, together with the findings of twin studies – which compare cancer risk in identical and non-identical twins to determine the relative influence of genetic and environmental factors – both point to the importance of non-genomic factors[21] – in other words, to the importance of environmental factors. I regard these as controllable risk factors that we can eliminate from our lives to prevent and treat cancer (Chapters 3–6).

FROM DNA DAMAGE TO DISEASE

There are now considered to be three main stages in the development of cancer (Figure 2.2). The initiation stage, which is characterised by the conversion of an ancestral, possibly stem, cell

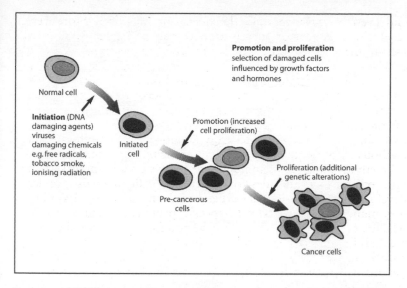

Figure 2.2 Initiation, promotion and proliferation of cancer cells (modified from Greenwald, Peter, 2002. Cancer chemoprevention, *BMJ*, 324, 714–718).

to a pre-cancerous condition in response to agents that damage DNA. As discussed above, some cancers are caused by inherited cells which have already been damaged, but in most cases the damage is caused by something in our lifestyle or environment.

The initiation stage is followed by the promotion stage, in which the initiated cell is transformed into a population of pre-cancerous cells, associated with further DNA damage and cell proliferation. Thirdly, there is the progression stage, involving the further transformation of pre-cancerous cells to a population of cancer cells.[22]

The body has many mechanisms and checks and balances for eliminating damaged cells. The fact that cancer cells not only survive but proliferate faster than normal cells suggests that some agent is preferentially fostering their growth relative to normal cells. The promotion and progression stages are thus extremely important in understanding, preventing and treating cancer.

INITIATION, OR BAD BEGINNINGS

Of the factors that damage DNA, environmental contaminants and chemicals such as tobacco smoke are considered further in Chapter 6, Lifestyle Factor 6. Viruses are also able to change DNA in human cells, by many different mechanisms. They can convert normal grow genes into cancer genes, which stimulate uncontrolled cell growth and division by various means. It has been suggested that the marked differences in the prevalence of some types of cancer between different countries reflect differences in the importance of chemical contaminants and chronic infection.[23] Thus the developed world has the highest incidence of cancer overall and is mainly affected by the so-called 'cancers of affluence', such as cancer of the breast and prostate, colorectal cancer and the less common cancers of the bladder, kidney and pancreas. It has been suggested that these reflect, at least in part, the widespread use of man-made chemicals. In contrast, the developing world is more affected by cancers of the stomach, liver and cervix. These cancers are thought to reflect chronic infection by agents such as *Helicobacter pylori*, hepatitis B and human papilloma virus.

Ionising radiation, including that from radiotherapy and other medical X-rays, can also change the nature of chemicals in the body, including DNA, and cause genetic mutations that can be passed to offspring. Some of the principal sources of ionising radiation were discussed in the previous chapter.

There is increasing emphasis on the role of free radicals in causing damage to DNA. Free radicals are highly reactive molecules that typically have very short lifetimes. The best way to think of the effect of free radicals in the body is to imagine a pat of butter or a piece of meat or some nuts going rancid. This occurs because of a chemical process called oxidation caused by free radicals. More technically, free radicals are defined as chemical species that possess an unpaired electron in the outer (valence) shell.[24] This means, in practice, that they are very short-lived, because they generally attack any nearby molecules, including proteins, fats, carbohydrates and DNA, to 'steal' electrons to make up for their missing electrons. The attacked molecule that loses its electrons then becomes a free radical itself, beginning a chain reaction that, once started, can become a cascade that results in cell disruption. Free radicals are produced continuously in cells, including as by-products of normal metabolism.[25]

The best-known defence against the generation of free radicals and the damage that they cause is the activity of antioxidants that we take in from food and drink. Sources of antioxidants are discussed further in Chapter 5, where I examine the role of diet in the chemoprevention of cancer.

It is worth re-emphasising that of the tens of thousands of genes in the normal cell the principal genes that are altered in cancer cells are just a tiny subset comprising the grow, don't-grow and fix-it genes. What we are looking for, therefore, are factors which encourage the growth of cancer cells by damaging these types of genes, so that we can eliminate such factors from our lives.

PROMOTION AND PROGRESSION OF CANCER, OR SURVIVAL OF THE UNFIT

Many scientists now think that the extent to which initiated cancer cells turn into established tumours depends on the promotion stage of the disease. This theory is supported by the observation that promotion may be accomplished years after initiation (as a result of exposure to a carcinogen, for example). Professor T. Colin Campbell, drawing on his extensive studies using experimental animals, likens initiated cancer cells to seeds that won't grow unless they are watered and fertilised, i.e. promoted. In study after study, he shows that, however cancer was initiated, whether by a virus or a chemical carcinogen, its ability to form tumours depends on the promotion stage, and this in turn depends on diet. Let us look at promotion more closely in the case of prostate cancer, before considering, in Chapters 4 and 5, how men can change their diet to reduce their risks of developing or advancing the disease.

Since reliable cancer registers began to be kept in the 1950s and 1960s, the age-standardised incidence of hormone-dependent cancers (breast, prostate, endometrial (lining of the womb), testicular and ovarian) have increased in most industrialised countries, over and above that which can be attributed to the introduction of screening.

Cancers of the prostate have generally been considered to be sex-hormone dependent.[26] The strongest link has been a positive association with androgen status, especially with testosterone.[27]

Hormonal and other influences on the prostate

The male hormone system is orchestrated by the hypothalamus gland at the base of the brain, which sends signals to the body's master gland, the pituitary gland, immediately beneath it. The whole process is controlled by gonadotrophin-releasing hormone, also called luteinising hormone-releasing hormone (LHRH), produced by the hypothalamus. The most significant hormones produced by the pituitary for male reproductive and sexual function are luteinising hormone (LH) and folical-stimulating hormone (FSH), which, respectively, control male hormone and sperm production in the testes. When LH and FSH are released from the pituitary into the bloodstream, they induce the production of testosterone and sperm in the testes. Approximately 95 per cent of testosterone in the blood derives from the testes, and a lesser amount from the adrenal gland. Testosterone is a relatively inactive hormone that becomes activated by a special enzyme to form dihydrotestosterone (DHT).[28] Androgens such as testosterone represent the primary steroid hormone affecting gene expression in the prostate.[29]

Although the prostate is clearly a sex-steroid-(androgen)-dependent tissue, there is much evidence to indicate the involvement of numerous other hormones, as well as growth factors and substances called cytokines (a unique group of growth factors normally involved in the body's immune response) in the development and progression of tumours affecting it. Factors such as IGF-I, fibroblast growth factor (FGF), members of the erbB family, and others, as well as their receptors and binding proteins, and other small bioactive hormones, are now also implicated in the development, growth and differentiation of the prostate.[30]

The use of hormone levels to identify individuals or groups of people at risk of developing reproductive cancer has so far proved unsuccessful, and several reasons have been used to explain these negative findings.[31] There is, however, much more compelling evidence of links between hormones and the progression of established cancers. For example, some prostate cancers may regress following hormone-deprivation therapy, including removal or ablation of the testicles, or as a result of the use of anti-androgens (*see* Chapter 1). Conversely, there is evidence that administration of steroid hormones increases the growth of reproductive tumours. In the case of prostate cancer, the most important seems to be testosterone (*see* p. 151). As discussed in Chapter 1, many drug treatments for prostate cancer are aimed at reducing tumour levels of testosterone. The main benefits of such therapy are for testosterone-receptor-positive cancers.[32]

The evidence that the two groups of biochemically powerful chemicals, hormones and growth factors, promote and progress prostate cancer that can eventually lead to metastatic cancer is considered further below.

CHEMICAL MESSENGERS

Hormones

As discussed above, hormones are secreted in special endocrine glands which contain a rich network of blood capillaries through which the hormones are released into the bloodstream. They circulate in the blood, usually in tiny amounts, until they interact with the target cell by way of highly specific receptors, located either on the cell surface or within the cell cytoplasm. This docking activates a series of intracellular reactions, including gene activation. By this means, hormones and growth factors enable the organism to exert control over a host of metabolic functions and to alter these functions in response to changes in conditions. The sex hormones, testosterone and oestrogen, for example, are involved in the onset of puberty in both males and females.

Hormones can be divided into two classes, peptides (proteins), which interact with receptors on cell membranes, and steroids (fatty or fat-soluble substances), which also interact with receptors but within the cell cytoplasm, through which they can directly affect the proteins released from a large number of target genes.

There is increasing concern now about man-made chemicals. It is thought that the most significant for prostate cancer and other cancers of the reproductive system are the chemicals that can disrupt the hormone system, in some cases because of their hormone-like behaviour. These are known as endocrine-disrupting chemicals or sometimes xeno (stranger) oestrogens.

Growth factors

The second class of chemical messengers – growth factors – also interact with cells by way of specific receptors and are increasingly strongly implicated in the promotion of prostate cancer.[33] They are generally less well understood.

The discovery of growth factors dates back to the early 1950s, when the Italian biochemist and 1986 Nobel laureate, Rita Levi-Montalcini, was working with tissue cultures of peripheral nerve cells. She found that, while the cultures would maintain themselves in a medium containing the right combination of nutrients, they did not grow much. However, when they were supplied with an extract derived from mouse salivary glands, they grew dramatically, extending towards the highest concentration of the extract. The substance was finally purified and characterised as a low-molecular-weight protein with chemical properties similar to that of insulin, which was called nerve-growth factor (NGF). NGF is now known to be just one of a large number of such small protein growth factors derived from a variety of tissues. They are generally named after the tissue from which they have been purified rather than that at which they act. They include, for instance, Brain-Derived Neurotrophic Factor (BDNF),[34] as well as IGF-I and IGF-II. The authoritative textbook, *Biochemistry* by Donald and Judith Voet,[35] states that EGF, which, like the IGFs, is implicated in reproductive cancers such as prostate cancer (*see* p. 139), is a hormonally active polypeptide that stimulates cell proliferation. IGF-I is very powerful and has profound effects on tissue such as that of the prostate, even when it is present in only tiny amounts in the blood (0.2 millionth of a gram per millilitre).[36] The IGFs, IGF-I and IGF-II, have a similar structure to that of insulin but circulate in the body at much higher concentrations because they are bound by specific binding proteins (insulin-like growth factor binding proteins, IGFBP-1 to -6)[37] which inhibit their bioavailability/bioactivity.[38]

There is now little doubt about the role of the IGFs in increasing the risk of prostate cancer. At a one-day meeting of the Royal Society of Medicine in London in October 2003, entitled 'Biology of IGF-I: its interaction with insulin in health and malignant states', eight papers were devoted to the topic of IGF-I and cancer. One paper by Grimberg, a distinguished endocrinologist from Philadelphia in the US, illustrated how IGF-I signalling may contribute to each stage of cancer progression, from enhancing the survival and proliferation of cancer cells, including by helping them to survive processes involved in apoptosis. She also presented evidence that IGF-I may promote cancer indirectly by interaction with other hormones, especially testosterone and oestrogen, the sex steroids long implicated in prostate and breast cancer.

In their review of more than three hundred publications on the role of IGFs in cancer progression, Professor Yu of Yale University and his colleague Professor Rohan stated that the IGFs play a pivotal role in regulating cell proliferation, differentiation and apoptosis.[39] Their binding proteins can inhibit or enhance the actions of the IGFs and the evidence consistently shows that IGFs exert strong effects on cancer cells and prevent their apoptosis. They also act together with other growth factors and steroid hormones in promoting cancer growth. According to Yu and Rohan, also, high circulating levels of IGFs and low levels of its binding protein IGFBP-3 are associated with increased risk of several common cancers, including those of the prostate, breast, colorectum and lung.[40] Many other researchers have studied the role of IGF-I in prostate and other cancers and their findings are considered more fully in Chapter 4.

As discussed earlier in this chapter, most human tumours develop by a multi-step process in which cells with damaged genes (mutations) grow more than normal cells. Spontaneous gene mutations occur frequently and naturally throughout life, and such events may be increased by viruses or chemicals in the environment.[41] It is increasingly recognised that the body's sophisticated defence mechanisms to eliminate such damaged cells, including apoptosis, must be overridden by some kind of external 'survival' signals to the initiated cancer cells. The most potent survival signal for many such cell types appears to be IGF-I.[42]

New work also concludes that the recent findings about IGF-I provide a potential mechanism through which an array of previously identified risk factors (*see* Chapter 1) may act.[43]

We have always used euphemisms for cancer: it is now 'neoplasms', but in my younger days it was 'growths' – and what a clue that was, given all the new findings on the role of growth factors! Indeed, the emerging evidence suggests that growth factors are to an initiated cancer cell what oxygen is to a spark or, as Campbell suggests, water and fertiliser to a seed. Dramatically lowering the levels of growth factors circulating in our bodies appears to be crucial to reducing the risk of cancer or of its recurrence.

Additional information on the role of diet, including limiting exposure to foods with high levels of hormones and/or growth factors likely to promote prostate-cancer cells, is considered in Chapter 5, together with food and drinks protective against the disease. Reducing risks from exposure to hormone-disrupting chemicals is considered further in Chapter 6 on lifestyle factors.

CHAPTER 2 IN A NUTSHELL

- The scientific evidence shows that, with a few exceptions, prostate cancer is not caused by inherited faulty genes but by environmental factors that translate into avoidable risks.
- The word cancer, from the Greek 'karkinos', meaning 'crab', conjures up visions of a creature that won't let go. This image of cancer is totally wrong; cancer cells are just some of our own cells that have started to behave badly.
- To understand what cancer is we must consider that our bodies make new cells almost constantly to replace older, dead or damaged ones. The new cell should inherit an *exact* replica of the types of genes in exactly the same sequence as the parent cell. Cancer can result if mistakes are introduced in the genes controlling this process.
- Genes can be thought of as knitting patterns or computer programs which, in cancer cells, have somehow been damaged and had a few mistakes introduced into them.
- Out of the more than 26,000 genes identified in the human genome, damage to only three sets of genes is thought to lead to cancer. These are the 'grow' genes that tell cells to make new cells, the 'don't-grow' genes that inhibit cells from entering the replication cycle, and the 'fix-it' genes that send out DNA repair kits to mend the damaged genes and, if they fail, tell the cell to commit suicide.
- One of the main results of these findings has thus been to show that there are only minimal differences between cancer cells and normal cells. This explains why it is extremely difficult to devise treatments against cancer that will not damage normal tissue as much as cancerous tissue and hence cause unpleasant side effects.

- Until recently, most scientists thought that the cells in a cancer were descended from a common ancestral cell, which had been a fairly normal cell until inappropriate reproduction was initiated by damage to the genes controlling cell renewal.

- Recently, other scientists have suggested that tumours arise from more specialised cells, called cancer stem cells, which have the properties of normal stem cells, particularly the ability to self-renew and differentiate into multiple cell types. This would explain why cancers frequently contain many different cell types and why they are so genetically unstable, rapidly becoming resistant to treatment.

- There are now considered to be three main stages in the development of cancer. **The initiation stage** is characterised by the conversion of an ancestral, possibly stem, cell to a pre-cancerous condition in response to DNA damage. A small proportion of cancers are caused by inherited damaged cells but usually the damage is caused by something in our lifestyle or environment. **The promotion stage** is the stage which many scientists now think is crucial in determining whether initiated cancer cells turn into established tumours. **The proliferation stage** is the stage at which cancers metastasise.

- Two groups of powerful biochemicals, hormones and growth factors, are implicated in promoting prostate cancer, eventually leading, in some cases, to metastatic cancer.

- Growth factors and hormones are important in regulating processes such as growth, differentiation and proliferation in normal cells, but an increase in their activity and expression can promote initiated cancer cells and help them to proliferate.

- It is increasingly recognised that the body's sophisticated defence mechanisms to eliminate cells with damaged genes are sometimes overridden by some kind of external 'survival' signals to initiated cancer cells. The most potent survival signal for many such cell types appears to be a growth factor known as IGF-I.

3. THE THIRD STRAWBERRY

In this chapter, I explain how I used my science, knowledge and experience of working in China and Korea, and with scientific colleagues from Thailand and Japan – as well as a large dollop of good luck – to identify what I believe to be the main factor that promotes prostate and breast cancer. I compare recent information on the incidence and death rates for prostate cancer between low-risk oriental and high-risk Western countries. Such comparisons, together with migration and twin studies, support the evidence that prostate cancer is closely associated with the Western diet and lifestyle. Despite this association, the conventional medical advice continues to be based on the same old risk factors such as age and family history of cancer. This may be because so many studies have been carried out within countries rather than between countries, although the latter comparison shows much more significant differences in prostate-cancer rates.

I return to my own story. Once the panic and fear had subsided after my cancer returned for the fifth time, I began to realise that the only thing that could save me was my scientific knowledge and approach.

It was all too clear from what my doctors said, and from reading medical textbooks, that chemotherapy treatment alone was unlikely to cure me. For five years, I had done everything my doctors had advised and undergone all the treatments that they had prescribed. I had followed to the letter the anti-cancer diet and lifestyle then recommended in the famous Bristol diet.[1]* Nevertheless, I now had a hard, cancerous lump in my neck that looked like half a small boiled egg sticking out above my collar bone, and this had grown in only ten days. Clearly, my lymph system was badly affected by breast-cancer cells. It is important to realise that, when cancer spreads from its original location to another part of the body, the new tumour has the same kind of abnormal cells and therefore the same name as the primary tumour. For example, if prostate cancer spreads to the bones, the cancer cells in the new tumour are still prostate cancer cells. The disease is metastatic prostate cancer; it is not bone cancer.[2] This is very important because it means that reducing risk factors for prostate cancer can help even when the disease has spread to other organs.

Years before I had cancer, I had worked with an American doctor who specialised in multiple sclerosis (MS). At that time, he had described the disease to me as a 'slot machine disease'. It was a strange expression, and the first time I heard it, I asked him what he meant.

'Think Las Vegas,' he replied. 'You're playing the slot machines. You get one strawberry – no big deal. You get two strawberries in a row – still nothing special. But if you get three strawberries, then you've hit the jackpot big-time.'

What he was saying is this: if a person had two out of the three factors that he thought were implicated in multiple sclerosis (or as he put it more graphically, two strawberries and a lemon) they would not develop any symptoms. But in the comparatively rare event of three strawberries coming up, then you would have problems – you would develop the disease. In the case of MS my colleague had suggested that the three factors were a genetic predisposition, an infection – and at the time slow viruses were the fashionable scientific interpretation – and an environmental or lifestyle factor. (My involvement in his work had been an attempt to identify potential environmental factors, particularly in the Orkney Islands and other parts of northern Scotland where the incidence of MS is unusually high.)

---

* The Bristol Cancer Help Centre diet is now closely similar to the one in this book.

Cancer, like MS, is a multi-factorial disease. This thought gave me my first real glimmer of hope: although there was nothing I could do about whatever might originally have *initiated* my own cancer (probably many years previously), there might be a lot I could do to eliminate whatever might be *promoting* it right now.

Since cancer develops at different rates over different periods of time in different people, it seemed likely that something maintains an environment in the body that promotes the cancer cells, enabling them to multiply out of control and eventually allowing them to invade other organs. Such a model could explain why, in some individuals, cancer goes into remission for long periods of time, or even fails to recur. On that basis, I had to identify and eliminate that something, that one 'strawberry', in order to overcome my disease.

So here I was – a scientist about to embark upon the most vital piece of research I had ever faced in my entire life. Like a plot straight out of a nightmare, the deal was starkly, exquisitely terrible: if I got it right, I could have my life back; if not, then it would be the last piece of research I would ever do.

THE SCIENTIST WITHIN

Now, I want to tell you something about myself which greatly benefited me at the time. As an earth and environmental scientist I am trained to observe natural phenomena such as rocks, fossils, volcanoes and earthquakes and to piece together observations to develop theories to try to understand how the Earth and its systems have developed.

Natural scientists like me work in a very different way to biological and medical scientists. If you think about it, we have to: the time scales of earth processes are so vast (up to thousands of millions of years) that it is impossible to carry out experiments in test tubes or under controlled laboratory conditions.

Instead, natural scientists work by piecing together fragments of, often very sparse, information; producing, synthesising and refining their theories from observations, observations and yet more observations.

This approach has been astonishingly successful. In less than a century and a half, such methods have allowed the amazing story of the Earth and the evolution of its life forms to be pieced together. We now know, for example, that the Earth was formed about 4,500 million years ago. It has been transformed by a complex interplay of physico-chemical and biological processes from a hot ball of dust spinning through space into a planet with a cool and varied surface environment where abundant water and an oxygenated atmosphere are capable of supporting complex and diverse life forms. We also know that the outer layer of the Earth is divided into huge plates. These move on million-year time scales in a complex interrelationship with convection currents deep in the Earth; with volcanoes and earthquakes concentrated along the plate margins. Life began more than 3,500 million years ago, since when various diverse life forms have evolved and become extinct, or survived, in response to changes in environmental conditions.

The findings of natural scientists have often been opposed by the orthodox scientific establishment. For example, in the second half of the nineteenth century, the famous natural scientist Charles Darwin suggested, on the basis of careful and extensive observations of rocks and fossils in relation to the modern world, that the Earth and its life forms had required more than 3,000 million years to evolve. At the time, Darwin's views were vehemently opposed by many other scientists. Lord Kelvin, in dismissing Darwin's findings, used physical calculations to show that the Earth was only 20 million years old. Kelvin was wrong by a factor of approximately one hundred and fifty in his calculation – an enormous error for a physicist to make! He made this mistake because he had failed to take account of the heat generated within the Earth by its own natural radioactivity. Darwin, the careful observer, was eventually proved right and the orthodox physical scientist was proved wrong.

Later, the earth scientist Alfred Wegener proposed the then heretical theory that the continents had once formed one large land mass that had split apart to form the present-day oceans and continents. Despite being founded upon careful observation, Wegener's theory was vehemently rubbished by orthodox scientists, who said there could be no mechanism for such a process. Again, as evidence mounted and Wegener's ideas became irrefutable, the theory of plate tectonics finally became widely accepted by the entire scientific community.

More recently, the suggestion of American scientist Walter Alvarez that there have been mass extinctions of life forms during the history of the Earth (such as the death of the dinosaurs because of the impact of a large meteorite) was ridiculed. Again, this suggestion is now widely accepted by the scientific establishment.

So, having no alternative but to die or find a way out myself, I determined to take control of my situation using my training as a natural scientist. I would work in the way that had taken me to the top of my career.

I reminded myself that, despite the billions of dollars spent on cancer research worldwide, little had been achieved in combating the global upward trend in the cancer death rate and certainly not in stemming the inexorable rise in the incidence of prostate and breast cancer in Western industrialised countries. Despite the dedication of doctors working to treat patients with cancer, the tools that they had at their disposal were essentially the same as those of twenty years earlier. If any other area of scientific research had produced so little benefit for such a high cost, it would have been closed down long ago. I would reject the orthodoxy that predicted – on the basis of a classification of the type of cancer I had and the stage that it had reached – that I would die in, at most, three to six months. I decided that, instead, I would look at my cancer in a detached way as a natural scientist, and try to understand the disease as a type of natural phenomenon. I would try to look at it in a holistic way in the tradition of Darwin. This, therefore, was to be my initial approach: look at the facts, the figures, the statistics, and the data and observe, observe, observe.

THE RIGHT HAYSTACK

When you're looking for a needle in a haystack, you must first find your haystack, which can be as difficult as finding the needle.

That was the problem. Current thinking at the time was that the factors involved in breast cancer were a genetic predisposition, total lifetime exposure to the female hormone oestrogen, total animal fat consumption, personality type and stress. I therefore had five major factors to evaluate. And, of course, not much time in which to do it. Quickly, I made preliminary assessments of each factor, as it seemed to apply to me. This is how my initial thinking proceeded:

Genetic predisposition The first thing I did was to remind myself that none of my parents or grandparents nor any of their sisters or brothers, at that time, had suffered from any kind of cancer. They had all lived to a ripe old age. There was therefore no evidence that I was genetically predisposed. As discussed in the previous chapter, inherited mutations of some genes are significant in the development of breast and prostate cancer.[3] However, only a small percentage of such cancers develop because of inherited genetic defects.[4] Inheritance of a mutated copy of a 'cancer gene' certainly does not guarantee that prostate or breast cancer will develop. I decided that, for me, this didn't present a promising line of investigation.

Oestrogen The female hormone oestrogen has been implicated in breast cancer since the nineteenth century when a Scottish surgeon, George Beatson, observed that breast tumours regressed in women whose ovaries were removed. The first attempts at hormonal treatment of prostate cancer date from the late nineteenth century, when an English surgeon found that castration of men with prostate disease led to symptom relief. The work was rediscovered in the 1940s by two Americans, Huggins and Hodges, who received a Nobel Prize for their work.[5]

It has always seemed most unlikely to me that a woman's natural oestrogen, or a man's natural testosterone, could be an important factor in them developing breast or prostate cancer. Otherwise, why is it that the older the man or woman (and hence the lower their testosterone or oestrogen levels), the higher the risk? As a natural scientist, it seemed to me then, as now, more likely that these sex hormones promote cancer only when another more fundamental factor, or factors, has caused the body's chemistry to malfunction. I decided to look into this in greater detail and I discuss my findings further in Chapters 2 and 4.

Fat Many scientists continue to link increased risk of prostate and breast cancer (*see* Chapter 1, p. 11) to the Western diet and suggest that the factor is total fat consumption, especially the amount of animal fat in the diet. In my own case, I'd eaten well below official guidelines for fat intake for years, consuming only lean meat dishes and low-fat cheeses, skimmed milk and yoghurt. My fat intake, I felt sure, wasn't the factor I was looking for. The role of good and bad fats in the diet is discussed further in Chapter 5, Food Factor 4.

Personality type and stress The American psychotherapist Lawrence LeShan has gone so far as to suggest that there might be a cancer 'personality type'. (In contrast, aggressive go-getting individuals – the stereotypical personality type-A people, are more likely to die of heart attacks or strokes.) On the question of stress, I, and many other women who have suffered from breast cancer, were under stress in our daily lives or had suffered tragic events. However, so have most people – and not everyone develops cancer. Recently, large well-controlled studies have suggested that there is little evidence to support the widespread belief that emotional factors whether caused by incidents associated with grief or because of an anxious or depressive personality, cause cancer.[6] Nevertheless, at the time it seemed to me to be a good idea to develop coping strategies for stress, and this is discussed further in Chapter 6.

Having completed my preliminary assessment, I was sure that none of the orthodox risk factors, with the exception of stress, seemed to fit my situation. For example my periods had started late, I had never taken contraceptive or HRT pills, I had given birth to three children and breast-fed each of them although for different lengths of time. I had consumed very little animal fat and none of my relatives had died before the age of 85 (other than by accidental death) and then not of breast cancer (remember my mother's reaction (Chapter 2): 'We've never had anything like *that* in our family!')

I felt that there had to be another factor. And I had to find it.

THE GAME'S AFOOT

'Come, Watson, come!' Sherlock Holmes used to cry when he was on the trail of a particularly exciting case. 'The game is afoot. Not a word! Into your clothes and come!!'

There's a certain kick you get when you're doing scientific detective work, even when it's a rather grim race against time. Even though I was, at that time, undergoing chemotherapy and so from time to time feeling desperately sick, I still felt the thrill of the chase as I started to use my brain for my own survival. But I still wasn't sure where to start looking.

Scientists are supposed to be logical, dispassionate types who labour long and hard for their results, but you'd be surprised how many real scientific breakthroughs would never have happened without a healthy dollop of good, old-fashioned luck. And that's what happened to me.

The first clue to understanding what was promoting my breast cancer came when my husband arrived back from working in China while I was being 'plugged in' for a chemotherapy session. He had brought with him cards and letters as well as some amazing herbal suppositories sent by my friends and colleagues in China. The suppositories had been sent to me as a cure for breast cancer. To this day I do not know what they contained but they looked like firework rockets. I gave them to Charing Cross Hospital for their research, but I was never able to obtain the results. Despite the awfulness of the situation, we both had a good belly-laugh and I remember saying that if this was the treatment for breast cancer in China, then it was little wonder that Chinese women do not get the disease!

Those words echoed in my mind. *Why* didn't Chinese women living in China get breast cancer? My mind flashed up the image of an atlas called *The Atlas of Cancer Mortality in the People's Republic of China*, which I had been given by Chinese colleagues when I had been working with them a few years earlier. The atlas had been prepared in the mid-1970s at a time when Premier Zhou En-lai was dying of cancer. He thought there should be more information on the disease, and about one million doctors and medical workers were recruited to document the incidence of cancer all over China. The exercise produced an extremely valuable research tool, especially for a population as genetically homogeneous as China where more than 85 per cent of the people are Han Chinese.

At the time I was presented with the atlas I had been helping to develop a collaborative project between Britain and China, aimed at examining the links between soil chemistry and disease. Specifically, we were examining how low levels of the chemical element selenium might be related to the occurrence of a type of heart disorder called Keshan disease, and also a crippling condition characterised by enlargement and deformity as a result of the degeneration of cartilage called Kashin-Beck disease (nicknamed 'big-bone' disease). It is now accepted that Keshan disease is a selenium-responsive endemic condition, which mainly affects children and women of child-bearing age and which, untreated, results in heart failure and death. Subsequent field trials of selenium supplementation involving thousands of children proved that selenium could effectively prevent Keshan disease.[7]

Initially, Western doctors and scientists had been highly sceptical of the findings of the Chinese scientists. It was not until organisations such as the famous Rowett Research Institute of Animal Health in Aberdeen, Scotland, replicated Keshan disease in laboratory animals by feeding them selenium-deficient diets, that the findings of the Chinese scientists were accepted. The scientific community, just like the wider community, can often be very chauvinistic when it comes to accepting the results of 'foreign' scientists from certain countries. I call this the Raffy Syndrome: Refuse to Accept Foreign Facts Yet.

More recently, the British Geological Survey (BGS), where I worked until 2005 as Chief Scientist, has worked with Chinese colleagues to develop methods to mitigate the problem of selenium deficiency caused by crops grown on certain soils, and the incidence and death rates of Keshan disease in China are now greatly reduced. There is also a greater understanding of the risk factors for Kashin-Beck disease, which include selenium and iodine deficiency in crops. It is perhaps worth emphasising again that without an understanding of the fundamental cause of such problems – which lay in the environment – there would have been little or nothing that conventional Western medicine could have done.

THE NEWS FROM CHINA

The Atlas of Cancer Mortality in the People's Republic of China had always intrigued me. It shows the markedly different distributions of the various types of cancer over the country. The distribution of lung cancer, for example, shows the disease to be concentrated mainly in urban areas (consistent with research in the West, which indicates that lung-cancer rates in polluted cities exceed those in rural areas, especially among smokers); and locally in areas of tin or uranium mining, where inhalation of radioactive aerosols is likely to be a factor. Overall, the mortality rate for stomach cancer in China is high; but the atlas shows that it occurs almost entirely in the cooler, wetter and mountainous areas of the north, while levels are extremely low in the southern, tropical areas of the country. This is consistent with the idea that this type of cancer is caused by infection with the *Helicobacter pylori* bacterium which mainly affects people who live in cold, damp, mouldy, overcrowded houses. In contrast, cancer of the nose and mouth is concentrated in south China, in a well-defined region north of Hong Kong and Hainan Island. The data in the atlas underline the view that cancer is not one disease but many different diseases with different distributions and causes.

What struck me the first time I looked through the atlas was the amazingly low rate of breast cancer shown *throughout* China. The background rate on the map is 1 cancer death in 100,000 women – an amazing 10,000 times lower than the rate in the UK at the time, which, at about 1 in 10 women, was similar to that in many other Western countries. I knew, however, that data from different countries could not be compared as simply as this. They must first be converted to fit a model age distribution for the population, using a method developed by Professor Sir Richard Doll of Oxford University (the man who first demonstrated the link between smoking and lung cancer). Otherwise, false assumptions might be made. For example, if a type of cancer affects mainly middle-aged and elderly people, as prostate and breast cancer do, and population A has many more young people than population B, then the overall cancer rate would appear to be much lower in population A than in population B – an erroneous impression. Therefore, statisticians have developed a simple method for adjusting data that takes these age differences into account. Data adjusted this way are termed 'age-standardised'.

Nevertheless, even using the age-standardised rates of incidence for prostate and breast cancer for China and Japan, compiled by the International Agency for Research on Cancer (part of the World Health Organisation) the prostate cancer rates are *extremely* low compared to Western countries (*see* p. 116).[8]

The difference between the incidence of prostate cancer in the West and in oriental countries is spectacular. The current official figure for 'lifetime risk' of prostate cancer among men in the UK is one in fourteen. In 2002 there were approximately 20,000 cases in the UK. However, the figures are confused by the issue of BPH. Men in their seventies and eighties will almost certainly have an enlarged prostate, and it has been estimated that at least one in three of these will be cancerous. 95 per cent of prostate cancers diagnosed are in men over 60. One study in the US of men over the age of 50 who had died of other causes reported that 40 per cent were found to have prostate cancer in autopsies[9] (others suggest a figure of 50 per cent, see box below).

Prostate cancer incidence has been increasing dramatically over the past 40 years throughout the West. It is now the second most common life-threatening (non-skin) cancer in men in most Western countries,[10] and it is rapidly overtaking the first – lung cancer. In the US the incidence more than doubled between 1973 and 2000.[11] The number of new cases of prostate cancer in the US was estimated to be 235,500 in 2006.[12] As discussed in Chapter 1, the only risk factors widely accepted by the orthodox medical profession continue to be age, family history and ethnicity, but none of these even begins to explain the rapid increase in the rate of prostate cancer – especially in affluent Western countries. The explanation is clearly not genetic: genes simply do not change in entire populations within one generation!

Prostate cancer does run in families, and men who have a father or brother with the disease have a five- to twenty-fold increased risk, depending upon which study you read. According to the University of Michigan Health System, Comprehensive Cancer Centre,[13] the risk increases in men of any age who have a first-degree relative (father, brother) with prostate cancer. Men who have a first-degree relative with prostate cancer, it is claimed, have approximately a two-fold increased risk of developing prostate cancer during their lifetime, and an individual who has two first-degree relatives with prostate cancer has five-times the risk.

In America, African-American men, more especially those of a Sub-Saharan African descent, have an incidence of prostate cancer that is 1.5 times that of whites. It has been suggested that there are complex differences between the DNA on the Y chromosome of Afro-Caribbeans and Caucasians (white people of European descent), but the low incidence of prostate cancer in rural areas of Africa throws doubt on this hypothesis. Interestingly, although Japanese immigrants to the United States have a higher incidence of prostate cancer than Japanese living in Japan, their rate is still about half that of US whites.[14]

By far the greatest differences in risk of prostate cancer are between men living a Western lifestyle and men in the Far East (Japan, China, Thailand, Korea and south-east Asia generally)

TWELVE FACTS ABOUT PROSTATE CANCER IN THE USA

- Prostate cancer is the most common form of cancer in men.
- Prostate cancer is the second leading cause of cancer death after lung cancer.
- The risk of developing prostate cancer increases with age.
- 80 per cent of men over the age of 65 who have cancer have prostate cancer (American Cancer Society Data).
- One in five men will develop prostate cancer in their lifetime.
- Approximately 335,000 men will be diagnosed with prostate cancer each year.
- Nearly 42,000 men will lose their lives to prostate cancer each year.
- African-American men have the highest prostate cancer incidence in the world.
- African-American men are twice as likely to die from prostate cancer as other men.
- Approximately 71 per cent of men diagnosed with prostate cancer and treated will live more than five years.
- For every man diagnosed with prostate cancer, there are two men with prostate cancer who are not diagnosed.
- Autopsies performed on men over the age of 50 who died from other causes showed approximately 50 per cent had undiagnosed prostate cancer.

From http://www.fgcu.edu/chp/deadlytomen/info.html

(Tables 3.1 and 3.2), who have the lowest incidence (though this changes if they move to the West).[15] The incidence of prostate cancer is generally agreed to be lowest in these parts of Asia (5 per 100,000).[16]

Interestingly, even in Japan, for long one of the most Westernised oriental countries, prostate cancer detected at autopsy is only about 1 in 2800, which contrasts with about 1 in 570 in white men in the USA.[17]

The number of deaths from prostate cancer increased in the 1970s and 1980s, according to researchers from Oxford

University, but then fell by 20 per cent in the European Union, and 30 per cent in America in men aged 50 to 74; this is attributed by the same sources to earlier detection and hormonal treatments.[18]

The fact that survival rates are higher in the United States has been attributed to the more frequent use of radical prostatectomy. More conservative treatments based on radiotherapy plus endocrine therapy tend to be used in Britain,[19] but comparison is difficult because incidence rates are so much higher in the US (Tables 3.1 and 3.2), possibly reflecting the greater use of the PSA screening test there (*see* Chapter 1).

The data I used to look at the incidence and mortality rates of prostate cancer for *Your Life in Your Hands* – which are also the data that I use now – are those of the WHO. The age-standardised data on the incidence of prostate cancer (Table 3.1) that I used in the first edition of the book (also included in the second edition) show that the lowest age-standardised prostate-cancer rate was only 1.7 per 100,000 males in rural China (Qidong county). The

Table 3.1 Age-standardised rates (ASR) of incidence (per 100,000)

	Prostate cancer in males
China, Qidong county (rural)	0.5
China, Shanghai (urban)	2.3
China, Tianjin (urban)	1.9
Hong Kong	7.9
Japan, Hiroshima	10.9
Japan, Miyagi	9.0
Japan, Nagasaki	9.1
Japan, Osaka	6.8
Japan, Saka	6.7
Japan, Yamagata	7.9
England and Wales	28.0
Scotland	31.2
USA (whites)	100.8
USA (blacks)	137.0

Data from *Cancer Incidence in Five Continents*, 1997. Vol. VII, published by the IARC (International Agency for Research on Cancer).

rate approximately quadrupled in Chinese cities (such as Shanghai and Tianjin) and at the time I was initially looking into the different rates of breast and prostate cancer I thought this was probably because of the serious urban pollution problem, the severity of which is rapidly overtaking anything the West can produce.

In highly urbanised Hong Kong, the rate for prostate cancer was approximately four times that in the rest of China – still only approximately 8 men in 100,000. The Japanese cities of Hiroshima and Nagasaki have rates of prostate cancer similar to those of Hong Kong: and remember, both cities were attacked with nuclear weapons so, in addition to the usual pollution-related cancers, one would also expect to find some radiation-related cases of cancer.

The conclusion I drew from the data at the time struck me with some force. If a Western woman were living a Japanese lifestyle in industrialised, irradiated Hiroshima, *she would slash her risk of contracting breast cancer by half*. If an American man were to do the same, he would slash his risk of contracting prostate cancer by a staggering factor of between 9 and 12!

The conclusion is inescapable. Clearly, some lifestyle factor not related to pollution, urbanisation or the environment is seriously increasing the chance of contracting breast or prostate cancer in those living a Western lifestyle.

The latest data from the WHO for 2002 show that the crude background rate for prostate cancer rates in China remain so low that they are not mapped.[20] The latest age-standardised rates (ASR) of the incidence of prostate cancer in males, in China and other oriental countries, with their distinctive diets and lifestyles, are compared with those of a range of Western countries in Table 3.2. The countries presented are all countries I have worked in and I have been able to discuss the data with local doctors. I have talked to doctors in China who hardly remember treating a case of prostate cancer in their entire careers (though this is changing now, as the Western diet becomes fashionable). I have also selected the countries where data are available for migrant communities (e.g. Chinese or Japanese migrants to America or Australia). These studies show that within a generation or so such communities acquire the same rates of prostate cancer and breast cancer as their host populations – indicating that dietary and

3.2 Age-standardised rates of incidence and mortality in males, per 100,000, year 2002

Country	Incidence of prostate cancer	Mortality
China	1.7	1.0
Thailand	4.5	2.9
Korea (South)	7.6	2.8
Japan	12.6	5.7
New Zealand	100.9	20.3
Australia	76.0	17.7
Canada	78.2	16.6
UK	52.2	17.9
USA	124.8	15.8
Iceland	81.0	23.0

lifestyle factors, rather than genes are the key factors: these are the strawberries that can be eliminated.

Migration studies such as those published by Kolonel into cancer incidence in different ethnic populations of first-and second-generation migrants to Hawaii[21] add considerable weight to the evidence of earlier migration studies that most cancers are environmentally determined. Professor Kolonel's research is now focusing on the interaction of diet with genetic susceptibility in determining cancer risk because the potential for understanding cancer through studies of ethnic and migrant populations has, he states, never been greater.[22] Migration studies of cancer incidence in migrants between different continents indicate large dietary influences on the incidence of epithelial cancers generally, including prostate cancer.[23]

It is difficult to compare the data in Table 3.1 with those in Table 3.2 directly because of changes in the groupings and methods used by the WHO IARC. Moreover, it is no longer possible to compare data for Hong Kong separately from China or individual Chinese or Japanese cities. Nevertheless, the most recent age-standardised data from the WHO (Table 3.2) still clearly show that incidence rates of prostate cancer are much higher in Western countries than in oriental countries. It is worth emphasising that many oriental countries, such as South Korea and Japan, are densely populated and have been highly industrialised and urbanised for many years, yet their rates of prostate cancer remain much lower than in the West. The rates are highest in Japan which was the first oriental country to come under Western influence at the end of the Second World War.

Compare the data for oriental countries with the USA, where, as indicated above, by 2002 prostate cancer was the most frequently diagnosed non-skin cancer. It has been estimated that in 2006 the 235,500 newly diagnosed prostate-cancer cases in the USA accounted for 33 per cent of all newly diagnosed cancers in males. This may be compared with newly diagnosed cases of lung cancer and colorectal cancers, which accounted for 13 per cent and 10 per cent, respectively, of cancers affecting men.[24] In the UK prostate cancer is also now the most commonly diagnosed cancer in men, with almost 32,000 cases diagnosed in 2003 which was 23 per cent of all newly diagnosed non-skin cancers.[25] Such evidence continues to indicate strongly that it is an environmental or lifestyle factor that promotes the disease and that the effects of that factor are becoming increasingly powerful.

The death rate from prostate cancer (Figure 3.1) shows two quite distinct groupings: Western countries, such as Germany, the UK and the USA, with high mortality rates (prostate cancer accounted for over 31,000 deaths in the USA alone in 2000[26]); and oriental countries, such as Thailand and China, with very low rates. (The death rate in Japan is rising, however, as the Japanese become more and more Westernised, while that in some Western countries, including the UK, is falling.[27] It has been suggested that the difference in the likelihood of surviving cancer between black and white men in the US, may stem from the difference in access to chemotherapy, or even to the doctors who prescribe it.

Interpretation of the data is complicated, however, by the extent to which some prostate cancers are slow growing and cause no problems during a normal lifetime while others are potentially life-threatening – metastatic cancers. From autopsies performed on men who have died of other causes, it is known that small amounts of cancer can be found within the prostates of many men. These lesions can first be detected shortly after the onset of puberty, with the frequency increasing steadily with age. By the time men reach the age of 70 and above, 80–100 per cent will

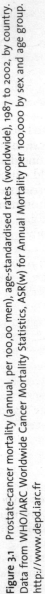

Figure 3.1 Prostate-cancer mortality (annual, per 100,00 men), age-standardised rates (worldwide), 1987 to 2002, by country. Data from WHO/IARC Worldwide Cancer Mortality Statistics, ASR(w) for Annual Mortality per 100,000 by sex and age group. http://www.depd.iarc.fr

have such lesions. While these numbers are high, only approximately 0.3 per cent of these patients will develop metastatic prostate cancer in any given year. Because it is only metastatic prostate cancer that is potentially lethal, it is important to understand what stimulates the cancer to spread beyond the confines of the gland.[28]

One clue to the puzzle of why some cancers metastasise comes from studies done in Japan and other Asian countries. There, localised prostate cancer increases with age, just as it does in the United States and Europe. However, the occurrence of metastatic disease in Japan is approximately 1/10th that in the United States. The incidence of prostate cancer varies by 120 fold when third world countries are compared with the United States and Europe. As discussed previously, migration studies strongly suggest an environmental rather than a genetic cause to explain the large variation in the incidence of metastatic prostate cancer. For example, when Japanese men move to America, their risk of developing metastatic prostate cancer increases in proportion to the number of years they have lived there, and the risk continues to rise with each succeeding generation born there. The implications of this finding are profound: it suggests, for example, that if Americans could adopt aspects of the Japanese life-style, they might reduce the death rate from prostate cancer by as much as 90 per cent.[29]

This evidence is supported by the fact that, when oriental people adopt a Western lifestyle in Hong Kong or as some wealthy Chinese do in Malaysia and Singapore, the rates of prostate and breast cancer approach those of the West.

The slang name for breast cancer in China translates as 'Rich Woman's Disease'. This is because, in China, only the better-off could afford to eat what used to be termed 'Hong Kong food'. The Chinese used to describe all Western food, including everything from ice cream and chocolate bars to spaghetti and feta cheese, as 'Hong Kong food' because of the availability of Western food in the former British colony and its scarcity, in the past, in mainland China.

Finally, let me just remind you that the statistics we have been examining aren't simply the abstract results of some obscure laboratory experiment. They are real-world, real-life body counts. The knowledge that these studies give us has been obtained at an extraordinarily high price: for example, the neat little graph in

Figure 3.1 reflects the loss of hundreds of thousands of individual lives. The least we can do, as scientists, is to study these figures with all our attention and to learn everything we can. From all the data, it seems a fair bet that the environmental lifestyle factor – the 'third strawberry' – that I was looking for when I had cancer is probably related to a long-standing cultural difference between oriental and Western countries.

I remember saying to my husband: 'Come on Peter, you have just come back from China. What is it about the Chinese way of life that is so different? Why don't they get breast cancer?'

Over the next couple of weeks Peter and I examined the results of the China study described below (*see* Chapter 5).

So the Chinese ate a low-fat diet: but so did I. The diet I had been living on for years before I contracted breast cancer was very low in fat and high in fibre.

Peter and I persevered and discussed the suggestions made by some scientists that it was the high levels of soya consumption in oriental countries such as China that gave the female population protection against breast cancer. Soya, provided it is organically grown and not genetically modified, is an excellent source of protein and it has many other benefits, especially for menopausal women.[30] The protective value of soya is discussed further in Chapter 5. However, at that time I had been consuming so much soya in various forms that I did not believe that this could be the factor that I was looking for.

A BELL RINGS

Then one day a couple of weeks later something rather special happened.

Peter and I have worked together so closely over the years that I am not sure which one of us first said:

'The Chinese don't eat dairy produce!'

It is hard to explain to a non-scientist the sudden emotional and mental 'buzz' you get when you know you have had an important insight. It's as if you have had a lot of pieces of a jigsaw in your mind and suddenly, in a second, they all fall into place and the whole picture is clear. Whenever that has happened to me in the past, I have always been proved right – even if, initially, my suggestions were regarded as controversial.

This is precisely the feeling I experienced. I felt the same 'buzz' or to use the German-derived word which sums up the feeling so well: *gestalt*. Suddenly, I recalled how many Chinese people were lactose-intolerant, how the Chinese people I had worked with had always said that milk was only for babies, and how one of my close friends, who is of Chinese origin, always politely turned down the cheese course at dinner parties. I knew then of no Chinese people who lived a traditional Chinese life who ever used cow's milk or other dairy food to feed their babies. The tradition was to use a wet nurse but never, ever dairy products.

Culturally, the Chinese used to find our Western preoccupation with milk and milk products very strange. I remember entertaining a large delegation of Chinese scientists shortly after the ending of the Cultural Revolution in the 1980s. On advice from the Foreign Office, we had asked the caterer to provide a pudding that contained a lot of ice cream. After enquiring what the pudding consisted of, all of the Chinese including their interpreter, politely but firmly refused to eat it and they could not be persuaded to change their minds. At the time we were all delighted and ate extra large portions!

In 1996, I attended an international conference in Beijing and was having lunch with two senior Chinese women scientists. A man smelling strongly of spices and garlic walked past, and I suppose my reaction showed. One of my companions giggled, and shyly asked me 'What do Chinese people smell of to you?'

I thought about it carefully and replied honestly, 'Nothing in particular.' Then, deciding that I could legitimately ask the question in reverse, I said:

'And what do we Westerners smell of to you?'

There was considerable laughter – usually reflecting embarrassment in Chinese people – but after encouragement on my part, they finally said:

'Westerners smell to us of sour milk!' – 'But', they added reassuringly, 'you don't.'

Recently I checked several Oriental (Chinese, Japanese, Korean and Thai) cookbooks. None mentioned dairy produce at all.

Since I wrote the first edition of *Your Life in Your Hands*, the evidence has continued to indicate strongly that the distinctive difference in rates of prostate and breast cancer between Western and oriental countries relates to diet.

The differences between the Chinese and American diets were thoroughly investigated and documented in 1994 by Campbell and Junshi,[31] and are shown as pie charts in Figure 3.2. The advantages of the Chinese diet include the following:

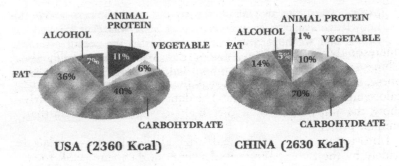

Figure 3.2 Comparison of American and Chinese diets

- It is low in fat. Only 14 per cent of calories in the average Chinese diet were from fat, compared with almost 36 per cent in the American diet, and most of the fat in the Chinese diet was healthy polyunsaturated fats from fish and vegetables, not the artery-clogging saturated fat from butter, cheese and meat that most Americans eat.
- It is high in fibre, which helps to eliminate excess hormones and toxins from the body. Fibre is also protective against hormone-dependent cancers such as prostate cancer and is one of the most protective components in the diet against colorectal cancer. Animal protein contains no fibre whereas all plant foods, including plant proteins, contain lots. Animal protein was found to make up only 1 per cent of an average Chinese diet, compared with 11 per cent of the average American diet. Vegetables are the main source of protein in China, giving an average fibre intake of 34 g per day, compared with the average US fibre intake of only 10–12 g per day.
- The low content of acid-generating animal protein does not give rise to the high levels of acidity in the body that favour the spread of cancer. Cheese is one of the most acid-generating foods known, generating three times as much acidity, weight for weight, as roast beef.[32] The typical American diet is very acid generating.[33]

- It is high in phyto-oestrogens, which are protective against prostate and breast cancer. Vegetables rich in phyto-oestrogens, such as soya, are the main source of protein in China.
- Traditionally Chinese people did not eat dairy produce, whereas in the West this can account for up to 40 per cent of the diet.[34]

Interestingly, the study by Campbell and Junshi showed that the Chinese took in more calories than Americans, but were much less obese, strongly suggesting that it is the type of food and not the calorie intake that is important. The data in Figure 3.3 also clearly show the importance of a diet high in vegetable, rather than animal, protein.

Unfortunately, the traditional oriental diet is being replaced widely by the typical Western diet, high in dairy and junk food. Peter Carey in his book *Wrong about Japan* describes how even

Figure 3.3 Relationship between prostate-cancer incidence and the ratio of vegetable protein (VP) to animal protein (AP) in the diet. Age-standardised cancer data from WHO/IARC, IARC Cancer Epidemiology Database. GLOBOCAN 2000, Cancer incidence, mortality and prevalence worldwide. Ferlay, J., Bray, F., Piesci, P. and Parkin, D.M. (eds). http://www.dep.iarc.fr/globocan/database.pdf. Diet data from Frassetto, L.A., Todd, K.M., Morris, R.C., Jr and Sebastian, A., 2000. Worldwide incidence of hip fracture in elderly women: relation to consumption of animal and vegetable foods. *J Geront: Med Sci*, 55A, (10), M585–M592.

the name of milk there, which translated literally as liquid from a cow's udder and elicited a YUK reaction, has been changed to the marketeer's word 'Miruku'! A French dairy group recently reported an 8 per cent rise in sales of probiotics in Asia, which totalled 14 billion euros in 2006.[35] According to Chinese colleagues, dairy is being marketed, just as in the West, as being essential for strong bones – an idea completely refuted by informed and distinguished doctors and scientists,[36] and more recently by my book *Understanding, Preventing and Overcoming Osteoporosis*, written with Gill Tidey, which is based on an in-depth analysis of the peer-reviewed medical and scientific literature.[37] As this book shows, osteoporosis is very rare in China and the Chinese have little cause to worry about it – unless they change to a dairy-rich Western diet!

Figure 3.3 shows the proportion of vegetable to animal protein in the diet of 33 countries (compiled from FAO food fact sheets[38]) plotted against prostate-cancer incidence. There is a clear relationship between diets with a high ratio of vegetable to animal protein and low prostate-cancer risk. The critical ratio of vegetable to animal protein is about 1 to 1. Put more simply, the data suggest that you can decrease your risk of developing prostate cancer by eating similar amounts of vegetable and animal protein, but note that this refers only to protein, and I recommend eating masses of vegetables and fruits as well (*see* Chapter 5).

Nevertheless, despite the mounting evidence of the links between the Western diet and prostate cancer, most conventional medicine continues to promulgate the same old risk factors (*see* Chapter 1). Much of the information on these risk factors may be relevant within countries such as the USA or the UK, but it ignores all the epidemiological evidence of the much lower rates in China and other oriental countries, evidence which strongly implicates the Western diet and lifestyle as the main causative factor.

One of the problems, it seems to me, is that researchers tend to look at their own populations: for example just people in Finland, or in Holland. Using Figure 3.1 as an example, they are frequently looking at minor perturbations in the lines at the top of the graph (i.e. rates within individual Western countries), while ignoring the much more significant differences between prostate-cancer and breast-cancer rates in different countries. These differences between Western and oriental countries have been clear and sustained ever since reliable standardised cancer registers were first kept. The data strongly indicate that differences in diet and lifestyle are at the root of the problem of the increasing incidence of prostate, breast and other reproductive cancers in the West – a trend now being followed in the East as they strive to become more and more Westernised.

A very high proportion of non-Caucasian human populations, as well as some Caucasians, become lactose intolerant after weaning, when the child's body stops producing lactase, the enzyme needed to metabolise lactose. This is a clear signal from nature that, as the Chinese used to say, 'milk is for babies' – and they meant human milk. Five thousand years of milk drinking has masked some of the most obvious ill effects of dairy consumption in Western countries.

Another clue that milk drinking by adults is unnatural is that no other mammal drinks the milk of another species. Wildlife programmes show animals eating the flesh and eggs of other species, and living on vegetable matter, but I have yet to see an example of an adult mammal suckling an adult mammal of another species for food.

We all know the old maxim 'you are what you eat'. In the West, the idea of using diet to treat illness goes back to the Hippocratic School of Medicine which originated in Greece in about 400 BC. Hippocrates scorned the belief that disease is caused by magical or supernatural forces, and said that everything had a rational origin. He also noted the body's ability to heal itself, given the right conditions. Interestingly he took most of his patients off milk.

THE FINGER POINTS

In my years of exploring alternative health systems – since I first had breast cancer – I have learned that many naturopaths believe that the part of the body that is diseased provides a clue as to the cause of the illness. This seems to be particularly the case for cancers for which we know the cause. For example, lung cancers reflect inhalation of cancer-causing cigarette smoke, radioactive aerosols such as the naturally occurring radioactive gas radon, or asbestos dust. Skin cancers frequently reflect excessive exposure to sunlight whilst cervical cancer is associated with infection by the sexually transmitted human wart (or papilloma) virus. It seemed highly likely that consuming a powerful biochemical solution from the mammary gland of one species of animal (milk) could be sending the wrong signals to my own mammary glands – my breasts.

And I'd certainly been a big milk drinker. Before I had breast cancer the first time, I had consumed a lot of dairy produce as skimmed milk and, particularly, as low-fat cheeses and yoghurt, which I had used as my main source of protein. I also used to eat some cheap but lean minced beef (which I have since realised was probably often ground up dairy-cow) as hamburgers with my children, especially when we went out for treats, or made it into spaghetti bolognese or other low-cost meat dishes.

At the time of my last recurrence of cancer in the lymph nodes in my neck, I had been eating yoghurt and some skimmed organic milk which I boiled before drinking, as allowed in the Gerson and Bristol diets. The original Bristol diet by Forbes[39] recommended Indian-style ghee (clarified butter) for cooking and one of the salad dressings for which a recipe is given is based entirely on yoghurt. A detailed case history describing a breast cancer cure in the Bristol diet book also refers to the extensive use of yoghurt. I had been careful to choose only those brands of yoghurt labelled as 'live' and 'organic' or I had often made my own yoghurt using milk labelled as 'organic'. In order to cope with the chemotherapy, I had initially been eating organic yoghurts as a way of helping my digestive tract to recover and repopulate my gut with 'good' bacteria.

However, following Peter's and my insight into the Chinese diet, I decided to give up all dairy produce immediately. Cheese, butter, milk and yoghurt and anything else that contained dairy produce – it all went down the sink or into the rubbish bin. It is surprising how many products, including commercial soups, biscuits and cakes, contain some form of dairy produce. Even many brands of margarine marketed as soya, sunflower or olive-oil spreads contain significant quantities of dairy produce. Many prescription and herbal drugs are in a lactose base. I therefore became an avid reader of the small print on food and drug labels.

I discovered that as far back as 1989 yoghurt had been implicated in ovarian cancer.[40] Dr Daniel Cramer of Harvard University studied the diet of hundreds of women with ovarian cancer and compared the data with those for a group of women who were similar in age and other factors but had not developed cancer. There was one thing that distinguished the two groups: the women with cancer had eaten much more dairy produce, especially supposedly 'healthy' yoghurt, than women without cancer. This finding has been confirmed recently at the famous Karolinska Institute in Sweden where researchers showed that for every glass of milk drunk the risk of ovarian cancer increases by 10 to 15 per cent.[41]

Dr Cramer suggested that the problem was the milk sugar, not the fat, so yoghurt and cottage cheese produced using bacteria, which increase the production of galactose from lactose (milk sugar), were of most concern. Although I am not sure that I agree with the underlying explanation proposed by Dr Cramer or with the chemical he implicated, the link he so clearly demonstrated certainly explained my situation and my observations and hypothesis. How I wish Dr Cramer's information had been more widely publicised at the time. If it had been, I believe I could have avoided any recurrence of my cancer. I examine the reasons why we are not told about such findings in Chapter 7.

I BECOME A HUMAN GUINEA-PIG

Up to this point, I had been steadfastly measuring the progress of my latest and greatest lump with callipers and plotting the results. Despite all the encouraging comments and positive feedback from my doctors and nurses, my own precise observations told me the bitter truth: the first chemotherapy sessions had produced no effect – the lump was still the same size.

Then I eliminated dairy products.

Within days, the lump started to shrink. About two weeks after my second chemotherapy session and one week after I gave up dairy produce the lump in my neck started to itch, and then it began to reduce in size. The line on the graph, which had shown no change, was now pointing downwards as the tumour got smaller and smaller. And, very significantly, I noted that instead of declining exponentially (a graceful curve) as cancer is meant to do, the tumour's decrease in size plotted on a straight line heading off the bottom of the graph, indicating a cure: not suppression or remission of the tumour.

One Saturday afternoon after about six weeks of excluding all dairy produce from my diet, I practised an hour of meditation (more of that later) and then felt for what was left of the lump. I could not find it. I went downstairs and asked my husband to feel my neck. He could not find any trace of the lump either. On the following Thursday, my cancer specialist examined me thoroughly, especially my neck where the tumour had been. He was initially bemused and then delighted as he said, 'but I cannot find it'. He was as overjoyed as I was. When I saw the same specialist for my annual check-up in 2001, he told me that my chemotherapy treatment had been only the same basic type that has been used for breast cancer for the past twenty years. None of my doctors, it appeared, had expected someone with my type and stage of cancer (which had clearly spread to the lymph system) to have survived, let alone be so hale and hearty.

When I first discussed my ideas with my cancer specialist he was understandably sceptical. But I understand that he now uses maps from *The Atlas of Cancer Mortality in the People's Republic of China* in his lectures and recommends that his other patients read my books.

I now believe that the link between dairy produce and cancer of the prostate, breast and ovary is as well established as that between smoking and lung cancer, as discussed further in Chapters 2 and 4.

I believe that what cured me was identifying the link between breast cancer and dairy produce and then developing a diet based on my findings. Initially, it was difficult for me, as it may be difficult for you, to accept that a substance supposedly as 'natural' and wholesome as milk might have such ominous health implications. In the next chapter, I want to tell you about some of the particular substances in dairy products that I believe are to blame.

At the beginning of this chapter I used the idea of a slot machine and its combination of lemons and strawberries to communicate the idea that prostate cancer and breast cancer are what scientists call multifactorial diseases, involving several different risk factors. I explained that, while there is little that we can do about some of our risk factors – or strawberries – such as our genes, if we eliminate some controllable risks, by changing at least one strawberry to a lemon, we can prevent prostate cancer or breast cancer (*see* p. 105). Indeed, even when we have one of these cancers, we can put the disease into remission by eliminating one of the strawberries – as I have done for the last fourteen years.

Most of the people who have followed my dietary and lifestyle recommendations (*see* Chapters 5 and 6) have also put their cancer into remission (see the stories at the end of Chapter 1).

CHAPTER 3 IN A NUTSHELL

- Prostate cancer is a multi-factorial disease. You can visualise what this is by thinking of a slot machine. You get one strawberry (a gene) – no big deal. You get two strawberries in a row (a gene and exposure to a carcinogen) – still nothing special. But if you get three strawberries in a row (a gene, exposure to a carcinogen and a bad diet?) then you could develop the disease. I was trying to find the strawberry (modifiable risk factor) that I could eliminate from my life to put my cancer into remission.
- *The Atlas of Cancer Mortality in the People's Republic of China* prepared in the mid-1970s at a time when Premier Zhou En-lai was dying of cancer gave me the best clue to identifying the third strawberry for my breast cancer. It shows the markedly different distributions of the various types of cancer across China and underlines the view that cancer is not one disease but many different diseases with different distributions and causes.
- The atlas shows high rates of some cancers in parts of China but the background rate of breast cancer shown *throughout* China is 1 cancer death in 100,000 women – **10,000 times lower** than the rate of 1 in 10 women in the UK – and what about prostate cancer? The rate was so low they did not even bother to map it!
- Even using the age-standardised rates of incidence for prostate and breast cancer for China and Japan, compiled by the International Agency for Research on Cancer (part of the World Health Organisation) the rates for both types of cancer are *extremely* low compared to Western countries; data for 1997 showed that America had an incidence of prostate cancer more than 260 times that of China!
- The death rate from prostate cancer also shows two quite distinct groupings: Western countries, such as Germany, the UK and the USA, with high mortality rates; and oriental countries, such as Thailand and China, with very low rates.

- Migration studies (e.g. Chinese or Japanese migrants to America or Australia) clearly show that the difference is not due to genetic differences. Within a generation or so such immigrant communities acquire the same rates of prostate cancer and breast cancer as their host populations – indicating that dietary and lifestyle factors, rather than genes, are the key factors. Hence there are strawberries that can be eliminated.

- Prostate cancer rates are increasing dramatically throughout the West and it is now the second most common life-threatening (non-skin) cancer in men in most Western countries and it is rapidly overtaking the first – lung cancer. In America it already has! It has been estimated that in 2006, 33 per cent of all newly diagnosed cancers in males were prostate cancers with lung cancers and colorectal cancers, accounting for 13 per cent and 10 per cent of cancers respectively.

- Such evidence continues to indicate strongly that it is an environmental or lifestyle factor that promotes the disease and that the effects of that factor are becoming increasingly powerful.

- The only risk factors for prostate cancer widely accepted by the orthodox medical profession continue to be age, family history and ethnicity, but none of these even begins to explain the global variation or the rapid increase in the rate of prostate cancer – especially in affluent Western countries such as the USA.

- Since I wrote the first edition of *Your Life in Your Hands*, the evidence has continued to mount that the distinctive difference in rates of prostate and breast cancer between oriental countries such as China and Western countries relates to diet.

- The important differences between oriental and Western diets mainly reflect the much higher proportion of plant foods relative to animal foodstuffs in the former. Hence the Chinese diet is low in fat, especially animal fat and animal protein but naturally high in vitamins, minerals and live enzymes as well as fibre and phyto-oestrogens. Traditionally Chinese people do not eat dairy produce, whereas in the West this can account for up to 40 per cent of the diet. Hence the traditional Chinese diet has little or no food containing powerful animal hormones, saturated fats or cholesterol or food that generates excess acidity in the body.

4. MILK IS A FOUR-LETTER WORD

In this chapter I explain much of the compelling scientific evidence that has accumulated over the years, even since I wrote Your Life in Your Hands *in 2000, suggesting that prostate cancer and breast cancer are associated with the Western diet and its high proportion of dairy produce. Milk contains hormones, such as prolactin and oestrogen, and growth factors, such as IGF-I and IGF-II, substances which, according to leading international experts, promote prostate cancer and other types of cancer. The chapter also explains why giving up dairy is unlikely to cause any health problems, but, on the contrary, is likely to cut your risk of suffering not only from prostate cancer, testicular cancer and other types of cancer, but from many other diseases as well.*

Just as oriental people used to be astonished when they saw Westerners consuming so much dairy produce, many of us have found it difficult to understand how anyone could possibly live healthily without it. Certainly I was one of those who had bought into the message, pushed by the industry, that dairy produce, especially yoghurt, was essential for good health.

It is all a matter of perception. One person's milk is another person's bowl of cockroaches. The reaction of both groups is 'yuk'.

In most of Western society, milk is promoted as a healthy, natural food: vital for babies, full of protein for active adults, and essential for older women, at risk of osteoporosis. Yoghurt (now probiotics) continues to be promoted as being essential for keeping the gut flora in balance. In short, dairy continues to be marketed as all things to all people. But this image is just that – a carefully crafted marketing image. The lowing cows roaming lush green pastures used to advertise dairy are a far cry from modern industrialised dairy production systems.

In fact there is no scientific evidence that we need to consume milk after weaning – indeed, we're the only species that intentionally does so. Even stranger is our obsession with the milk of other species: the cow or goat. Can you imagine drinking dogs' milk, pigs' milk, or rats' milk? Just the thought fills us with disgust – maybe that's how we ought to feel about cows' or goats' milk, too.

Drinking the milk of another species is a fairly recent practice, dating back only about 6000 years in Europe and central Asia,[1] a practice not followed until recently by most of the rest of the world. Seventy per cent of people in the world, more than 90 per cent of the populations of some Asian countries, remain lactose (milk-sugar) intolerant. There is still an enormous variation in the consumption of dairy products. People in most Western countries consume more than 250 kg a year, compared with at most a few kg in oriental countries, such as China, Vietnam and Thailand, and many African countries.[2]

Cows' milk isn't intended by nature for consumption by any animal other than baby cows. If we compare its profile of nutrients with that of human breast milk, you'll see some major differences.[3] The vertical line on Table 4.1 represents the nutritional profile of human milk; the horizontal bars show how cows' milk compares. It is clear that cows' milk contains about three times as much protein as human milk, and about four times as much calcium – both of which can place an excessive burden on the human kidney. The high calcium in dairy also causes other problems (see Chapter 6). One particular concern about cows' milk lies in its low levels of essential polyunsaturated acids compared with human milk. This is thought to reflect nature putting a higher priority on increased body size in cows and on the development of the brain in humans.[4] Attempts have been made to increase the nutritional value of cows' milk for humans by feeding cattle on fish meal and soya[5] and flax seed.[6]

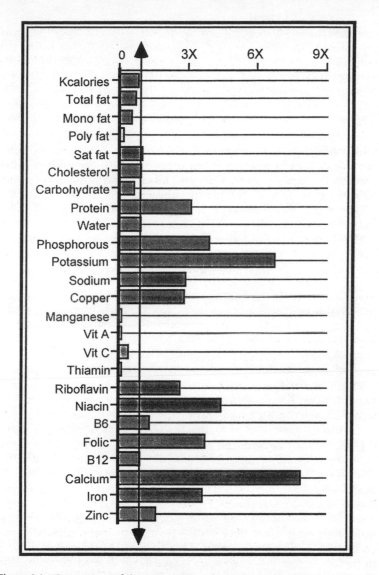

Figure 4.1 Comparison of the composition of typical cows' and human milk. The vertical line represents the composition of typical human milk.

Anything naturally good in dairy produce comes from plants or the action on them of microbes in the gut. Surely it is better to eat salads and vegetables, which are not unlike the grasses that cows are supposed to eat in the first place – after all, they are the real source of the immensely strong bones of animals designed to be totally vegan, such as cows and hippopotamuses. It has even been suggested recently that the highly promoted conjugated linoleic acids that occur in dairy fat have a pro-carcinogenic effect.[7]

One best-selling supposedly anti-cancer diet recommends consuming meat and dairy produce to protect against cancer, and another book still available in the UK continues to recommend yoghurt as part of an (anti-breast-) cancer diet. Even ICON, the magazine of the charity, CANCERactive, now carries articles suggesting that probiotics – the new marketing name for yoghurt – protect against cancer. This is advice I shall strongly refute.

THE CHANGING QUANTITY AND QUALITY OF DAIRY

Many scientists believe that the amount of dairy produce in our diet is now far too high and that its quality has changed greatly. It has been calculated that the average weekly consumption of dairy by people in the UK is now about the same as the petrol consumption of our cars – approximately 5 litres a week per person! Recently the Royal Society,[8] Britain's most authoritative scientific organisation, suggested that routes of human exposure to oestrogen that changed in the latter half of the twentieth century included increased consumption of dairy produce. They went on to point out that dairy practices have changed since World War II, in that pregnant cows continue to be milked, increasing the oestrogen content of the milk. Indeed, in today's large-scale intensive dairy farms cows are pregnant and milked for most of the year.[9] During pregnancy the cow's ovaries secrete high levels of progesterone and the placenta secretes high levels of oestrogen – and the hormone levels in milk from both Holstein and Jersey cows have been shown to have increased markedly.[10]

Milk products now supply between 60 and 80 per cent of female sex steroids such as oestrogen and progesterone in the diet, the remaining 20 per cent being derived from other animal products such as meat. Significant concentrations of the male hormone testosterone also occur in cheese, milk and milk products,[11] and androgen precursors also occur in dairy.[12] Particular concern has been expressed about the oestrogen content of cow's milk by Gamaa and Sato,[13] whose study into cancer incidence and food intakes in 40 countries showed an increase in hormone-dependent cancers with increasing cheese and milk consumption. Moreover, selective breeding and high-protein feed to replace grass has increased the average milk yield per cow from nine litres (16 pints) a day to a staggering 22 litres (39 pints) a day.[14]

The United States Department of Agriculture has estimated that the average American's diet comprises more than 40 per cent dairy produce, more than double most official guidelines[15] – which distinguished nutritional scientists think are already set too high.[16] The American diet is certainly not a healthy one.

INCREASING FIGURES

It is estimated that a staggering 60 per cent of Americans are now overweight enough to begin experiencing health problems as a result. About 25 per cent of all Americans under 19 are overweight or obese, a figure that has doubled in 30 years.[17]

In Bill Bryson's book *The Lost Continent* he repeatedly refers to the obesity of the American population:

> Iowa women are almost always sensationally overweight – you see them at Merle Hay Mall in Des Moines on Saturdays, clammy and meaty in their shorts and halter tops, looking a little like elephants dressed in children's clothes, yelling at their kids, calling out names like Dwayne and Shauna.

Another book called *Fat Land: How Americans Became the Fattest People in the World*[18] has been described as a well-written report on the obese American, and how they got that way. And the question was asked 'if America is out in front, can the United Kingdom be far behind'?[19] Some of the latest data from the UK Food Standards Agency (FSA) answer this question. In 2004 the FSA reported that the number of obese men in the UK had risen from 8 per cent in 1987 to 25 per cent; in women the number had increased from 12 per cent to 20 per cent. The influence of vested interests, including the dairy industry, in giving misinformation to consumers is discussed further in Chapter 7.

MILK – WHAT A COCKTAIL!

Let us now look at a list of the incredibly powerful biochemicals that are contained in milk.

Why are they there? Mammals developed fairly recently in the history of the Earth (they have existed for only about 200 million years, out of the 4,500 million years of the age of the Earth) and are the most evolved and intelligent creatures on the planet. Their high degree of development is achieved by a long period of gestation in the womb, where they are fed a complex cocktail of chemicals, including hormones and growth factors, which bring about cell growth, differentiation and proliferation, including the migration of embryonic stem cells to different parts of the developing foetus. Following birth, infant mammals are suckled (ideally in humans for about one and a half years) because milk carries similar chemical messengers to maintain growth and differentiation. The transport medium for the chemical messengers – plasma – simply changes from red blood to white milk, known as 'white blood' in some cultures.

Milk from every mammal contains hormones, growth factors and other powerful biochemicals. The reason why all mammals, other than humans, stop drinking milk at a certain age is because by then they produce all the hormones, and growth factors they need. The production, secretion and levels of these substances are regulated through a complex, delicately balanced system of interaction. The concern is that by absorbing extra quantities of highly bioactive substances from cows' milk, goats' milk and/or the meat of animals used for dairy production there could be undesirable growth and differentiation of tissues in the human body, leading to cancer.

In fact cows' milk has been shown to contain over 35 different hormones and 11 growth factors![20] Indeed, growth factors for laboratory research studies are normally obtained from milk or cheese whey.[21]

Some of the growth factors, hormones and peptides in milk include the following[22] [my bold]:

- bombesine (a neuropeptide).[23] Milk contains both bombesine and GRP (bombesine-like peptide).[24] Bombesine levels in milk are three times higher than in blood,[25] and GRP and bombesine have been implicated in prostate cancer[26] and breast cancer.[27]
- GRP (Gastrin-releasing peptide).[28]
- substance P (a neurotransmitter),[29] which increases vascular permeability[30] and stimulates histamine secretion,[31] causing allergic reactions.
- CGRP (calcitonin-gene-related peptide, also a neurotransmitter).[32]
- **IGF-I and IGF-II**[33] **(insulin-like growth factors)**. IGF-I and IGF-II are quite resistant to decomposition by enzymes.[34] They promote both prostate[35] and breast cancer.[36] See also the work of He[37] and Perks and Holly.[38]
- **EGF (Epidermal growth factor)**.[39] Like IGF, EGF is quite resistant to decomposition by enzymes.[40] EGF enhances prostate cancer[41] and breast cancer,[42] and was the first growth factor to be shown to be absorbed by the blood through the gut wall.[43] It is to be strongly avoided by those with tumours over-expressing the HER 2 protein. EGF has been implicated in androgen-independent prostate cancer.[44]
- NGF (Nerve growth factor).[45]
- **Oestrogen**. There is particular concern about the oestrogen content of cows' milk,[46] which is the most important source of dietary exposure to animal oestrogen. Hartmann and others[47] found that milk products now supply 60–80 per cent of female steroid hormones such as oestrogen in the diet, the remaining 20 per cent coming from other animal produce such as meat.
- **Prolactin**. To be able to breastfeed, the female body is better equipped to cope with temporarily increased prolactin production. Males are not, and prolactin-producing tumours in men are therefore larger, more active and resistant to treatment.[48] Prolactin enhances prostate[49] cancer and breast cancer.[50]
- PRP (Prolactin-releasing peptide).[51]
- **LHRH** (or: GnRH, stimulates secretion of LH and FSH).[52]
- **progesterone**.[53] Hartmann and others[54] found that milk products now supply 60–80 per cent of female steroid hormones such as progesterone in the diet, the remaining 20 per cent coming from other animal produce such as meat.
- peptide YY.[55]
- peptide histidine methionine.[56]

- neuropeptide Y (stimulating appetite).[57]
- TRH (stimulating TSH secretion).[58] TRH stimulates prolactin[59] and growth hormone (GH) secretion,[60] through T3.[61]
- TSH (stimulating T3 and T4 secretion).[62]
- T3 (Triiodothyronine).[63] T3 increases the number of oestrogen receptors, increasing oestrogen-influence.[64]
- GHRF (Growth-hormone-releasing factor).[65] GHRF stimulates GH and hence IGF-I and IGF-II secretion.[66]
- ACTH (regulating cortisol secretion).[67]
- neurotensine.[68]
- cortisol.[69]
- insulin (regulating blood-glucose level).[70]
- beta-endorphine (opioid peptide).[71]

Since many of the powerful chemicals contained in milk are known to have an important role in the development of young mammals, including cell division, and milk is designed for this purpose, it is worth asking the question: what happens if the chemicals which are intended by nature to stimulate cell growth in newly born animals such as cows and goats send similar signals to adult tissue in humans? Much recent scientific evidence reviewed below supports the link between dairy consumption and breast and prostate cancer and other hormone-dependent cancers.

Many of the growth factors, hormones and other biochemicals contained in dairy milk are implicated in the production and development of other cancers, including ovarian and testicular cancer.[72] It has been suggested that different growth factors increase cancer-risk of different tissues. Excessive LHRH, which is concentrated in milk, stimulates secretion of LH and/or FSH, which, in turn, have been implicated in prostate,[73] ovarian[74] and testicular cancer.[75] It has also been suggested that different growth factors promote types of cancer not associated with the reproductive system. There is evidence for the role of milk in promoting lung cancer. For example, in Japan, in 1996 people consumed more than three times as many cigarettes as in Norway,[76] but in Norway lung-cancer mortality in men was higher.[77] Also, in countries such as Russia, UK, France, Canada, USA and Australia fewer cigarettes are smoked,[78] but lung-cancer mortality in men is higher than in Japan.[79] In all these countries more milk, containing lung-cancer-promoting substances, is consumed,[80] again suggesting that dairy contains substances that select for and promote damaged or initiated cancer cells.

The insulin-like growth factors (IGF-I and IGF-II) and prostate cancer

Let us look at the role of the insulin-like growth factors, especially IGF-I, for which evidence of its role in prostate, breast and other cancers continues to mount.

Why should these substances cause problems such as prostate or breast cancer?

In humans, free or circulating IGF-I levels decline with age consistent with their role in growth. IGF-I levels are higher in teenage girls than boys, and the difference extends into adulthood. Levels are elevated in pregnant women. Although IGF-I is essential for growth, its levels do not correlate closely with growth rates; supporting other evidence that some IGF-I is of dietary origin. It was suggested some years ago by distinguished biochemists that IGF-I levels may reflect nutritional status.[81]

The levels of IGF-I in the blood are highest during the years of puberty, which is, of course, a time of rapid growth. Indeed, at the onset of puberty, IGF-I sends signals to prostate and breast cells to begin dividing so that the prostate and breasts will grow in adolescent boys and girls.

Both insulin and the IGFs cause cells to increase in size. Insulin has a simple short-term action of cleaning excess nutrients from the circulation and storing them in cells. In contrast, the IGFs are involved in cell proliferation and differentiation, and a complex set of factors has evolved to ensure that IGF activity occurs only when conditions are optimal for growth. Zinc levels are particularly important in the case of prostate cancer,[82] which seems to store zinc.[83] See Chapter 5 and Lifestyle Factor 1 in Chapter 6 for healthy and unhealthy sources of zinc.

In 1990, researchers at Stanford University reported that IGF-I promotes the growth of prostate cancer cells. In 1995 researchers at the US National Institute of Health reported that IGF-I plays a central role in the progression of many cancers, including that of the prostate. According to Hans R. Larsen, the evidence of a strong link between cancer risk and a high level of IGF-I is indisputable.[84]

Pollack[85] has suggested that the relation of IGF physiology to carcinogenesis will become relevant in cancer-risk assessment and chemoprevention, although he continues to emphasise the potential value of drugs that target the IGF-I receptor and indicates that several candidate pharmaceuticals are being proposed for clinical trials. Lonning also recommends that future therapeutic strategies in treating breast cancer should consider total blockade of the IGF-I receptor.[86] Yee and Sachdev state that there are abundant data from human, animal and laboratory studies supporting a role for the IGFs in cancer and that interactions with their receptors have been shown to stimulate cancer proliferation, prevent cell suicide and enhance metastasis. Again, their research centres on targeting the IGF-I receptor.[87] Pollack raises particular concern about the use of IGF-I and GH in anti-ageing preparations for humans.[88]

Several prospective studies, using stored blood collected up to 14 years before the onset of disease, have shown associations between IGF-I and prostate cancer.[89] The associations remain when people whose blood samples were taken soon before diagnosis are excluded from statistical analysis, suggesting that the observed relationships do not reflect release of the growth factor by pre-clinical cancers.[90] The effects are sizable, and stronger than the effects of most previously reported risk factors.[91]

This study and that of Chan and others, 1998,[92] into IGF-I levels and prostate cancer, discussed further below, are both prospective studies whereby symptomless groups of patients are followed for years and data for those who develop disease are compared to data for those who do not. Evidence for causal relationships is generally considered to be more convincing when it is obtained from prospective studies than when it is derived from retrospective studies (i.e. carried out after the disease has developed), because in the latter there is a chance that the high measured levels of IGF-I could be caused by the disease.

Researchers from McGill University and the Harvard School of Public Health in the United States have also found increased levels of IGF-I circulating in the blood to be a strong predictor of prostate cancer.[93] Men with the highest levels of circulating IGF-I had a 4.3-fold increased risk of developing prostate cancer compared with those with the lowest IGF-I levels. In the article in the magazine *Science*, Pollack writes that 'until now, researchers interested in prostate cancer have focussed on male hormones such as testosterone, but these (IGF-I) results open up a whole new direction of research. This is of the same order of magnitude as the relationship between cholesterol levels and the risk of heart disease.' Also according to Pollack, most recent population studies and laboratory investigations support initial prospective studies linking risk of future diagnosis of prostate cancer with levels of circulating IGF-I.[94] Yet another recent study from 1998 confirms that increased IGF-I levels in blood are associated with large relative risks for common cancers.[95] Other studies have also linked high circulating levels of bioavailable or bioactive IGF-I with an increased risk of developing prostate[96] and other[97] cancers. A study carried out by the University of Texas, for example, showed that high circulating levels of IGF-I increased the risk of lung cancer,[98] and a study carried out by Harvard Medical School showed that high circulating levels increased the risk of colorectal cancer.[99] IGF-I has also been linked to an increased risk of childhood cancers, melanoma and pancreatic cancer.[100] Indeed, Campbell and Campbell suggest that IGF-I should be used as a predictor of certain cancers in much the same way as cholesterol is used to identify those at risk of heart disease.[101]

In summary, the scientific literature strongly supports the link between high circulating IGF-I levels and several types of cancer (including prostate cancer). Let us look more closely at what this has to do with consuming dairy produce.

The link between IGF-I and dairy

There is no doubt that the established medical view now is that growth factors promote cancers directly, but much of conventional medicine assumes that growth factors such as IGF-I are made in the body. It would also be true to say that we manufacture our own cholesterol, but cholesterol-related disease (e.g. heart disease) is caused by consuming *extra* amounts of the substance from dairy and other animal products. There is increasingly strong evidence that the same applies to IGF-I.

IGF-I is exactly the same chemical whether it is in the milk of goats, sheep, cows, humans or other mammalian species. Levels of IGF-I are naturally higher in cows' milk (and in that of sheep and goats) than human milk, because these animals grow more rapidly. As pointed out by John Robbins in his book *A Diet for a New America*,[102] while a human normally takes 180 days to double its birth weight, a cow takes only 47 days and a goat even less – just 19 days – so such milk is likely to be particularly bad for us because it will contain more growth factors than human milk.

The dairy industry tries to argue that IGF-I has no effect in the human body because it is destroyed during digestion and does not cross the gut-blood barrier. Independent studies, however show that substances contained in milk closely similar to IGF-I are not destroyed by the digestive system because of the protective effect of casein (the principal protein in milk).[103] The 1999 report of the EU Scientific Committee states 'there is clear evidence that orally ingested IGF-I reaches the receptor sites in the gut in its biologically active form.'[104] Moreover, research published by the Cancer Epidemiology Unit at Oxford University[105] has shown that serum IGF-I was 9 per cent lower in vegan men than in meat eaters (also thought to consume dairy produce) and milk-consuming vegetarians. More recently, studies have confirmed that serum IGF-I levels in European women increase significantly with increasing consumption of dairy; levels also increase with increasing intake of animal protein from meat, poultry, fish and eggs but these relationships were not statistically significant. There was no relationship with vegetable protein from pulses or cereals and the more vegetables consumed the lower the serum IGF-I levels.[106]

IGF-I is not destroyed during pasteurisation of milk. In experiments, after being treated at 175°C for 45 seconds (longer than the US Department of Agriculture Pasteurisation Protocol), the concentration of IGF-I was not reduced.[107]

IGF-I has growth-promoting effects in response to concentrations as low as 1 ng/ml. Milk contains approximately 30 ng/ml, so two 8-oz glasses of milk a day would contain 200 ng of IGF-I per kilogram of body weight per day for a person weighing 70 kg.[108] Also, milk secretions of mammals contain special forms of IGF-I which are ten times more potent than normal IGF-I. In normal cows' milk, 3 per cent of the IGF-I is reported to be in this form.[109] Interestingly, one study reported a 10 per cent increase in circulating IGF-I levels in people consuming low-fat milk.[110]

There are now many scientific studies into the links between diet, circulating IGF-I levels and cancer. In one study, Dr Chan and her colleagues investigated the relationship between dairy calcium and prostate cancer in the 20,885 men in the Physicians' Health Study.[111] The results clearly showed that men consuming more than 600 mg a day of dairy calcium had a 32 per cent higher risk of prostate cancer than men consuming less than or equal to 150 mg of dairy calcium a day, even after adjusting for other risk factors such as age, smoking, exercise levels and body mass index. Chan concluded that the results support the hypothesis that dairy products and calcium are associated with a greater risk of prostate cancer.[112] The study also found that those who ate the most dairy produce had 17 per cent less vitamin D in their bloodstream than those who consumed the least. This vitamin is known to play a protective role against prostate cancer[113] (see further in Chapter 6, Lifestyle Factor 1). The Harvard study is the largest to date, by arguably one of the most respected epidemiology teams in the world.

Evidence of a dose-response relationship between dairy consumption and prostate cancer has also been noted by Barnard.[114] He goes on to say that mechanisms that may explain the association include the deleterious effect of high-calcium foods on vitamin D balance, increased serum IGF-I concentrations and the effect of dairy products on testosterone concentration or activity.

Another researcher, E. Giovannucci, concludes:

> For prostate cancer, epidemiologic studies consistently show a positive association with high consumption of milk, dairy products and meats.[115]

and

> Diets high in dairy products and meats are related to higher risk of prostate cancer incidence or mortality in most ecologic, case-control and prospective studies.[116]

A recent Scandinavian report also links the volume of dairy consumption to the level of risk of prostate cancer. High dairy consumption was reported to increase risk by 50 per cent.[117] Morimoto and others also reported that milk consumption is linked to increased serum IGF-I levels,[118] and Hoppe and others reported that an increase in daily milk consumption from 200 ml to 600 ml increased circulating IGF-I levels in Danish boys by a massive 30 per cent.[119]

In *Your Life in Your Hands*, I quoted other studies that suggested such a link, including that of Outwater and others,[120] which was based on a review of more than 130 peer-reviewed publications. I also quoted the findings of an EU scientific committee that concluded that excess levels of IGF-I in milk posed an increased risk of prostate and breast cancer.[121] Strong evidence of a causal association between higher levels of milk consumption and IGF also came from a comparison between people whose diets were supplemented with milk and a control sample of people whose diet was not supplemented.[122] Associations of calcium, milk and dairy products with IGF-I also suggest a link between diet and prostate cancer.[123]

Together, the evidence suggests that the association between IGF-I and cancer incidence complies with many of the accepted criteria for causality:[124] the association is strong and specific, it demonstrates the correct temporal sequence, it is dose responsive, it has biological plausibility, and it has coherence with other documented associations. According to Holly and others, the last remaining criterion of causality to be satisfied would then depend on interventions, showing that reducing circulating IGF-I levels reduces cancer incidence.[125] They go on to suggest that the fact that circulating IGF-I concentrations are strongly dependent on nutrition raises the prospect of being able to reduce cancer risk by less aggressive interventions. Investigation of nutritional interventions aimed at reducing serum IGF-I concentrations would be warranted if such reductions were confirmed to reduce the risk of cancer.

There are no specific data on the effects of reducing dairy consumption, but one study of prostate cancer sufferers who had chosen not to undergo treatment for early prostate cancer clearly demonstrated the importance of diet. The group who followed a vegan diet, including soya rather than dairy, had PSA levels 10 per cent lower than the control group, and another test indicated that prostate-cancer-cell inhibition in the experimental-diet group was eight times that of the control group.[126]

Gunnell and others, from a consortium of British universities including Bristol and Cambridge, examined the association of diet with the IGFs in healthy middle-aged men. They found that raised levels of IGF-I, relative to the binding protein that prevents it locking onto receptors, were associated with higher intakes of milk, dairy products, calcium, carbohydrate and polyunsaturated fats, while lower levels were correlated with high vegetable consumption, particularly tomatoes. They found no evidence of an association with red meat. Their findings that vegetable intake was weakly related to lower bioavailable/bioactive IGF-I is consistent with the observation that vegetable-rich diets protect against prostate, breast and colorectal cancer.[127] Their findings were not affected by socioeconomic status or other lifestyle factors such as smoking.[128] These associations, with the exception of carbohydrates, support all the factors I proposed as limiting levels of circulating IGF-I in *Your Life in Your Hands*. Unfortunately, Gunnell and his co-workers looked at carbohydrates as a whole; in YLIYH I advised against refined carbohydrates but not against others, based on scientific evidence that refined white bread increases circulating IGF-I levels whereas whole-grain cereals contain chemopreventive chemicals active against prostate and breast cancer (*see* further in Food Factor 6, Chapter 5). Other studies had previously reported reduced levels of IGF-I in those on vegan diets,[129] and with increased tomato consumption.[130]

Thus, scientific investigations by leading scientists in some of the world's most prestigious universities and research centres show that consuming dairy products increases circulating levels of IGF-I,[131] and this in turn increases the risk of prostate cancer,[132] breast cancer,[133] and other cancers. There are a few studies that purport to show the opposite, and, as discussed in the final chapter, their validity has been questioned.

TIME TRENDS OF IGF-I LEVELS IN MILK

Following the development of fixed farming communities, Western man has consumed milk and this has always contained growth factors such as IGF-I. Prostate and breast cancers have also existed in Western populations for a long time. A mid-seventeenth-century painting (*see* p. 148) by Rembrandt entitled *Bathsheeba at her Toilet* (1654), which hangs in the Louvre in Paris, clearly shows that the model Rembrandt painted had a large tumour in her right breast.

Modern practices such as the use of genetically modified hormones have dramatically increased the levels of IGF-I in milk. The average concentration of IGF-I in milk from cows treated with genetically modified recombinant bovine growth hormone, rBGH, is *significantly (2 to 5 times) higher* than in untreated milk, and there is about twice as much IGF-I in the meat of treated cows as in that of untreated cows.[134] In the US, the rBGH is available under the trade name Posilac without veterinary prescription, but its use is banned in the EU, although under the GATT it has not been possible to ban milk products imported from the US.[135] One of the most important effects of rBGH, as far as prostate and breast cancer studies are concerned, is that it increases the amounts of IGF-I and IGF-II in milk. Also, the long-term treatment of cows with the hormone implant oestradiol as a growth promoter increases secretion of IGF-I.[136]

Over the years, the dairy industry in most Western countries has chosen to increase the average milk yield by feeding the cows on protein concentrate rather than grass and selectively breeding from cattle which are higher milk producers. This has resulted in the selection of cows such as the Holstein which have higher levels of naturally occurring BGH, so that even before the era of rBGH, levels of IGF-I in milk were increasing. The practice of milking cows when they are pregnant has also increased IGF-I levels in milk, as well as steroid hormones.[137]

IGF-I is only *one* of the powerful chemicals in milk which may have a significant role to play in the development of prostate and breast cancer. What about all of the others? Here are some of them.

IGF-II AND EGF

According to Outwater and others,[138] IGF-II is also a potent mitogen (a substance that induces cell division) present in dairy milk. The US Food and Drug Administration reported that IGF-I levels are approximately 30 ng/ml. Those of IGF-II are approximately 350 ng/ml – more than ten times greater. Most studies have concentrated on IGF-I because of the effects of rBGH on its concentration, and there is little about IGF-II in the literature. One experiment, however, which involved increasing IGF-II levels in transgenic mice 20–30 fold, indicated the development of a wide range of tumours after eighteen months.

Epidermal growth factor (EGF), which is also a mitogen (promoting cell division), also occurs in milk. It is well established that it stimulates the proliferation of epidermal and epithelial tissues generally and that it crosses the intestinal wall and enters the bloodstream.[139] EGF is implicated in promoting several types of cancer, including HER2-receptor-positive breast cancer and some types of lung cancer.

PROLACTIN

Both the long and short form prolactin receptors have been demonstrated in the glandular secretory epithelium of the rat prostate, the long form being regulated by testosterone, prolactin and oestrogen. The researchers suggest that since prolactin increases the synthesis of epithelial-cell DNA it may have implications for prostate-cancer progression. Research in Finland into prolactin receptors in the prostate also concluded that prolactin may increase prostate cancer progression because it increases the synthesis of epithelial-cell DNA.[140]

The hormone prolactin is a key milk-supporting hormone in mammals and it is found in all milk. It has been linked to prostate and breast cancer by several research groups. For example, Clevenger and others[141] from the University of Pennsylvania, writing in the *American Journal of Pathology* in 1995, suggested a role for prolactin in the pathogenesis of breast cancer. The ability of bovine prolactin to act as a mitogen in cultures of rodent breast-cancer cells is undisputed. Struman and others in 1999[142] also showed that the human prolactin/GH family are angiogenic – that is, they promote the development of microvascular structures. Remember from Chapter 2 that cancers need to develop a blood supply system and scientists are trying to develop anti-angiogenic substances to effectively starve cancers. The same molecules however, can have anti-angiogenic properties. These properties are thought to be important in the development of the vascular connections between the mother and developing foetus (stress and some drugs, including some for treating psychotic disorders, increase the body's circulating prolactin).

Most amazingly, in the lab prolactin is actually measured by adding milk to cultures of a type of cancer cell (rat lymphoma) and weighing the increase in the mass of the cancer to calculate the concentration of prolactin! This technique has been shown to be a sensitive bio-assay method (relies on biological rather than chemical reaction) for determining the levels of prolactin in milk, and it depends upon prolactin's ability to stimulate cancer cell growth. I actually first discovered this in a book entitled *Breast Feeding – A Guide to the Medical Profession*.[143] Genetically engineered prolactin is also marketed and sold for experiments on prolactin-dependent tumours.[144]

Prolactin in milk has been described as biologically potent and in new, suckling infant mammals it influences the transport of fluid, sodium, potassium and calcium. Again, we manufacture our own prolactin. Is it not likely that, as in the case of cholesterol, triglycerides and IGF-I, disease could be caused by consuming foods (especially in large quantities over many years) in which extra amounts of this chemical is concentrated?

Hence, at least one hormone (prolactin) and a potent growth factor (IGF-I) contained in milk and the meat from slaughtered dairy cows have been shown to be cancer promoters. There is evidence that IGF-II is also a cancer promoter, and these are only three of the many powerful biochemicals in milk designed to influence development of the newborn of the same species. If prostate tissue is frequently bathed in fluid with elevated levels of growth factors used in nature to signal to young males to develop their prostate glands during puberty for the production of semen, and also with high levels of a hormone for which the prostate has been shown to have receptors, is it surprising that prostate cells make mistakes that can lead to cancer?

TESTOSTERONE AND OESTROGEN

Testosterone is widely thought to be one of the main hormones to affect prostate cancer, just as oestrogen is considered to affect breast cancer.

It has been suggested[145] that two of the potential mechanisms that might explain the strong associations between circulating IGF-I levels and cancer incidence are: IGF-I could be affecting steroid levels and/or amplifying sex steroid actions in the prostate and breast; or IGF-I levels could be having a direct effect on the development of cancer in these tissues. The association between IGF-I levels and prostate cancer is difficult to reconcile with the argument that IGF-I levels are just a reflection of steroid activity.[146] The association between prostate cancer risk and IGF-I is stronger in men over 60 years of age, when androgens are likely to have less influence.[147] The strength of the associations between IGF-I and prostate and breast cancer also suggests that they are unlikely to be due to IGF-I acting merely as a surrogate of steroid status. An alternative explanation might be that IGF-I determines steroid levels or actions, enhancing the production of gonadal steroids from both the testis[148] and the ovary.[149] The proliferative effects of steroids in the prostate and breast can also be made worse by IGF-I[150] – indeed it has been reported that IGF-I is able to activate the androgen receptor even in the absence of androgens in prostate cells.[151] Increased circulating levels of IGF-I could therefore enhance and add to the effects of steroids on the prostate. A combination of such potential interacting mechanisms involving IGF-I effects on steroids is a plausible explanation of the associations of testosterone with prostate cancer and oestrogen with breast cancer.[152] Put more simply, the evidence suggests that high circulating levels of IGF-I stimulate the body to produce levels of oestrogen or testosterone more appropriate for teenagers than post-menopausal women or post-andropausal men.

HORMONES, GROWTH FACTORS AND PROSTATE CANCER AS A DISEASE

As indicated in Chapter 2, DNA can be damaged by many factors, although the body is well equipped to repair or eliminate damaged cells. The problem of cancer developing into a disease is more likely to reflect the influence of factors favouring the growth of damaged, relative to normal, cells over the longer term. Absorbing growth factors and hormones through the diet will preferentially favour such damaged cells – those least able to deal with growth factors – and hence promote cancer. Eventually, tumours can start producing more growth factors, stimulating their own reproduction, but probably only in very advanced cases. Even so, some natural substances can help to block their activity (see Chapter 5).

Let me finish this section on the connection between dairy and prostate and breast cancer by quoting from the conclusions of the review paper by Outwater and others who studied the findings of about 130 peer-reviewed publications: 'The existing evidence indicates possible cancer risks associated with the consumption of dairy products. Bovine GH has not been considered to be of health concern because subsequent increase in bovine milk IGF-I levels are within the "normal range" based on untreated cow's and human breast milk. However, it is possible that the "normal range" could be carcinogenic when milk is ingested regularly over a lifetime. Hormones and growth factors in milk, such as IGF-I, are consumed in nature by the fast-growing infant; it may be that regular milk ingestion after the age of weaning produces enough IGF-I in mammary tumours to cause the cell cycle to supersede its boundaries of control, increasing the risk of cancer.'[153] Although the statement specifically referred to mammary tumours, it would appear to apply equally to prostate cancer.

This same point is made by the EU Scientific Committee on Veterinary Measures Relating to Public Health.[154] They state 'The physiological actions of IGF-I and IGF-II relate to growth and development of the embryo and foetus and to cellular differentiation, proliferation and cancer.' Is this not just a modern, high-technology way of saying what the Chinese have always known: that milk (and they meant human milk) is just for (human) babies?

All these findings provide compelling evidence that dairy consumption is one of the key factors contributing to prostate cancer, breast cancer and some other types of cancer – though all of the other dietary factors in Chapter 5 are important too.

I RECOMMEND

I recommend that all men who wish to prevent or treat prostate cancer should *totally eliminate all forms of dairy produce from cows, goats or any animal source from their diet and make the other dietary and lifestyle changes indicated in Chapters 5 and 6.* Those with active cancer, particularly, should cut down their intake of foods of animal origin as much as possible.

THE RISK WE RUN

I know that there will be many people who will read this book and say that they have consumed dairy produce all their lives with no ill effect – just as there are people who point out that someone they know has smoked 40–60 cigarettes a day and lived to be 100. The problem is one of increasing risk to those in the population who, for genetic or other reasons, are more vulnerable. Risk is a difficult idea to explain. Many scientists who are specialists in risk (which is a concept based on statistical probabilities) point out that no one would buy lottery tickets if they understood the subject, but human behaviour is based more on personal experience and emotions than mathematical concepts.

The best way of explaining cancer risk is perhaps the aeroplane analogy, which I use to try to persuade people to stop smoking. According to this example, you should think how you would feel if you were going to fly in an aeroplane and you knew with certainty that one out of every ten flights was going to crash. Would you fly? I don't think you would! Perhaps because they understand risk, very few scientists smoke.

I have never smoked and knowing that I am vulnerable to breast cancer I will no longer eat any dairy produce (including meat from animals used for dairying) in any form, at any time. I have lived without any dairy produce whatsoever in my diet for fourteen years. Since then, a large cancer in my neck that was thought to be incurable, shrivelled and disappeared and has not returned. My previously brittle nails are now long and strong, my skin is in excellent condition and I have no signs of osteoporosis. Most people think I am younger than my 62 years. Similar advice to give up dairy is given by Dr RM Kradjian, MD, the Chief of the Breast Surgery Division at the Seton Medical Center, Daly City, California, in his book, *Save Yourself from Breast Cancer*,[155] and in a letter entitled 'The Milk Letter: A Message to my Patients'.[156]

I believe that I, and those who have suffered from prostate cancer or breast cancer and shared my advice, have avoided death by dairy. New evidence is also emerging that the consumption of dairy products is an important risk factor for testicular cancer and confirms that consuming dairy produce increases the risk of ovarian cancer. There are many other diseases which are helped by avoiding dairy, as detailed in *Eating for Better Health*.[157] Some of these are described below, and many of the beneficial effects of a dairy-free diet have been confirmed over and over again by communications from followers of the dietary and lifestyle factors outlined in this book.

SOME OTHER PROBLEMS WITH MILK AND HEALTH

An increasing amount of scientific evidence shows that dairy milk is not the wonder food the dairy industry would have us believe. Indeed, scientists are now linking cows'-milk consumption to a wide range of human diseases. Here are some of them.

Babies who are fed cows' milk in the first year of life are at risk of developing iron deficiency. The iron in cows' milk isn't easy for babies to absorb, and such milk also appears to interfere with the body's absorption of iron from other foods. Even worse, cows' milk has been shown to cause iron loss by producing gastrointestinal bleeding.[158] Many authorities, including the American Academy of Pediatrics Committee on Nutrition, recommend that whole cows' milk should be excluded from the diet in the first year of life.[159] The UK Department of Health has recently endorsed the resolution passed at the World Health Assembly in May 2001 that babies should be exclusively breast fed for the first six months of life.[160] Paediatricians learned long ago that cows' milk was often a cause of colic in young infants, and even breast-feeding mothers consuming cows' milk can have colicky babies.[161] This is how one British consultant paediatrician describes allergy to cows' milk in infants: 'An infant receiving cows' milk protein (CMP) may be persistently restless, screaming at intervals and appearing in pain. His appetite may be excessively greedy, he may regurgitate freely and he may have loose, mucousy stools in which blood and sometimes sugars are detected. There may be impaired weight gain and anaemia is common. Infants, especially if their parents or siblings suffer from eczema, hay fever or asthma, may develop facial or generalised eczema, persistent nasal congestion and noisy wheezing when CMP is introduced, or these symptoms may be accentuated at that time, with or without gastrointestinal disturbance.'[162]

Milk is one of the commonest causes of food allergies. It is the single commonest cause of allergy in infants,[163] and CMP has frequently been implicated in causing eczema, asthma and migraine. It has been suggested that some of the thousands of cases of cot death that occur in the USA every year might be caused by cows' milk allergy.[164] Respiratory problems, canker sores, skin conditions, and other subtle and not-so-subtle allergies can all be caused by dairy products. Over 70 per cent of the world's adult population are unable to digest the milk sugar, lactose, suggesting that this is the normal condition for adults, not some sort of deficiency.[165] The symptoms, which include abdominal pain, flatulence and diarrhoea, are relieved by taking the enzyme that breaks down lactose, called lactase. Lactose intolerance would seem to be nature's early warning system!

According to the website of the US Food and Drug Administration (FDA),[166] a food allergy, or hypersensitivity, is an abnormal response to a food triggered by the immune system. Many people often have gas, bloating or other unpleasant reactions to something they eat, but this is not a true allergic response. Such a reaction is called 'food intolerance'. Lactose (milk sugar) intolerance is very common, especially among non-Caucasians. This is of particular concern since it is used as the matrix or filler for many orthodox and herbal tablets. The FDA continues:

> The food protein fragments responsible for an allergic reaction are not broken down by cooking or by stomach acids or enzymes that digest food. These proteins can cross the gastrointestinal lining, travel through the bloodstream and cause allergic reactions throughout the body.
>
> The timing and location of an allergic reaction to food is affected by digestion. For example, an allergic person may first experience a severe itching of the tongue or 'tingling lips'. Vomiting, cramps or diarrhoea may follow. Later, as allergens enter the bloodstream and travel throughout the body, they can cause a drop in blood pressure or eczema, or asthma when they reach the lungs. The onset of these symptoms may vary from a few minutes to an hour or two after the food is eaten.

Over 170 foods have been documented in the scientific literature as causing allergic reactions.[167] Most sufferers are affected by the so-called 'big eight': milk, eggs, soya, wheat, peanuts, shellfish, fruits and tree nuts, which between them account for the great majority of food allergies.[168] Cows' milk is known to be a risk factor for many allergic conditions such as asthma and eczema.[169] The most common foods linked to eczema are cows' milk and eggs.

Pending legislation on allergens in manufactured foods, the UK Institute of Food Science & Technology makes the following recommendations for label warnings (to take the example of dairy): 'where calcium caseinate is the MSA (major serious allergen) concerned, the warning should read "Contains MILK PROTEIN". It would be helpful to the purchaser to add to this category of warning the words "to which some people may be allergic".'[170]

Let me quote from an article in the *Sunday Times*[171] on the role of milk in allergies.

> Hippocrates, the father of medicine, swore by milk-exclusion diets for curing all sorts: enfeebled babies, diarrhoea, skin

complaints, wheezing, painful joints ... As Hippocrates suspected, the white stuff [milk] is the commonest cause of childhood allergies. Standard medical advice is that such allergies usually desist by the age of three. But in a recent Finnish study, two thirds of a group of 56 infants diagnosed with cows'-milk allergy were still allergic and highly symptomatic at the age of 10. Other studies show that many children are milk allergic but don't know it. Reactions include runny noses, wheezing, coughing, ear infections, rashes and stomach upsets. When milk is withdrawn from their diet, symptoms improve or clear altogether, and reintroducing it leads to relapse in the majority. The chief culprits appear to be lactose and bovine protein.

Diabetes

Insulin-dependent diabetes (Type 1 or childhood-onset) is linked to dairy products. Epidemiological studies of various countries show a strong correlation between the use of dairy products and the incidence of insulin-dependent diabetes. This disease, which tends to strike in early teenage years and accounts for many deaths a year in the UK alone, starts with the immune system destroying the beta cells in the pancreas that produce insulin. It has been suggested that there may be a genetic predisposition, but mounting evidence suggests that the disease is linked to an allergy to bovine (cow's) serum protein.[172] More recent studies also strongly support a link between early and adolescent exposure to cows' milk and type-1 diabetes.[173]

Dirty milk and infectious illnesses

Milk is an excellent culture medium for the growth and transmission of many bacteria and micro-organisms. Pasteurisation was originally developed to destroy *Coxiella burnetii* (the organism responsible for Q-fever) and *Mycobacterium tuberculosis* (the organism responsible for tuberculosis), which were thought to be the most heat-resistant pathogens likely to be present in raw milk. However, new studies suggest that a microbe called *Mycobacterium paratuberculosis* (MAP) may survive pasteurisation if it is present in high numbers prior to heat treatment.[174] In cows, the microbe causes chronic enteritis, known as Johne's disease, which is an incurable, chronic, infectious disease characterised by diarrhoea, weight loss and debilitation. It is one of the most widespread bacterial diseases of domestic animals throughout the world, and is believed to be associated with Crohn's disease in humans[175] (which affects 20 per cent of the population in the USA[176]). This problem has made headlines in prestigious newspapers in Britain. For example, an article entitled 'TB bacteria found in treated milk' (*Sunday Times*, 20 February 2000) discussed links between *Mycobacterium paratuberculosis* and Britain's 80,000 cases of Crohn's disease. Recent new molecular studies support a causal link between MAP and Crohn's disease.[177] Moreover, up to 7 per cent of samples of pasteurised milk in the UK have been found to contain MAP, increasing at times to 25 per cent.[178] In the UK the FSA has responded by introducing a strategy to reduce the risk of consuming dairy, but this does not consider other routes of exposure. It has been suggested that drinking water or inhaling particles contaminated by cows' faeces was responsible for a cluster of cases of Crohn's disease on watersheds around Cardiff.[179]

The *Sunday Times* article mentioned above goes on to describe serious outbreaks of food poisoning also involving pasteurised milk which, in one case, affected sixty people, killing one child and requiring a second child to have a kidney transplant. Hugh Pennington, Professor of Microbiology at Aberdeen University, who traced the outbreak to milk contaminated by manure-related *E. coli* 0157 bacteria, is quoted as saying 'There have been enough problems with milk in recent years to show there is an issue here. Most of the time farmers will get away with dirty milk, but when things go wrong it can be disastrous.' As with Crohn's disease, there is evidence that exposure to *E. coli* is increasingly from cows and sheep via the environment, as a result of contact with animal faeces or water contaminated with faeces.[180]

Drinking milk contaminated with bovine tuberculosis can cause infected glands in children's necks. Bovine tuberculosis now affects more than 700 herds annually in the UK, following the fiasco of the Krebs trial into the extent that badgers are responsible for spreading the disease. There is a simple answer to the problem: remove all the cows and save the health and wealth of the nation. Keep the badgers instead, as there appears to be no evidence of transmission of tuberculosis to humans.

Listeria monocytogenes is a bacterium which can occur in soft cheeses and cause very serious illness, including meningitis and septicaemia; the mortality rate can be as high as 30 per cent in those affected by Listeriosis.[181] The most vulnerable people include those who are immunosuppressed, which of course includes those on chemotherapy. The incubation period before the development of the disease can be as long as ten weeks, causing considerable difficulty in identifying the source of infection.

Most food poisoning cases in the UK are caused by consuming contaminated meat or dairy products.[182] The dairy industry also contributes to the spread of many other nasty infectious illnesses such as brucellosis, leptospirosis (Weil's disease) and crypto-sporidium (a malaria-like parasite resistant to normal water disinfection processes that is now affecting even some of our major groundwater sources), not to mention BSE and new-variant CJD.

As if these allergies and unpleasant infectious illnesses were not bad enough, a wide range of chemicals can be administered legally to dairy animals.[183] These chemicals include antibiotics to treat infection and for use as growth promoters, and anti-parasitic drugs including those active against worms. In the USA and some other countries, hormones, including oxytocin, are used as veterinary prescription drugs. It is claimed that their use in cows does not pose any concerns regarding the safety of human food, provided that they are used according to directions. They can, however, be misused – for example oxytocin can be used to increase milk production – and effective policing is needed to ensure that milk does not contain excess residues of hormones administered by dairy farmers.[184]

The trend towards intensive farming means that cows are being unnaturally forced to produce more and more milk. In the USA, for example, there has been an almost constant annual increase in milk yield per cow of 1.5–2 per cent. One of the consequences of this artificial, high-pressure milking regime is an increase in infections of cows' udders, which can cause pus to be present in milk. Even in the EU, milk for human consumption can be sold legally even when it contains up to 400,000 somatic pus cells per ml (EU directive 92/46/EEC), so one teaspoon of milk can contain 2 million pus cells. Because increased pus diminishes the value of milk, dairy farmers use antibiotics on their animals. In 1990, a survey by the FDA found antibiotics and other drugs in 51 per cent of 70 milk samples taken in 14 cities.[185] There is growing concern that residues such as these may increase the human allergic response to milk, as well as increasing the immunity of bacteria to antibiotics, making human diseases more difficult to treat. It is estimated by the EU that 3–10 per cent of the human population is allergic to penicillin and the other antibiotics most commonly used to treat mastitis in cows. Their report also states that increased use of anti-microbial substances in treating mastitis might lead to the selection of resistant bacteria.[186]

Milk is designed to be a concentrated source of chemicals which ensure the growth and well-being of newly-born and young mammals. Unfortunately, many harmful man-made chemicals which the body cannot distinguish from natural substances also become concentrated in milk. See further in Chapter 6, Lifestyle Factor 6.

Osteoporosis and dairy

Dairy is strongly and wrongly promoted as protecting against osteoporosis. Indeed, the most commonly asked questions from those recommended to adopt a dairy-free diet are 'Won't I get osteoporosis?' or 'Won't my osteoporosis get worse if I stop eating dairy products?' or 'Where do I get my calcium from?' The marketing of dairy produce as an essential source of calcium has been so strong that even some medical professionals, who should know better, insist that eliminating dairy produce from the diet will lead to calcium deficiency and hence increase the risk of osteoporosis. For many people, however, cheese is likely to be part of the cause, not the cure, of osteoporosis. The widely available scientific evidence on the real causes of osteoporosis, presented in *Understanding, Preventing and Overcoming Osteoporosis*,[187] appear to have made little impact on conventional thinking. We were unable to find a single website from an orthodox medical source, national or international agency or charity that does not recommend dairy as a source of calcium and protection against osteoporosis. Our book presents evidence from the peer-reviewed scientific literature which strongly and convincingly refutes this.

I shall quote here from John Robbins' best-selling book *Diet for a New America*:[188]

The [US] National Dairy Council has spent tens of millions of dollars to make us think that osteoporosis can be prevented by drinking more milk and eating more dairy products. **But the only research that even begins to suggest that the consumption of dairy products might be helpful has been paid for by the National Dairy Council itself.**

Hegsted's work published in 1986[189] showed a clear link between excessive amounts of calcium consumed as dairy produce in the diet and increased osteoporosis. He showed that excessively high intakes of calcium consumed over a long time impair the body's ability to control the activity of the activated form of vitamin D, calcitrol. This in turn controls calcium absorption from food, how much is laid down in bones and how much is excreted. According to Campbell[190] ruining the body's calcium regulatory mechanism in this way is a recipe for osteoporosis in menopausal and post-menopausal women.

The WHO advises that osteoporosis is not a disease of calcium deficiency and Campbell in his book *The China Study* gives the same advice that I give; that staying physically active, keeping salt to a minimum and eating plant foods, while avoiding animal produce, especially dairy, is the best way to prevent osteoporosis.

Other problems

There have been several studies recently that link dairy to a wide range of other illness and conditions. In 2005 a paper published in the *Journal of the American Academy of Dermatology* linked teenage acne directly to the consumption of dairy.[191] Moreover, dairy produce such as cheese, butter and whole-milk products supply so much saturated fat that they are now officially classified as junk foods in the UK (*see* Chapter 5) and no dairy products contain any fibre at all. It is therefore perhaps not surprising that recent research has confirmed the link between the consumption of cows' milk and constipation.[192] For the same reasons, vegans have healthier levels of cholesterol, LDL and HDL in their blood than vegetarians who consume dairy products[193] and are therefore at significantly lower risk of cardiovascular disease. Recent research also shows that milk intake is associated with increased risk of developing Parkinson's disease. There was a 2.3-fold excess of Parkinson's disease in those consuming more than 16 oz of dairy a day compared to non-milk drinkers.[194]

Let me finish with a statement from a review of *Your Life in Your Hands* posted on the Amazon.com website by a physician in the USA: 'In my practice I see so many patients with acid reflux disease, asthma, frequent migraine headaches, feeling tired all the time. As soon as we stop the milk and related products their improvement is remarkable. I think it does not make sense that millions of our citizens take medications for the above-mentioned disorders and do not follow a common sense approach by discontinuing milk products and giving themselves a chance to feel better naturally. I switch all my patients from milk to soy on their first visit and in one week they feel the difference.'

For further information on the problems of dairy foods you may wish to update yourself regularly using the website of the AntiDairy Coalition, http://www.antidairycoalition.com.

CHAPTER 4 IN A NUTSHELL

- There is no scientific evidence that we need to consume milk after weaning – indeed, we are the only species that intentionally does so.
- Drinking the milk of another species is a fairly recent practice, dating back only about 6,000 years in Europe and central Asia, a practice not followed until recently by most of the rest of the world.
- Seventy per cent of people in the world, and more than 90 per cent of the populations of some Asian countries, remain intolerant to lactose (milk-sugar).
- There is still an enormous variation in the consumption of dairy products. People in most Western countries consume more than 250 kg a year, compared with at most a few kg in oriental countries, such as China, Vietnam and Thailand, and many African countries.
- Milk from every mammal contains hormones, growth factors and other powerful biochemicals.
- Cow's milk has been shown to contain over 35 different hormones and 11 growth factors, including IGF-I and EGF. Casein, the main milk protein, has been shown to protect such substances contained in milk from being broken down during digestion.

- The concern is that by absorbing extra quantities of such highly bioactive substances from milk and/or the meat of animals used for dairy production on a daily basis there could be undesirable growth and differentiation of tissues in the human body, leading to cancer.
- Research now shows convincingly that circulating levels of IGF-I reflect the diet, especially high dairy intakes.
- Absorbing growth factors and hormones through the diet preferentially favours initiated cancer cells, which have damaged 'grow' and 'don't-grow' genes – those least able to deal with growth factors – and hence promotes cancer.
- Many of the growth factors, hormones and other biochemicals contained in dairy milk are involved in the production and development of prostate cancer as well as breast cancer, testicular cancer and ovarian cancer and non-reproductive cancers such as colorectal cancer.
- Many scientists believe that the amount of dairy produce in our diet is now far too high and that its quality has changed greatly.
- In today's large-scale intensive dairy farms, cows are pregnant and milked for most of the year. During pregnancy, the cow's ovaries secrete high levels of progesterone and the placenta high levels of oestrogen, with the result that hormone levels in milk have increased markedly.
- Moreover, intensive dairying has increased the average milk yield per cow from nine litres (16 pints) a day to a staggering 22 litres (39 pints) a day, also greatly increasing levels of IGF-I in dairy produce.
- Much research, including several prospective studies, using stored blood collected many years before the onset of prostate cancer, has shown associations between IGF-I and prostate cancer. The effects are sizable, and stronger than the effects of most previously reported risk factors.
- The link between consuming dairy, increased IGF-I levels and prostate cancer is clear. In one study, Dr Chan and her colleagues investigated the relationship between dairy calcium and prostate cancer and showed that men consuming more than 600 mg a day of dairy calcium had a 32 per cent higher risk of prostate cancer than men consuming less than or equal to 150 mg of dairy calcium, even after adjusting for other risk factors such as age, smoking, and body mass index. The study

also found that those who consumed the most dairy had 17 per cent less vitamin D than those who consumed the least. This vitamin is known to protect against prostate cancer.

- Evidence also suggests that high circulating levels of IGF-I stimulate the body to produce levels of oestrogen or testosterone more appropriate for teenagers than post-menopausal women or post-andropausal men, increasing cancer risk.
- Consuming dairy products is implicated in many other diseases, including allergies, auto-immune disease, diabetes, osteoporosis and Parkinson's disease.

5. THE FOOD FACTORS

Let your food be your medicine and your medicine be your food.

Hippocrates

In this chapter I explain the dietary factors that can help you to prevent and overcome prostate cancer.

THE POTENTIAL OF PREVENTION

L et me begin by stating the potential for cancer prevention, as presented in the major report *Food, Nutrition and the Prevention of Cancer: a Global Perspective*, published by the World Cancer Research Fund and the American Institute for Cancer Research.[1] The report reviewed more than 4,500 research studies and involved more than 120 scientists, including from the WHO, the FAO and the US National Cancer Institute.

- Eating right, plus staying physically active and maintaining a healthy weight, can cut cancer risk by 30 per cent to 40 per cent.
- Recommended dietary choices, coupled with not smoking, have the potential to reduce cancer risk by 60 per cent to 70 per cent.
- As many as 375,000 cases of cancer, at current cancer rates, could be prevented each year in the USA through healthy dietary choices.

- A simple change, such as eating the recommended five servings of fruits and vegetables each day, could by itself reduce cancer rates more than 20 per cent.

All this agrees closely with the advice of the American-based Physicians Committee for Responsible Medicine,[2] of distinguished nutritional and medical scientists such as T. Colin Campbell and John Macdougall in the USA, and of nutritionists such as Patrick Holford in the UK. It also agrees with the science-based recommendations on diet and lifestyle in this and my other books.[3] Quite simply, a healthy diet is based on pulses, whole-grain cereals, nuts, seeds, fruit and vegetables, and other foods of plant origin.

The evidence that a diet with lots of fruit and vegetables is preventive against cancer continues to increase. One review of more than 250 studies found that the data overwhelmingly support an inverse association between consumption of fruit and vegetables and cancer risk.[4]

Research in this field is currently focused on identifying biomarkers, such as DNA damage, rather than overt cancer, to allow less expensive trials of shorter duration to be carried out. An example of a useful biomarker for diet is the level of carotenoids in a person's blood as a measure of their fruit and vegetable intake.[5] This is important because the carotenoid lycopene (see p. 187), significantly reduces diffuse, high-grade prostate cancer.[6]

Even the Beef USA factsheet,[7] aimed at promoting beef and dairy as sources of conjugated linoleic acid (CLA) as anti-carcinogens, states, 'Of the vast number of naturally occurring substances, demonstrated to have anti-carcinogenic activity, all but a very few are of plant origin.'[8] Another source states that CLA is the *only* known antioxidant/anti-carcinogen associated with animal foods.[9]

The numerous components in vegetables and fruit thought to contribute to the reduced risk of cancer include dietary fibre, vitamins, minerals and various phytochemicals (i.e. plant chemicals) including those that act as anti-oxidants. Many fruits and vegetables from beetroot to pomegranates and from mandarin oranges to watercress are now being marketed as superfoods! In contrast, animal foods lack any fibre and contain saturated fat, cholesterol and, of course, animal protein, as well as hormones and growth factors, all of which are associated with increased risk of cancer.[10]

Table 5.1 shows the relationship between phytochemicals in plant foods and their suggested modes of action.

It has been known for the last 20 years that prostate cancer has a significant dietary basis. The China study[11] showed a reduction in risk in those consuming typical oriental diets. Moreover, people from the Mediterranean region are much less likely to develop prostate cancer than other Europeans. One reason for this may be that their diets are rich in cooked tomato products.[12] Another reason may be their use of olive oil to replace butter. Also, in Chapter 3 we showed the clear relationship between a low ratio of vegetable to animal protein in the diet and increased risk of prostate cancer.

All of this evidence supports the case for a change to a predominantly plant-based diet to prevent prostate cancer and other types of cancer, as proposed in this book and elaborated in *The Plant Programme*.

DIET AS TREATMENT

When I wrote the first edition of this book, some conventional doctors agreed that the available evidence suggested that the risk of men developing prostate cancer could be reduced by changing to a regime like the Plant Programme. They maintained, however, that once cancer had developed, changing diet would not help to treat the cancer or prolong survival, and that to do so could be detrimental.[13] I disagree with this advice strongly, based on the correspondence I continue to receive from prostate-cancer sufferers and my experience of working with people with the disease, even at an advanced stage. The conventional medical view fails to understand that removing the factors that favour the promotion of cancer will help treatment. Moreover, evidence is accumulating that dietary changes can help to treat cancer. T. Colin Campbell in his book *The China Study*[14] reports animal experiments published in some of the most prestigious scientific journals in which diets rich (more than 20 per cent) in protein (specifically the cows' milk protein, casein), promoted several types of cancer after initiation, but the disease regressed dramatically when the

Table 5.1 Food sources of phytochemicals and proposed mechanisms of action

Phytochemical	Food	Proposed mechanism(s) of action
Allicin Diallyl sulphide S-allyl-L-cysteine	Garlic Onions	Inhibits enzymes that activate cancer-causing chemicals (carcinogens) Stimulates enzymes that detoxify carcinogens
Catechins	Tea (green)	Antioxidant
Ellagic acid	Grapes Strawberries	Antioxidant
Flavonoids: *Citrus* – Diosmin and Hesperidin	Grapefruit juice Orange juice	Decreases levels of biochemicals that influence cell growth and proliferation
Noncitrus – Genistein and Daidzein (phyto-oestrogens)	Apples Grapes (red) Soya	Antioxidant Blocks oestrogen and androgen hormones from binding to their receptors (retarding cell proliferation)
Indoles	Cabbage Turnips	Increases conversion of oestrogens to inactive forms Stimulates enzymes that increase carcinogen detoxification
Isothiocyanates	Cruciferous vegetables	Inhibits enzymes that activate carcinogens Stimulates enzymes that detoxify carcinogens

Lignans	Flaxseed and grains	Prevents oestrogen and prostaglandin hormones from binding to their receptors (retarding cell proliferation)
Lutein and Zeaxanthin	Kale Okra Romaine lettuce Spinach	Antioxidant
Lycopene	Tomatoes Watermelon	Antioxidant
Monoterpenes: Limonene	Lemon peel Orange peel	Decreases cell proliferation by decreasing activity of ornithine decarboxylase (ODC), an enzyme that helps trigger cancer Decreases activity of growth-promoting proteins Prevents expression of oncogenes Stimulates enzymes that detoxify carcinogens
Phenols	Berries Grapes Mustard Tea Turmeric Sesame seeds	Antioxidant Inhibits formation of carcinogens such as nitrosamines Stimulates enzymes that detoxify carcinogens
Phytate	Grains Nuts Seeds Soya beans	Inhibits cell proliferation and the spread of cancer cells (metastasis)

Table 5.1 *Continued*

Phytochemical	Food	Proposed mechanism(s) of action
Polyphenols	Artichokes	Antioxidant Stimulates enzymes that detoxify carcinogens
Protease inhibitors	Dried beans Lentils Soya beans	Antioxidant Inhibits transformation of normal cells into cancerous ones Inhibits expression of certain genes and cellular processes that promote cancer
Sulphoraphane	Broccoli	Stimulates enzymes that detoxify carcinogens

Adapted from the MD Anderson Practice Guidelines on Nutrition and Cancer Risk Reduction http://www.mdanderson.org/departments/nutrition/display.cfm/id51f759d8-98b2-11d5-813005o8b603a14&methoddisplayfull&pn

dietary intake of animal protein was reduced to less than 5 per cent. Campbell states in his book 'Like flipping a light switch on and off we could control cancer promotion merely by changing levels of protein, regardless of initial carcinogen exposure'. A study of the effects of changes in diet and lifestyle in people with early prostate cancer who were not undergoing conventional surgery, chemotherapy or radiotherapy was carried out at the Preventive Medicine Institute in California. This showed clearly that those who changed to a diet consisting mainly of fruit and vegetables, whole grain cereals and legumes, supplemented with soya, had a 10 per cent lower PSA level than the control group and the level of cancer inhibitors in their blood was eight times higher than that of patients keeping to a typical Western diet.[15]

Nevertheless, I would emphasise that the Plant Programme is meant to complement, not replace, conventional medical treatment.

JUNK SCIENCE AND SOUND SCIENCE

No intelligent doctor should object to any of the scientifically based recommendations of the Plant Programme. It includes a diet packed with healthy, natural, nutritious food. So why is it that when you mention using diet to complement your treatment for cancer there can be such a negative[16] or at best a lukewarm response from many doctors?

I think there are several reasons for this. First, some people follow diets that are so strict and extreme that they become undernourished at a time when they need all their strength. In extreme cases they may even have been persuaded to use diet instead of conventional medicine to treat their cancer – advice I strongly disagree with. Frequently, cancer patients have been recommended by their alternative practitioner to follow a diet that eliminates all wheat products, potatoes, tomatoes, peppers and other vegetables belonging to the deadly nightshade family and all fruit on the grounds that it contains sugar; increasingly they are told not to have soya products. None of this has any scientific basis. The same practitioners that recommend such diets frequently sell their own synthetic chemical versions of vitamins and minerals and a range of wacky extracts often at exorbitant prices (see further in Chapter 6, Lifestyle Factor 1.) Such an approach is likely to be unhelpful and even make matters worse, and the advice to cut down on vegetables such as tomatoes and fruit demonstrates their total ignorance of the peer-reviewed scientific literature.

There is also much confusing advice in anti-cancer diet books and magazines. One such book suggests avoiding parsnips, broad beans, pumpkins, honey, watermelon, pineapple, couscous and muesli (all excellent foods as part of an anticancer diet) because they are said to promote cancer by stimulating insulin production. This is nonsense! Other books claim that yoghurt is protective, while others group soya, rice and vegetable milks with goat's milk.

All this is junk science and it causes serious problems in using diet to prevent and treat cancer. First, it eliminates cancer-protective foods from the diet: for example, tomatoes which contain lycopene, shown in many studies to be anti-cancer and especially effective against prostate cancer. Secondly, it diverts attention from the real culprit foods such as dairy products that internationally renowned nutritional scientists and doctors agree promote cancer. Thirdly, it causes confusion, which is used by producers of cancer promoting foods to keep pushing their dangerous produce (see further in Chapter 7).

The Plant Programme is based on sound science from the peer-reviewed scientific literature and it follows the principles of diets that have been studied by teams of internationally renowned scientists from universities that are centres of excellence such as Oxford in the UK and Cornell in the USA.[17] Such diets have been found to prevent not only prostate and breast cancer and the other 'cancers of affluence' such as colorectal cancer and pancreatic cancer but also a host of other diseases. These include type 1 and type 2 diabetes, cardiovascular disease and strokes, osteoporosis, food poisoning, kidney disease, and a whole range of auto-immune diseases including hyperthyroidism and multiple sclerosis as outlined in *Eating For Better Health*.[18]

BACKGROUND TO THE DIET

The food factors that follow page 174 are based on the principles of the Chinese diet. The recipes in *The Plant Programme* and *Eating for Better Health*, are designed to accompany the food factors, with recipes adapted to suit Western tastes. All the recipes contain high levels of foods known to be protective against prostate cancer and other types of cancer and to contain no foods known to promote these diseases. The recipes are delicious – and are also practical and easy to make for busy people.

Before discussing the food factors further, I want to tell you a little more about the Chinese diet. This has evolved over thousands of years of observation and practical experience and has been thoroughly documented and referenced. It is not a new fad diet based on the latest single-issue biochemical theory, but has evolved over more than 5,000 years as a sustainable system of nutrition and agriculture by one of the most biologically successful people on Earth.

In Japan, where the traditional diet is similar to that of China, a healthy diet is believed to be based on eating at least thirty different ingredients a day. Compare this with the diet of the average American, for whom 40 per cent of all they consume is dairy.

THE CHINESE WAY

In some parts of China less than 3 per cent of the population under 65 years of age die from any form of cancer, and prostate cancer is almost unknown. Although cancers such as stomach cancer are more prevalent in China,[19] they are attributed to chronic infections rather than diet.

The Chinese diet has been handed down from generation to generation using the pictogram system of writing, which was developed early in their history. Chinese writing has evolved progressively into the sophisticated system in use today (an educated person in China is expected to know at least 10,000 different pictograms) and, like the diet that is recommended here, continued to evolve.

Legend in China describes how Emperor Shen Nung, revered as the founder of Chinese agriculture, set out in 3494 BC to discover the healing properties of plants. Each day he would taste various plants to determine their properties – poisoning himself several times in the process, so that he also had to find many antidotes. This story of Emperor Shen Nung may well be a metaphor for the trial and error method of the discovery of the properties of plants, but there is little doubt that Chinese agriculture and medicine are derived from knowledge accumulated over the last 5,000 years. It is worth recalling that China had reached a considerable level of sophistication while the British Isles were emerging from the Stone Age.

To those used to modern Western science and medicine, some concepts basic to the Chinese approach to diet, such as balancing yin and yang foods, may sound strange, but the observations provide excellent responses to nutritional and environmental problems and have sustained the Chinese population for thousands of years. The Chinese diet has been shown to be one of the healthiest diets in the world.[20]

It is this kind of well-tried, observation-based depth of tradition, particularly from China and other parts of South East Asia that are the basis of the food factors described here.

FOOD FACTOR 1: FROM DAIRY TO SOYA

Soya consumption has been shown to be inversely related to prostate cancer risk.[21] As discussed below, it contains a wealth of anti-cancer agents and helps to prevent the spread of cancer generally, but first we need to learn about the different types of oestrogens that we are exposed to.

Phyto(plant)-hormones, xeno(stranger)-hormones and animal hormones – the good, the bad and the deadly

Unfortunately, the fact that soya contains phyto-oestrogens has been used to persuade people, including health professionals who really should know better, that it promotes hormone-dependent cancer such as prostate cancer and breast cancer and that it can feminise males. This is discussed in detail below (see Chapter 7), but it is worth noting here that the hormones to which we are exposed that are dangerous include just two groups: animal hormones such as oestrogen and testosterone, and man-made chemical hormone mimics known as xeno (stranger)-hormones. The former are overwhelmingly from dairy in our diet (see Chapter 4), while the latter are from pesticides, plastics and detergents in consumer products and contaminants in the environment (see further in Chapter 6, Lifestyle Factor 6).

It is also worth noting that in experiment after experiment, casein (cows' milk protein) has been shown to promote cancer whereas soya protein has no such effect. In *The China Study*, Campbell describes the powerful effects of casein on cancer promotion and then states 'So the next logical question was whether plant protein tested in the same way has the same effect on cancer promotion as casein. The answer is an astonishing "NO"' (the capitals are his). Neither soya nor wheat protein were found to promote cancer, even at the highest levels of intake. In fact, the phyto-oestrogens in soya are particularly helpful in all cases of hormone-dependent cancers, such as prostate cancer, because they block receptor sites for hormones and growth factors in the cell or on the cell surface. One report stated that consuming two glasses of soya milk a day cut the risk of prostate cancer by 40 per cent.

Prostate cancer is hormonally driven, and, as discussed earlier, dairy increases natural hormone levels.[22] One of the first and most essential things you can do to reduce your risk of prostate cancer is to remove **ALL** dairy products (whether from cows, sheep, goats or any other animals) from your diet. You can replace them with soya, oat, rice or any other vegetable substitutes. The important thing is to ditch the dairy.

By doing this you will immediately and dramatically reduce your body's exposure to a powerful cocktail of hormones and growth factors increasingly shown in scientific paper after scientific paper (*see* Chapters 2 and 4) to promote prostate cancer. You will also be reducing your exposure to antibiotic residues and other powerful biologically active chemicals (including man-made endocrine-disrupting chemicals, which can become particularly concentrated in milk – *see* Chapter 6). You will reduce your cholesterol and triglyceride intake, with great benefits for your heart and circulatory system, thereby reducing the possibility of developing thrombosis, to which patients undergoing surgery, chemotherapy and some other cancer treatments are especially susceptible.[23]

Ringing the changes: the benefits

Recent dietary studies into the effects of exchanging soya for animal products indicate a reduction in cholesterol levels of more than 20 per cent. Moreover, it is the levels of the 'bad' cholesterol – low-density lipo-proteins or LDLs – which are reduced. However, simply adding soya to a typical Western diet is unlikely to be sufficient to counteract high plasma cholesterol.[24] You must replace – not supplement – dairy with soya produce to achieve the benefits. Soya lecithin provides substances called choline and inisitol, which help to improve liver function, which is particularly important during chemotherapy. Soya also contains co-enzyme Q10. and has a good balance of calcium and magnesium.

Replace dairy milk with soya or other vegetable milk, replace cheese with tofu, and use soya ice cream (or water ices or sorbets) instead of dairy ice cream. There are no half measures and, as discussed previously, using skimmed milk or low-fat yoghurt is irrelevant and will not help to reduce your risk of cancer or your recovery from the disease, because the most likely cancer-promoting agents are proteins or sugars, not just fats.

Remember that soya contains plant oestrogens which protect the prostate and that one of the plant oestrogens – genistein – seems to prevent cancer through multiple mechanisms: not only is it phyto-oestrogenic, it is anti-angiogenic too, meaning that it actually prevents tumours from developing their own blood supply.[25] It is also a powerful antioxidant, increasing the activities of protective anti-oxidative enzymes in various organs, with an important role in the removal of free radicals. Also, soya isoflavones have been shown in animal and other laboratory substances to inhibit the growth of cancer cells by inhibiting their DNA replication, interfering with their signalling pathways, reducing the activity of various enzymes that they need to grow and inhibiting the actions of a range of growth factors and chemicals called cytokines that cancer cells need in order to develop.[26] Most experimental studies into soya and cancer show that soya products prevent the growth of a range of cancer cells.[27]

A gift from the wise men

The soya bean is one of the most nutritious vegetables known. It is said that the soya bean was a gift to all generations of humankind from the sages and wise rulers of China. The first commercial use for the soya bean in the West, however, was as a source of oil for the manufacture of soap. This pattern of usage, so different from that in Asia, is changing as more and more people appreciate the extraordinary health-giving properties of soya.

The soya bean is an environmentally-friendly crop, too. One acre of land cultivated by conventional Western agricultural practices will feed an average adult for 77 days if it is used to raise beef. That may seem impressive, until you learn that the same acre can feed an adult for 527 days when it is devoted to growing wheat. However, if soya beans are grown on the same land, then it will yield enough protein to feed a person for over six years! The protein content of the bean when harvested is about 40 per cent, which rises to 50 per cent after it has been processed. Soya also contains a full range of proteins whereas other plant foods contain only some. Hence many vegans depend on combining cereals and pulses to obtain the full range of the twenty amino acids necessary for good nutrition. The delicious traditional Jamaican dish of rice and peas, which I ate a lot of when I worked there, is a good example.

The best soya for health

There is only one problem with buying soya now: it has often been genetically modified. One of the reasons this has been done is so that it can withstand being treated with herbicides to destroy insects and weeds. So read labels carefully and buy only organically grown soya.

Most of us are now familiar with soya milk, which can be purchased from all supermarkets. Alternatively you can buy a machine and make your own from soya beans. There are many other traditional soya products which you can enjoy. Let me introduce you to some of them.

Tofu, or bean curd, is made from soya beans. It has a higher percentage of protein than any other natural food, is very low in saturated fats, is entirely cholesterol-free, and is inexpensive. It has been a staple food for millions of people in Asia for over four thousand years. Tofu is good for everyone, because it is so full of good nutrients, so low in bad nutrients and is easily digested. Puréed carrots and leeks with tofu can be used as a nutritious, easily digested food for babies and invalids.[28] Also, it can be cooked quickly in simple stir fries or simmered in soup. It is made by precipitating soya milk, normally using calcium or magnesium sulphates so it is also high in some of the most bioavailable forms of calcium or magnesium. In their classical treatise on the subject, William Shurtleff and Akiko Aoyagi explain its revered status in the East. They point out that when Japanese connoisseurs speak of tofu they use many of the same terms we employ when evaluating wines. And when the new crop of soya beans arrives at tofu shops, ardent devotees sample the first tofu with similar relish to that of French vintners.[29]

Commercially, tofu is available in either 'silken' form (suitable for making low-fat, high-protein dressings, deserts and sauces) and firm, which can be used in an infinite number of ways: scrambled, marinated, smoked, barbecued, crumbled into salads, in burgers, sandwiches and soups. Tofu may not taste good on its own but it is very good at absorbing almost any flavour or colour.[30] Tofu is ideal as a replacement for dairy cream or milk in many potato dishes. It can also be liquidised with a wide range of fresh juice with honey to make delicious sweets and puddings.

Tempeh (pronounced 'tem-pay') is a fermented soya-bean product, made in the traditional manner for centuries throughout Indonesia. You can buy it in health-food shops and a growing number of supermarkets. It is highly digestible, smells like fresh mushrooms and tastes remarkably similar to chicken or veal cutlets. Since the protein in tempeh is partially broken down by fermentation it is very digestible and particularly suitable for young children and the elderly. The easiest way to serve it is as wedge-shaped slices, pan fried until crisp and golden brown on both sides and served with rice and a selection of vegetables.

Natto can generally be found in Chinese or Japanese grocery stores, though it is less readily available than tempeh. Like tempeh, it is made by fermenting soya beans, but in this case, for less than 24 hours. The fermentation process makes the high-quality protein of the soya beans particularly easy to digest.

Miso, which is a fermented mixture of soya beans and other cereals, has a paste-like texture and is an important component of oriental macrobiotic diets. It has subtle, aromatic flavours and ranges in colour from brown to pale yellow. It is one of the staples of every Japanese and Chinese kitchen and is made by inoculating the basic ingredients with a mould before aging the mixture in cedarwood kegs for at least one year. It is commonly used as an ingredient in soups, sauces, dressings, spreads, casseroles and other vegetable dishes. In Japan, miso is used as a medicine in the same way that Jewish people use chicken soup; miso is much healthier, though. On no account should miso be boiled or cooked at high temperatures, because this will destroy its beneficial, health-giving substances. Unfortunately, synthetic misos, with various colourings and additives, have become widely available. Avoid such products and buy only traditional miso which is free of additives and contains many different beneficial enzymes and bacteria. Also buy only good reputable brands because fermentation in unhygienic conditions can lead to high concentrations of the micro-organisms thought to be responsible for stomach cancer. I buy miso only in waxed cartons, never in plastic (*see* p. 241).

Soy Sauce is an ancient and traditional Japanese seasoning which is now accepted the world over. It is a dark, rich sauce with a savoury, salty taste. Very little is required within a dish or serving. There are three types:

The first is the widely available commercial type, made by speeding up the fermentation process using chemical additives. It usually contains colourings and preservatives as well. I do not recommend this.

The second is called shoyu and is made by fermenting wheat and soya beans together for at least three years. It makes a delicious addition to most savoury meals and aids digestion. It is easy to find in health-food, macrobiotic or Japanese grocery shops.

The third is tamari, which is made by fermenting soya beans and salt for two to three years. It is less widely available than shoyu and has a very strong flavour.

Both shoyu and tamari contain enzymes, similar to those found in our saliva, which help in digesting proteins and starches.

Many of these soya products are widely available, not only in specialist health-food shops but also, increasingly, in supermarkets. Since there are so many different types and flavours, it is worth experimenting until you find the flavours you enjoy most. Your brain will adapt to the change in taste and you will soon find you do not want to go back to dairy produce.

So what about yoghurt, now marketed as probiotics, often with no mention of dairy, and all those healthy *Lactobacillus acidophilus* bacteria it contains which are so good for us? There is evidence that taking these bacteria increases immunity, prevents infections and increases vitamin production. Don't worry: it is easy to buy capsules of the bacteria, break them open, and sprinkle the contents on soya milk or other cold drinks. Hence you have the health benefits of the bacteria without the risk that consuming dairy products carries. Moreover, following the Plant Programme will favour the growth and survival of these helpful bacteria in the digestive tract.

If you do only one thing to cut your risk of prostate cancer, make the change from dairy to soya products. Remember that soya products reduce prostate cancer risk, while milk and the growth factors and hormones it contains have been shown in experiment after experiment to promote the growth of prostate and other cancer cells.

Anti-soya propaganda

Since the publication of the first edition of *Your Life in Your Hands* in 2000, there have been many attacks on soya (frequently on untraceable and unattributable websites), many suggesting that soya causes cancer. There have even been recommendations from health professionals that people who have prostate or breast cancer should not have soya.

Some men express concern to me that eating the phyto-oestrogens in soya will feminise them. Many of the questions put to me express concern about these issues. So what are the scientific facts?

Soya is a bean just like most other beans and peas which are also packed with phyto-oestrogens; and I do not know of any non-aligned scientists who believe that beans, especially soya beans, and peas in a diet such as the Plant Programme cause health problems. Moreover, despite exhaustive studies, there is no evidence that soya feminises males.[31] Certainly a lack of male potency and reproductive capacity does not appear to have been a problem in China or other oriental countries over the many centuries they have used soya. Rather the reverse. Man-boobs (gynaecomastia) are far more likely to reflect intake of animal oestrogens from dairy and other animal produce, or xeno-oestrogens from the environment, than eating soya. In all my years of working in China and other oriental countries I did not see a single man with boobs there although it is hard to avoid seeing men with them in the UK or US. According to a recent article in *The Times* 4,000 men had their man-boobs removed by plastic surgery in 2003 in the UK.

In fact much of the evidence used to attack soya is from animal experiments which appear deliberately designed to demonstrate some adverse effect of eating soya. For example in some experiments ridiculously large amounts of raw soya were fed to experimental animals. Marilyn Glenville[32] poses one of the key questions in relation to such 'research': 'who eats raw soya anyway?'

In other experiments, laboratory animals are fed extracts of soya processed in aluminium vessels in such a way that the soya absorbs aluminium. Such soya isolates can turn up in soya 'meat' or 'cheese' products and as flavour enhancers in soups and sauces and other processed foods such as cakes, bread and biscuits. They are not present in the traditional whole-soya products such as natto, tempeh or bean curd (tofu) recommended in the Plant Programme. The 'scientists' behind the scare stories seem unaware that the association of Alzheimer's disease and aluminium has long been discounted in favour of a link with a protein called beta amyloid which forms plaques in the brain. Most respected non-aligned scientists think that the plaques are in fact formed as a result of eating a diet too high in animal protein such as dairy and meat.[33]

It would make sense that the anti-soya campaign is led by vested interest groups such as the dairy industry. Marilyn Glenville in her book *The New Natural Alternatives to HRT*,[34] which recommends soya to treat menopausal symptoms states 'the good publicity for soya tends to alarm another section of industry, the pharmaceutical giants who stand to lose a lot of money if alternatives to HRT are found. The dairy industry, which would lose out if the population shifts to soya instead of milk and other dairy produce, is also affected.'

The argument that soya is carcinogenic centres on the fact that soya contains phyto-oestrogens – but the fact is that most vegetables naturally contain phyto-oestrogens or substances that are converted to phyto-oestrogens in the gut. Such foods include berries such as strawberries, cranberries and bilberries, wholegrain cereals, seeds and spices, peanuts, cabbage, hops, tea and, of course, peas and beans (the legume family, to which soya belongs).[35] In general, phyto-oestrogens are found in the seeds, stems, roots or flowers of plants, serving as natural fungicides and acting as part of the plant's defence mechanism against micro-organisms.[36]

Phyto-oestrogens are chemically and structurally similar to the mammalian oestrogen, oestradiol, and have oestrogenic properties. However, their oestrogenic activity is generally much less than that of human oestrogens (their oestrogenic activity ranges from 1/500 to 1/1000 of that of oestradiol), and they have been found to be protective against prostate cancer and other hormone-dependent cancers.[37] All the experiments on soya-bean phyto-oestrogens (isoflavones such as genistein) continue to indicate that such chemicals help prevent the growth of prostate and other cancers by a variety of mechanisms.[38]

Of course, the dairy industry have tried to fight back, and as their propaganda about the need for dairy calcium to prevent osteoporosis increasingly founders,[39] they have latched on to the presence of substances called CLAs (*see* p. 166) in dairy products and the meat of ruminant animals such as cows and sheep, which they claim to be preventive against cancer. CLAs are natural derivatives of the essential fatty acid, linoleic acid, which is found in vegetable seeds and the oils produced from them, such as soya. Interestingly, the dairy industry is trying to increase the amount of CLA in milk by adding extracted whole soya-bean and linseed oils to a corn-alfalfa diet.[40] As queried in an article in the *Sunday Times*,[41] how much artery-clogging saturated fat would we have to consume (as dairy) to have enough CLAs to be protected against cancer?

One final question

If soya is so bad for health why is so much used to feed dairy cows and why is it being used to improve the nutritional quality of cow's milk?

The Japanese rule

At this point I would like to re-emphasise that simply adding soya to a typical dairy-rich Western diet will *not* decrease prostate-cancer risk. It is absolutely essential to eliminate ALL animal dairy produce, including 'hidden dairy' such as casein whey and lactose. Other vegetable milks, creams and yoghurts, besides soya, are all OK, including coconut, rice, oat and pea milks, but I recommend only organically produced GM-free products.

I also emphasise that I am not advocating that people live on an entirely soya-based diet, and I continue to recommend the Japanese principle, on which *The Plant Programme* cookbook is based, of eating at least thirty different food substances every day. I also agree with the advice of the American Cancer Society that eating a balanced diet should include five or more servings a day of fruit and vegetables (though I think it should be much more – see Food Factor 2), along with foods from a variety of other plant sources, such as cereals, legumes, seeds and nuts; this is more effective than consuming one particular food in large amounts.[42]

Just one word of warning about soya; along with many other vegetables such as turnips, broccoli and brussel sprouts, it contains substances called goitrogens that can cause the thyroid to be underactive, so ensure that you take your kelp tablets (see p. 240) to counteract the effects of goitrogens on the thyroid and be especially careful if you have hypothyroidism. There is further information on goitrogenic foods and thyroid disease in *Eating for Better Health*.

MAKING THE BREAK FROM DAIRY

If You Used To Do This ...	*Now Do This!*
Take cows' milk in your tea or coffee	Use soya milk in tea, straight from the carton, or drink green tea with a slice of fresh lemon or lime. In coffee, heat the soya milk first to avoid curdling. Avoid dry 'creamers' or 'whiteners', which can contain synthetic chemicals or hidden dairy
Put cows' milk on your breakfast cereal	Use soya, rice, oat or coconut milk, or pour fresh fruit juice over your cereal instead (I always do this in hotels)

Tuck into a bowl of ice cream	Enjoy high-quality sorbets or water ices. Or try one of the growing range of delicious soya ice creams now on the market
Douse your desserts in cream or custard	Most supermarkets sell small cartons of a brand of soya cream; to make your own whisk soft, plain tofu with a little honey. One of the oldest brands of custard powder is dairy free! Simply prepare it using soya milk or another vegetable milk instead of dairy
Drink glasses of milk or milkshakes	There is now a wide range of naturally sweetened fruit soya, rice, oat or coconut milks in various carton sizes. Or make your own at home! See the recipes in *The Plant Programme*
Use dollops of butter in cooking or served onto bread or vegetables	Use organic, first cold-pressed extra-virgin olive oil in cooking. Try herb-flavoured olive oil drizzled over toast or baked potatoes, and lift your sandwiches with a spread such as tahini (sesame seed paste) or houmous to replace butter and enhance your nutrient intake
Eat masses of hard, soft or cottage cheeses	Several brands of dairy-free hard 'cheeses' are currently available in health-food shops which can be used in cookery as well as simply grated or sliced. Double-check the labels to ensure that the product is free from casein, lactose and other 'hidden' dairy ingredients. There are many soft soya 'cheeses' – available as tofu dips, spreads or patés. My favourite option is houmous! It has similar benefits to soya

Dive into a daily dose of yoghurt – now marketed as probiotics, often with no mention of dairy	Soya yoghurt is widely available in plain and fruit flavours and in a variety of carton sizes
Eat dairy (made from cow) meat products such as burgers, sausages, luncheon meats, patés and pastes	A huge range of products are now available to replace meat. Look in the dry mix, freezer, tinned or chilled food sections of your health-food shop or supermarket. Although some of the products are based on nuts, most are based on soya – but make sure that this is not as isolates.
Cook with dairy products	Soya milk or cream readily substitutes for dairy milk in recipes as varied as Béchamel sauce and creamed soups to rice pudding and quiche. Most recipes calling for butter succeed as well with olive oil or soya spread. The meat replacements mentioned above work well in traditional recipes, as do the cheese substitutes, but avoid products made with isolates.

FOOD FACTOR 2: VITAL VEGETABLES AND FREQUENT FRUIT

Vegetables and fruit are the energy foods we evolved to eat. They are packed with healthy antioxidants, vitamins and minerals, fibre, live enzymes and other good-for-health phytochemicals – which help to fight cancer. There is no dispute about their health benefits among mainstream scientists.

The US National Cancer Institute has launched a publicity campaign to boost men's fruit and vegetable consumption from the 'bare minimum' of five servings a day to nine servings a day. Only 4 per cent of men in the US consume nine servings. More than a third of the population eat only one or two servings, and 4 per cent eat less than that.[43] The official recommendation of five portions a day, especially when each portion can comprise a glass of (commercial) fruit juice and a tablespoon of dried fruit,[44] was always completely inadequate.

Based on this new information and many other findings described below, the second food factor is to increase is the amount of vegetables and fruit you consume. The evidence that an abundant intake of vegetables and fruit can play an important role in reducing cancer incidence is becoming overwhelming.[45] The only people who recommend elimination of either fruit or vegetables from the diet now are fringe practitioners ignorant of the scientific literature.

Anti-cancer chemicals

The list of anti-cancer chemicals identified in vegetables and fruit just keeps on growing (Table 5.1). The investigation of plant chemicals pioneered by Lee Wattenberg of the University of Minnesota in the USA has identified many agents that protect against cancer in laboratory studies.[46] Perhaps this is hardly surprising. I have always wondered why I have never seen or heard of a plant with cancer, despite all the poisonous chemicals we pour on them, so perhaps in the same way that humans discovered that some substances such as honey contain natural antibiotics because they do not readily 'go rotten', we should have realised long ago that plants contain anti-cancer agents. Indeed several chemotherapy agents are purified plant alkaloids.

In addition to the phyto-oestrogens discussed above, plant-derived foods contain thousands of other phytochemicals, many of which have been investigated in laboratory and clinical studies to determine their effects on cancer risk and their mechanisms of action.[47] The Division of Cancer Prevention of the US National Cancer Institute is currently sponsoring more than 65 chemoprevention trials, many of them concerned with food substances in relation to particular cancers. They include, for example, three trials of lycopene in preventing prostate cancer.[48] Salvesterol, which is concentrated in fruits such as tangerines, has been found to inhibit the enzyme CYP IBI which occurs in cancer cells but not normal cells, and this substance as well as bromelain in pineapple and papain in papaya are protease inhibitors which means they damage cancer proteins.

In general, the outcomes of studies into protective substances in fruit and vegetables highlight the difficulty of identifying single dietary components such as beta-carotene as chemopreventive agents (see further discussion in Chapter 6, Lifestyle Factor 1).[49] This may be because substances such as beta-carotene are simply biomarkers for other protective components of vegetables and fruit, or because it may not react in the same way when separated from the chemicals with which it is associated in natural food substances.

Eating your greens and other colours

Recent research has provided new evidence in favour of my rainbow rule of eating as many different coloured vegetables as possible.[50] Eat as many vegetables as possible, including salad vegetables, and make sure they are fresh and ripe. Most vegetables and fruit include such vitamins as beta-carotene (which is the precursor of vitamin A and is especially rich in yellow and orange vegetables such as carrots, saffron, red and yellow peppers, pumpkins and sweet potatoes, and fruit such as peaches, cherries and apricots (including the dried variety)). Beta-carotene has long been suggested to be protective against several forms of cancer, including by acting as an antioxidant. Other vegetables and fruit also contain other carotenoids such as lycopene, vitamin C (in most fresh or very lightly cooked vegetables and fruit) and vitamin E (in most fresh fruit and vegetables), which counteract the activity of free radicals and stop our tissues being damaged by them. Garlic and Brussels sprouts are also especially rich in antioxidants. The pigment in red vegetables and fruit – lycopene (which is enriched in tomatoes (especially cooked ones) pink grapefruit and red grapeskins) – is also a powerful antioxidant and may have other cancer-preventing properties.

Lycopene is the much-talked-about antioxidant where prostate cancer is concerned. It binds to fats and lipids in the blood stream, protecting against some of the worst aspects of Western diets. One study stated that seven to ten helpings of tomatoes per week reduced risks by 40 per cent; another suggested that 40 per cent of prostate-cancer sufferers eating these quantities showed relief of symptoms.[51]

Research reported from Israel in 1995 suggests that lycopene (the main tomato carotenoid) is a more potent inhibitor of proliferation in human cancer cells than beta-carotene.[52] In addition to its powerful antioxidant properties, it suppressed IGF-I-stimulated growth of (breast) cancer cells. More recently, associations of lower bioactive IGFs with increased consumption of tomatoes and products containing tomatoes[53] have supported the results of earlier findings reported for Greek men.[54] The findings of the protective effect of tomato intake on prostate cancer have been reported in several investigations.[55] Interestingly, a small trial of lycopene-only supplementation found no difference in IGF-I levels between those taking the tablets and the controls – whereas in trials of beta-carotene pills rather than carrots, which had been shown to be protective (see Chapter 6, p. 235), the pure chemical actually made matters worse.

Other good sources of natural lycopene include strawberries, red grapes, peaches, peppers and carrots. One large helping of freshly made tomato soup contains masses of lycopene (see the easy-to-follow recipe in The Plant Programme). I recommend against tinned or packaged tomato soup, since they frequently contain cream, whey or other dairy products and many tin cans are lined with a substance which can leach BPA, an endocrine-disrupting chemical (see p. 264). If you eat tinned baked beans, be very careful to read the label, because even some brands that claim to be in tomato sauce might be more accurately described as being in a milk or cream source.

Fresh red peppers, as well as being rich in lycopene, are a particularly good source of vitamin C, which strengthens the immune system and neutralises toxins. Other especially good sources of Vitamin C include papaya, berries, cherries and all citrus fruits. Salad vegetables, especially watercress, and raw or lightly cooked broccoli are also good sources.

Plants, especially green leafy vegetables, avocado, beans, carrots, pumpkins, apricots, melons and newly sprouted shoots such as bean sprouts and alfalfa are all good sources of folic acid, which is involved in making the copies of the chromosomes carrying our gene sequences when cells divide. This is the very point at which mistakes which could cause cancer are likely to happen. An adequate intake of folic acid is essential to protect your DNA during radiotherapy or chemotherapy. A great deal of evidence suggests that most Americans' diets are deficient in folic acid.[56] Deterioration in the elderly has also been attributed to folate deficiency.[57] Indeed, throughout the West, women wishing to become pregnant are advised to take folic acid pills to avoid birth defects such as spina bifida in their babies.

Surely we should *all* be eating a diet that has adequate quantities of folic acid without having to resort to taking pills. As discussed previously, some of the chemotherapeutic drugs used to disrupt breast cancer cells replace folic acid in cell division. I believe that it was drinking fresh juices high in folic acid as soon as I was able to after chemotherapy that helped me to recover so quickly and saved my hair from falling out. I drank about half a pint of green Bramley apple with fennel juice, about 50:50 apple-fennel, and about half a pint of carrot juice every day. I also ate lots of melon, which is especially rich in folic acid. People who were treated with me who took folic acid pills still lost their hair, but most of the people I have persuaded to use juices have kept theirs (though this does not work with some of the new chemotherapeutic agents with a different mode of action).

Protective phyto(plant)-oestrogens

I have mentioned plant oestrogens in the context of soya several times in the book because of their protective effect against prostate cancer. Plant oestrogens are found in almost all fruit, vegetables and cereals. Vegetables such as soya, lentils, peas and beans – which are all legumes capable of fixing nitrogen from the air to make proteins – are rich sources of isoflavones. Typical oriental, Mediterranean and Latin American diets include large quantities of legumes, and it has been calculated that a typical Western diet provides only about 3 mg of isoflavones a day compared to the 30–100 mg a day in oriental diets.

Red clover has particularly high levels of phyto-oestrogens called coumestans and, like chick peas (the basis of houmous) and lentils, it contains all of the four important dietary isoflavones. Sunflower seeds and alfalfa sprouts also contain substantial quantities of phyto-oestrogen compounds.

Other rich sources of protective phytohormones include wild yam or sweet potato, and fennel, which contain both phyto-oestrogens and phytoprogesterones. Flaxseed has a high content of lignans, which are converted in the digestive tract into substances that help to regulate endocrine function. Much research on flax has been carried out by the US Food and Drug Administration (FDA), the National Cancer Institute and the

Canadian Food Protection Branch.[58] The recommendation is to take about one tablespoon a day of flaxseed in your diet for each 100 pounds of body weight (but be prepared to go to the loo more often!).

Sowing the seeds and sprouting them

As well as being a good source of phyto-oestrogens, seeds can be good sources of zinc, selenium and vitamin E. Sunflower and sesame seeds can be particularly good sources of zinc, which helps vitamin C work and accelerates healing.

I eat sprouted seeds, including soya, pumpkin and sesame (all rich in zinc), sunflower, alfalfa and lentil. They are all rich in vitamin C and other vitamins and minerals as well as high-quality proteins. I generally buy mine already sprouted, but if you wish to sprout your own, here's how to do it:

- Buy organic seeds from health-food stores or supermarkets. Use only the clean, whole ones and discard the rest. NEVER buy seeds from agricultural merchants, because they may have been treated with chemicals which can be fatal if consumed.
- Use a jar large enough to hold at least half a litre of water with a piece of cheesecloth or muslin held in place around the top with a rubber band.
- For every 100 ml of water, use two to three tablespoons of seeds. First, soak them overnight in four times their own volume of (ideally filtered) water, until they have doubled in size. Then pour off the water.
- Keep the sprout container in darkness, and rinse the seeds two or three times a day. Make sure you drain them thoroughly by turning the container upside down, or they will rot.
- Throw away any seeds that have not sprouted after two days. The rest will be ready to eat after four or five days. On the last day they can be put into the light, but only for a few hours or they will become bitter.
- Most sprouts need a final rinse before being drained and stored in the fridge in a covered container. Some varieties have loose husks which need to be removed. Place such sprouts in a large bowl of water and agitate until the husks float to the top, then skim them off.

Some really powerful cancer-busters – are you getting enough?

Vegetables and fruit also contain compounds, or their precursor chemicals, which have no known nutritional value but which have anti-cancer properties (*see* Table 5.1). They include indoles, isothiocyanates, dithiolthiones and organosulphur components (some of which are thought to produce natural pesticides). About twenty years ago epidemiological studies showed that consumption of cruciferous vegetables, including bok choy, broccoli, Brussels sprouts, cauliflower, cabbage and kale, which contain dithiolthiones, was associated with a decreased risk of developing cancer. A synthetic dithiolthione called oltipraz has been shown to inhibit the development of tumours in laboratory animals. Like other beneficial plant chemicals, it interferes with cancer development in several ways including by activating the liver enzymes that remove cancer-causing agents from the bloodstream.[59] Sulforaphane, an isothiocyanate which is also found in cruciferous vegetables and is responsible for their sharp taste, is also thought to prevent cancer by activating detoxifying enzymes in the liver. In rats it blocks the formation of chemically induced cancers. Recently, research at Robert Gordon University in Aberdeen suggests that only raw broccoli offers any protective effect against colon cancer as measured by the amount of DNA damage in colon cells from laboratory pigs.[60] It is suggested that cooking destroys glucosinolates, which are the precursors of isothiocyanates produced in the colon, which are the substances protective against cancer. The degree of cooking of the broccoli is not described, however. It is best to eat vegetables which are as raw as possible (light steaming or stir frying), although it is important to cook all meat and fish slowly and thoroughly (*see* Lifestyle Factor on cooking, p. 241). All cruciferous vegetables also contain good amounts of fibre, which helps to eliminate toxins.

Garlic, onions, chives and leeks (the allium family) are important in helping to protect against cancer. They contain chemicals similar to those used in anti-radiation pills (cysteine-like amino acids) and are particularly useful in reducing the effects of diagnostic X-rays and radiotherapy in the body. They contain powerful antioxidants. Allicin, one of garlic's main biologically active components, created when garlic is crushed, has been shown to decrease proliferation of prostate-cancer cells in laboratory studies.[61] In addition to allicin, garlic also contains other powerful antioxidants such as selenium and germanium. Research into cancer at universities in Pennsylvania and Texas has identified two other compounds active against cancer in crushed garlic: diallysulphide and S-allyl cysteine. Current studies at the Memorial Sloan-Kettering Cancer Center in New York indicate that it is effective against prostate cancer, especially in the initial phases of the disease, partly by improving the cell's ability to eliminate carcinogens and partly reducing the ability of carcinogenic chemicals to bind to DNA. Preliminary studies at the same centre have indicated that garlic also prevents prostate (and breast) cancer cells from dividing, thereby limiting the growth of tumours.[62] Garlic is also a natural anti-microbial agent active against a wide range of fungi, bacteria and viruses and it was used for these purposes in the First World War. You should have at least two to three raw cloves of fresh garlic a day to prevent and treat prostate and other types of cancer, and to ward off infectious illnesses when your immune system is impaired from cancer treatment. Many people worry about smelling of garlic but if everyone eats it, no one notices – just as everyone who has dairy products does not notice that they and others smell of sour milk (a much more unpleasant smell to me)! I have a friend who kept telling me that I smelt of garlic. I simply put on a worried face and replied 'Oh dear that means you are not getting enough!' She doesn't comment any more.

Juices and smoothies

One of the problems if you have active cancer is in consuming the amount of fresh fruit and vegetables needed to deliver adequate quantities of anti-cancer chemicals to the sites of the tumours. The best way to overcome this problem is to extract juices from the vegetables and fruits. This way, the active compounds are separated from the large mass of fibre that you would otherwise have to chew through and the anti-cancer agents are made more biologically available to your body. Even if you do not like certain vegetables, you can hold your nose and simply drink the juice as if it is a medicine – it is! Naturopaths and some doctors have been treating patients with fresh juices and raw food to improve their health since the nineteenth century. The therapy was pioneered in Germany and Switzerland before being used by health clinics worldwide. Famous pioneers include Father Kniepp, Dr Kellogg, Dr Max Bircher-Benner and Dr Max Gerson. To make the quantities of juices needed you must invest in a juicer (*not a liquidiser*). There are several available, but when I had cancer I found that the cheaper ones burned out quickly and I therefore invested in a type normally used in commercial juice bars – which I still use.

Carrot juice is good, but do not drink more than a half-pint glass a day or you may turn orange (I did – with orange palms and an orange moustache, which was described grandly by one of my doctors as carotenosis!). Do not have too much cabbage juice either. Cabbage contains substances known as goitrogens which can cause problems with the thyroid gland if taken in too large quantities, especially if it is eaten raw. It increases the requirement for iodine which is essential for good nutrition (*see* p. 235) and for which the main source in the diet is seafood. The main green juice I drank every day when I was ill with cancer was made from green Bramley apple, celery and fennel, with small amounts of watercress.

If you're thinking of cheating by drinking bottled or frozen juices instead of freshly made ones, there is simply no point. If you cut an apple it immediately starts going brown (because it has oxidised) and you need the green unoxidised juice. The same is true for all juices. If you buy commercial juices they will be far more oxidised and chemically far less potent as anti-cancer agents. Also they may contain some type of preservative or have undergone some type of process to stop them going rotten (just think about it, how else could carrot juice be sold weeks after it is prepared?) so they will be chemically changed. The only exceptions are good frozen juices, not made from concentrates. I have discovered people with colon cancer changing the diet I recommend by eating vegetable pills instead of raw vegetables and their juices – a complete waste of time!

Smoothies have become very popular as a way of having fruit. They are delicious but make your own with banana not dairy yoghurt as a thickener. I buy them only if they are in glass containers or are freshly made at a juice bar.

Soups, salads and stir fries

In addition to juices, you should have masses of fresh salads and vegetables. I cook vegetables by lightly steaming them (not by boiling) or just wilting them in a little extra-virgin olive oil (essentially cooked for a few minutes without water). This is an especially good method of cooking spinach, which is delicious if a few onions are softened in the extra-virgin olive oil first. I also eat lots of vegetable soups. Stir fries are delicious and a good way of persuading young people to eat vegetables. Lightly sauté vegetables for just a few minutes in olive oil and then pop on a lid so they cook in their own juices

Let the wind go free

One of the problems people complain of when they start to eat lots of fruit and vegetables is the number of times they have to go to the loo. Sorry, but that is what is supposed to happen – two to three times a day is normal, not two to three times a week! Also by not suffering from constipation you will reduce your chance of suffering from diverticulitis, haemorrhoids (piles) and varicose veins. A good indication that your diet is correct is when your stools float rather than sink. You may also suffer from 'wind', but don't worry – after a few weeks of the diet recommended here the body will adjust and you will have no further problems. My late mother-in-law, a wonderful highland Scot with a great sense of humour who became Mayoress in the Borough of Southgate and a Justice of the Peace, knew a little rhyme that might help when you first change to the Plant Programme. It went like this:

Where'er ye be
Let the wind gang (go) free
Except at the kirk (church) or taking tea.

Eat fresh, whole foods, as nature intended

Whole foods are a complex package of essential nutrients with many benefits that cannot be found in bottles of pills. Whole foods really are greater than the sum of the parts. For example, natural foods contain enzymes that help break down the components of the food. Hence bananas are rich in carbohydrates and contain amylase, a carbohydrate-splitting enzyme. Natural carrot juice contains all sorts of substances that work with beta-carotene. Foods generally contain hundreds or thousands of substances (many of which have yet to be studied) that may be important for health. It has been suggested that the difference between natural vegetables and fruit and commercial juices or pills is similar to that between trees and paper. Be like Chinese people and eat everything when it is as fresh and ripe as possible. This is much healthier than eating dead junk food and trying to make up the difference with yet more synthetic chemicals sold as vitamin and mineral supplements.

Sea vegetables

Sea vegetables are especially valuable sources of nutrients such as calcium, magnesium and iodine. Seaweed is also protective against radiation. Alginate, a mucous material extracted from seaweed, is a standard protective agent against radioactivity, so kelp and other seaweeds help reduce the side effects of X-rays and radiotherapy. Agar-agar, which is widely used to replace gelatine in vegan foods, can also be used in your diet as a source of iodine. Other seaweeds which I use include: arame, hiziki, dulse and wakame (which I add to some soups immediately before serving). Nori, which is commonly sold in sheets, can be used to wrap rice balls, sushi and many other foods. A lunch box containing this is available from at least one supplier of ready-to-eat meals – much better for you than grabbing a sandwich or baguette!

One final question

With all this accumulated evidence on the beneficial effects of vegetables and fruit in protecting against cancer and other diseases, why did it take so long for us to be told? (*See* Chapter 7 for further discussion on this point.)

ORGANIC FOOD AND PESTICIDES

In the UK, organically grown food has its origins in the work of Sir Albert Howard who published *An Agricultural Testament* in 1940, advocating that Britain preserve the 'cycle of life' and adopt 'permanent agriculture' systems, using urban food waste and sewage to build soil fertility. The first person to apply the term 'organic' to food production was J I Rodale in his 1942 publication *Organic Gardening and Farming*. In 1946 the young Lady Eve Balfour was inspired by Howard to set up the Soil Association, a pioneering organic farming charity that is the major organic certification organisation in the UK today. In 1974 the Soil Association established the UK's first set of Organic Food Standards, which form the basis of EU regulation 2092/91 which lays down in detail how food must be produced, processed and packaged to qualify for the description 'organic'. The regulation also specifies detailed criteria for the inspection and certification of food producers and processors. In the USA, organic regulations have been developed on a state-by-state basis; currently there is no national organic legislation comparable with that in the EU.

The establishment point of view

Sometimes, people who advocate organic food are dismissed as middle-class food fanatics, with no rational or scientific basis for their concerns, a view often supported by establishment scientists. I'd like to tell you why this caricature is wrong and why it is so vitally important that you insist on as much high-quality organic food as possible, despite the efforts of organisations such as the Food Standards Agency when it was under the direction of Sir John Krebs to persuade us that there is no difference between organic and conventionally produced food.[63] The evidence of the presence of pesticide residues in conventionally produced food continues to mount, as do the beneficial effects of eating organic food. For example, a study published in 2006 demonstrated that an organic diet provides a dramatic and immediate protective effect against exposure to organophosphate pesticides commonly used in food production.[64] Moreover, the synthetic nitrogen fertilisers used in industrial agriculture leach into ground and surface water creating bacteria and toxins that may be linked to some types of cancer.

I believe it is particularly important to limit exposure to harmful chemicals. I believe the food industry contributes significantly to modern health problems with their widespread use of chemical fertilisers, pesticides, plant and animal hormones and other veterinary medicines, and genetically modified crops, designed to survive being dowsed with herbicides that kill other plants. Thus, even eating an apparently healthy diet can lead to an increasing burden of man-made toxins, many of which have not been properly assessed for their carcinogenicity, especially in the cocktail we are supposed to take in.

The establishment view was that a relatively small percentage of cancers are attributable to pesticides, following epidemiological studies which indicated that not more than 2 per cent of cancers are attributable to the use of pesticides.[65] If this is accurate, it is still a lot of cancers! However, this estimate preceded our knowledge of the endocrine-disrupting behaviour of certain pesticides (many of which are now banned or strictly controlled), so it is likely to be a serious underestimate of cases of, particularly, prostate and other hormone-dependent cancers. Moreover, it has emerged recently that one of the authors of the key 1981 paper on pesticides and cancer, Professor Sir Richard Doll, had a conflict of interest inasmuch as since 1979 he had been paid large sums of money by pesticide manufacturers, which he failed to declare.[66]

In July 2006 the EU stated 'Long term exposure to pesticides can lead to serious disturbances to the immune system, sexual disorders, cancers, sterility, birth defects, damage to the nervous system and genetic damage.'

Pesticides, endocrine disruption and cancer

According to Lang and Clutterbuck, animal studies have implicated about 50 pesticides as cancer-causing agents.[67] Many other pesticides are suspected of causing birth or genetic defects; and over 60 pesticides have been implicated in causing various reproductive effects. In 1993 a distinguished American scientist Theo Colborn coined the term endocrine-disrupting chemicals[68] to describe chemicals that interfere with the functioning of our hormone systems either by mimicking or blocking the action of hormones such as oestrogen or testosterone. Endocrine-disrupting chemicals are increasingly linked to hormone-dependent cancers such as prostate cancer. Recently more than 100 pesticides have been identified as having endocrine-disrupting properties[69] and these are just the active ingredients. Many pesticide formulations also contain other chemicals such as nonyl phenol ethoxylate (NPE) designed to achieve good dispersion of the active ingredients over crops. NPE is one of the most notorious endocrine-disrupting chemicals known,[70] and it is now being banned for use on food crops across Europe. One of the things that always occurs to me when this happens is how do all those who kept reassuring us that a substance was safe or that there is no benefit to eating organically produced food manage to keep their jobs when they are proved wrong? Because they are part of the establishment?

A new study on women aged 55 or younger in one of Canada's largest fruit- and vegetable-growing regions showed that women who have worked on farms are up to nine times more likely to develop breast cancer than those who have never been employed in agriculture.[71] These findings raise further suspicions that the array of fungicides, herbicides and insecticides used on many farms is a factor in the 'huge increase in the rates of breast cancer' in Canada and may be responsible for at least some cases of prostate and breast cancer in the population as a whole.

According to McMichael,[72] there has been a 30-fold increase in global pesticide use and a nine-fold increase in chemical fertiliser use since the 1950s. This has increased food yield, but it has also caused widespread chemical pollution, destruction of wildlife and disturbance of ecosystems. In Western countries, millions of kilograms of pesticides are used each year for agricultural and non-agricultural applications, including forestry, landscaping, gardening, food distribution and home pest control.

Fortunately, in the UK, more than seventy such products, including some that were in use for growing vegetables, have recently been cleared from garden-centre shelves because they have been banned by the EU – but why did it take so long?! After banning DDT in the 1970s, followed by other organochlorines including the drins and many, many other pesticides, it might have been expected that there would have been a speedier reaction to limit our exposure. I am still left with the question: What are we still using today that in the future we shall find evidence to ban?

Avoiding the chemical nightmare

The alternative to the chemical nightmare of industrialised agriculture is to buy organically produced food, ideally grown to the standards of and policed by the UK Soil Association – their symbol is a circle with the words 'SOIL ASSOCIATION' around the top and 'ORGANIC STANDARD' round the bottom, and a sort of curly, triangular design inside the circle. Also, I object to buying so-called organically produced food, produced to no particular standard, which is then expensively flown in to supermarkets from across the world – long-distance air transport causes pollution too.[73] Choosing food that carries symbols such as that of the Soil Association also means you will avoid genetically modified food. A recent report into the environmental performance of supermarkets by the UK National Consumer Council rated Sainsbury's and Waitrose best for organic food and responsible use of pesticides on non-organic produce. If you are unable to obtain good organically produced food at your local supermarket, use a search engine on the internet to identify local suppliers – who will often deliver to your door. If you cannot afford the additional expense of buying organically produced food for all your needs and cannot grow your own, make food that will not be cooked (such as salad vegetables and fruit) your spending priority, since at least some of the damaging chemicals in pesticides break down during cooking and processing.[74] See further in Chapter 6, Lifestyle Factor 3.

Peel fruit if it is not organically grown, because the skin, which is otherwise very nutritious, is often treated with chemicals and then waxed so the chemicals do not wash off. This is often the case with oranges, grapefruit and lemons and some heavily marketed commercial apples. Of course, it does not matter too much whether or not citrus fruit has been waxed if it is to be peeled, but it does if you are using it to make marmalade or other food which uses the skin or the rind of the fruit. I avoid eating apples that have been treated in this way. I stick to English Cox's and Bramleys which I have never found waxed. Just one important cautionary note: animal manure and waste are used as fertiliser in organic farming, so pathogens will remain on your foods unless you are particularly vigilant: wash all fruit and vegetables thoroughly before eating them.

Another problem with some organically grown food such as peanuts stored in hot, humid conditions, usually in developing countries, is that it may be contaminated with high levels of carcinogenic fungal substances called aflatoxins, which, it is claimed, are killed off by the use of pesticides. If buying peanuts, simply buy them in their shells and discard the shells. I have been eating organic for years and have never had a problem.

TEN KEY WAYS TO BOOST YOUR VITAL VEGETABLE INTAKE

If You Used To Do This . . .	*Now Do This!*
Boil your potatoes and cabbages to death	Buy a stainless steel or bamboo steamer, add an inch of water in the pan, put on the steamer and fill it with veg. It takes about the same length of time to cook and you won't believe how much better it tastes!
Think crudités mean celery sticks dipped in salt	Keep the celery sticks but add raw carrot sticks, raw broccoli and cauliflower florets, chunks of raw courgette and sweet pepper, cucumber, tomato, spring onions and on and on. Ditch the salt and add a dollop of houmous or soya yoghurt seasoned with chopped chives and herbs for dipping
Turn up your nose at any vegetable except frozen peas	Lightly cook chopped veg in a little vegetable stock, blend and serve as a soup, flavoured with pepper and herbs. You can add great quantities of greens into it, and it tastes delicious
Think a salad was a careful arrangement of limp lettuce, shrivelled cucumber, a slice of tomato and half a boiled egg covered in salad cream	Aim to create a salad with at least five ingredients. Here is the 'add list' for one of my favourite salads: grated carrot and turnip, chopped spring onion, diced cucumber and courgette, red kidney beans or tiny cubes of marinated tofu, watercress and parsley, rocket, radicchio and

	Cos lettuce. Mix and serve with sunflower seeds and a little walnut or sesame oil with a cider vinegar flavoured with herbs drizzled over each serving
Throw the parsley garnish away	Make garnish fresh and from finely chopped herbs, such as parsley, coriander and watercress, and vegetables, such as tomato, onion and courgette. This will add valuable nutrients as well as some colour to your meal.
Eat just one tablespoon of vegetables at each evening meal	I use the Rainbow Rule: fill one-quarter of your plate with white veg such as potato, parsnip, celeriac or turnip. These can be mashed, baked, roasted or steamed. Fill the next quarter with orange veg such as carrot, sweet potato or pumpkin; another quarter with yellow veg such as swedes, sweetcorn and sweet pepper; and the final quarter with greens. Alternatively use similar combinations to make into vegetable kebabs, roast vegetables, salads or stir-fries. Also, add red tomatoes and peppers to your cooking whenever you can.
Think garlic was for rubbing inside the salad bowls	Buy a garlic crusher and lots of garlic bulbs. Whatever recipe you are reading, double the amount of garlic listed. Add chopped garlic to soups, stir-fries and casseroles, and crushed garlic to salad dressings, houmous and savoury sauces.
Reach for a dictionary whenever you heard the word 'brassica'	Add all the edible members of cabbage family to your diet: broccoli, Brussels sprouts, cabbages of all sorts, cauliflower, collards,

	kale, kohlrabi. These are rich in calcium and phytochemicals known to be anti-carcinogenic. Eat some raw or lightly steamed every day.
Think vegetable juice meant gravy and that a pound of carrots would last a year	Push one half pound of organic carrots, well scrubbed, through your new juicer. Drink immediately. Tomorrow, do the same with celery and tomatoes.

FOOD FACTOR 3: HEALTHY NOT WEALTHY PROTEINS

The first thing to say about protein is that in the West we generally eat far too much of it. Protein is needed only to repair our cells and tissues and it is quite unsuitable for energy generation. It is estimated that only 5 to 6 per cent of our daily calorie intake should be protein, with a maximum intake of about 10 to11 per cent. Many people in the West consume much more, some people having an unhealthy 20 per cent or more, especially those who followed the infamous Atkins diet; too much animal protein such as cheese makes the body too acid, increasing the risk of a range of disease from cancer to osteoporosis.

To make matters worse, much of the protein consumed is animal rather than vegetable protein. The Western diet, with its high content of animal protein, is linked to many of the cancers of affluence, not only prostate cancer but also breast and ovarian cancer, colorectal cancer and pancreatic cancer.[75] These diseases all have the highest incidence and mortality in wealthy Western countries and increase as wealth increases in developing countries as they abandon their traditional diets in favour of the Western diet.

Undoubtedly one of the main differences between the Western and traditional oriental diets is the amount of animal protein in the former, while the latter is heavily based on foods of vegetable origin. Figure 3.3 shows how crucial this is to preventing and treating prostate cancer, so, if you wish to prevent prostate or other types of cancer, don't even think about going on a high-animal-protein diet to help weight loss. I advise people who have active cancer of the prostate (or breast or colon) to eliminate all animal produce from their diet until they are better, always ensuring that their diet is balanced. For other people, a small amount of animal protein in the diet is fine provided it is balanced by at least twice as much vegetable protein and lots of other vegetables and fruit as well.

It is worth remembering that all vegetable protein provides dietary fibre, whereas no animal protein has any. A good dietary fibre intake has been shown to be particularly important in preventing colorectal cancer as well as diverticulitis, haemor-rhoids and varicose veins. This was first proposed by Professor Dennis Burkitt in the 1950s, based on his studies of African diets, and has recently been confirmed by the European Prospective Investigation of Cancer study which found that those having the diets highest in fibre had a 43 per cent lower risk of developing colorectal cancer.

Soya has a complete range of amino acids, and other pulses such as peas and beans, cereals (see below) and nuts are good sources of protein – without the unhealthy animal fat. All pulses are also very good sources of fibre, including a type that binds and inactivates free radicals in the gut and bloodstream. As discussed above, they are also valuable sources of phyto-oestrogens. Eat at least one good-sized portion a day.[76] Cereals are a good source of vegetable proteins, complementing those in pulses, and are discussed further under Food Factor 6. Another good protein source is nuts. I eat lots (but never pre-shelled because they quickly become rancid; and groundnuts can be contaminated with carcinogens – *see* p. 199). I avoid brazil nuts, which can contain elevated levels of the radioactive substance radium-226. When one of my colleagues told me this because he was concerned that I was eating so many, I did not believe him. After leaving some of the nuts I had been eating in our radiation detector overnight, I could see that he was right!

Now my cancer is gone, I eat one small portion of animal protein such as an organic egg a day, although I always keep to a vegan diet for at least one day a week. I eat fish but no more than once a week and only if it is wild or organically farmed, since this is less likely to contain antibiotic residues and other man-made pollutants. Oily fish such as salmon, herring and mackerel are rich in vitamin D, essential for healthy bones, and omega-3 fatty acids.

Vitamins A and D, found in oily fish and in fish oils, may work to reduce the risk of prostate cancer and breast cancer by lowering blood levels of IGF-I. I particularly avoid farmed trout, which may have been treated with steroid hormones to produce only female fish. If I eat salmon, I buy that produced to the standards of the Soil Association. This is much paler than most farmed salmon on the market, because it does not contain the artificial colouring agent which make other farmed salmon so vividly pink; one such agent, canthaxanthin, has been implicated in damaging eyesight. The same additive is used to feed non-organically produced chickens to colour their skins and the yolks of their eggs.[77] Non-organically produced farmed fish can also contain antibiotic residues and toxic chemicals used to control sea lice and to prevent growth of other organisms on the cages in which the fish are kept. In the past, the latter have included tributyl tin, an appalling endocrine-disrupting chemical (see p. 264).

Fish-liver oil is a good source of omega-3 fatty acids and vitamins A and D – but ensure that you buy the ultra-pure varieties which have had harmful chemicals such as PCBs (see p. 263) extracted. I take a teaspoon of Seven Seas cod-liver oil a day, the type which is labelled 'original and ultrapure', which is slightly more expensive.

If I eat meat, I choose organically reared lamb or chicken, or wild game such as rabbit or venison. Game generally has higher levels of nutrients and far lower levels of fat than concentrate-fed animals which have led a sedentary life.

In the first edition of *Your Life in Your Hands* I wrote 'If I were an American, I would never eat beef or pork unless it was absolutely guaranteed to be organically produced.' In 2006 research carried out by some of the world's leading epidemiologists at Harvard showed that eating such meat was linked to breast cancer.[78] Growth-hormone implants based on male and/or female hormones have been used in beef production in the USA for about thirty years. According to the Institute of Agriculture and Natural Resources at the University of Nebraska, implants are available for all cattle except calves less than forty-five days old and breeding cattle. Some of the most potent hormone implants combine both male and female hormones. Such meat has higher levels of IGF-I than untreated meat.[79] A genetically engineered pig growth hormone – Porcine Somatotrophin (PST) –

is also available in the United States, but I can find no evidence of the use of such products in sheep meat production.

One physician has been quoted as saying 'it is very likely that hormone residues in American beef are a factor in the early onset of puberty among girls in recent decades.'[80] It has been claimed that PST is safer than any of the steroid hormones banned by the European Union (but still used in America) because cooking destroys PST. However, this doesn't take IGF-I levels into account, nor does it address the problem of undercooked meat. Although the use of all such hormones is banned throughout Europe, on a BBC Radio 4 programme, British pig farmers complained that European farmers were allowed to feed their animals on sewage sludge – a practice forbidden in Britain! The message is clear. If you wish to eat pork, bacon or ham, eat organically produced British products especially from traditional rare breeds such as Gloucester Old Spot and Tamworth pigs.

Other good sources of protein and essential trace nutrients include organically produced eggs. Eggs also contain high levels of the amino acid cysteine used in anti-radiation pills so, in moderation, egg consumption will help combat the effects of radiotherapy and diagnostic X-rays. The sulphur in cysteine is in a form thought to de-activate free radicals and hence protect cells.[81] I ate one small organically produced egg a day while being treated with radiotherapy; I often eat organic eggs now, but never more than one a day.

Populations such as the Eskimos living on a predominantly fish diet have long been known to have less hormone-dependent cancer than those eating other animal fats. If properly cooked, seafood also contains lots of iodine, and iodine compounds (like those of zinc) are involved in ensuring that mistakes (which could cause cancer) do not occur during cell division in the body.[82]

One valuable tip for those who like the taste of meat or fish but wish to cut down the amount they eat is based on my husband's experience as a young soldier in Nyasaland (now Malawi) in the 1950s. The African soldiers he was responsible for were very fit and healthy and ate a diet consisting mainly of 'Mzima' or mealy meal made from maize, flavoured with small amounts of Ndiwa which was a sort of stew made from rabbit, chicken or fish with lots of vegetables. At mealtimes the Mzima was just dipped in the Ndiwa so that the overall amount of animal food was low but it flavoured most meals. You can easily copy this idea, for example, by making fish stew or spicy chicken with tomato from the Plant Programme with extra vegetables and use the juice to flavour vegetable based rice or pasta dishes over a few days.

In summary, I try to maximise the amount of vegetable protein and minimise the animal protein in my diet to cut my risk of suffering from any of the cancers of affluence or other chronic degenerative diseases linked to the Western diet. As for eating cheese and yoghurt – I don't even consider it!

PREVENTION FOR ORDINARY MORTALS
For those without cancer but who wish to cut their risk or those who have recovered from cancer (like me).
Remember to keep total animal produce very low.

If You Used To Do This . . .	Now Do This!
Breakfast	
Processed refined cereals with milk and white sugar	Organic muesli or porridge with a tablespoon of flaxseed, moistened with fruit juice previously sweetened with honey, raw cane sugar or molasses, or use rice, soya or coconut milk
Fried sausage, bacon, scrambled eggs and fried bread	1. Grilled organic bacon or vegetarian alternative, tomatoes and mushrooms brushed with, or softened in, olive oil. Toast or lightly fry bread in olive oil, or 2. Haddock poached in 50 per cent soya milk, 50 per cent water, or 3. A boiled or poached egg on wholemeal, organic bread lightly fried in olive oil 4. Best of all, Bubble and Squeak – a tradional British breakfast of fried leftover potatoes and cabbage
Toasted white bread and butter with marmalade	Toasted organic wholemeal bread with soya spread and marmalade

Commercial orange juice	Freshly made melon and raspberry juice or any other juice you enjoy

Snacks and nibbles

Commercial biscuits, especially those containing whey, casein, lactose, milk powder or other dairy	Dried fruit, nuts, pumpkin seeds, bananas, dried coconut. Dairy-free sesame bars or other snacks from health food stores. Dairy-free ginger nuts

Main meals

Meat cooked in butter or lard eaten rare or undercooked	Roast or grill meat slowly and thoroughly using olive oil and black pepper, garlic and other herbs and spices to flavour

Fast foods

Hamburgers, sausage, paté, prepared dishes from supermarkets	Eat veggie burgers or veggie sausages. Fish or eggs are the ultimate fast food. Steam or poach fish in water or white wine flavoured with ginger, onions, fennel or dill, or simply grill after brushing with olive oil and seasoning with salt, black pepper and herbs
Eat mainly tinned peas	Lightly steam fresh peas, mange tout, asparagus, broccoli or any other vegetables and keep the juice to make soup or gravy. Don't add butter, use olive oil flavoured with herbs
Chips, buttered or roast potatoes. Baked potatoes with butter or cheese	Just scrub potatoes before baking or steaming, then rub in olive oil and garnish with chopped parsley before serving. Eat with houmous or taramasalata instead of butter and cheese
Milky sauces and cream soups	In sauces, replace the dairy with soya milk; or use potato as a thickener

Thin soups	Miso-based soups (*see* p. 178), or use simple vegetable broth
Puddings	Choose from fresh fruit salads, water ices or sorbets, soya ice cream, tofu fruit puddings or other delicious puddings described in *The Plant Programme*. Use soya or coconut cream rather than dairy
Cheese course	Substitute a salad course with pine nuts, sun-dried tomatoes and herb-flavoured olives, artichoke hearts and marinated tofu
Commercial mayonnaise, salad dressing or salad cream	Make a base of 3-1 virgin olive oil to wine, cider, raspberry or balsamic vinegar, season with black pepper to taste and use various herbs and garlic to ring the changes
Cheesy or yoghurt-based dips	Replace with houmous, tahini or taramasalata
After-dinner chocolates	Buy the organic, dairy-free, dark chocolate version
Milky tea or coffee	Substitute from lists in Food Factors 1 and 8
Late-night milk-chocolate or malt drink	Check that it contains no dairy, then make it with soya milk instead of dairy, using raw sugar, vanilla or other flavourings you enjoy

FOOD FACTOR 4: OILS AND FATS

One clue to the puzzle of why prostate cancers metastasise in those on a Western diet but not in Oriental men eating their traditional diet was discovered when death rates from prostate cancer were compared with the annual fat consumption of men in a wide range of nations around the world. The nations included in the study ranged from Western industrialised nations to third world countries in which most of the population lived a rural agrarian existence. The results showed that the death rate from prostate cancer was directly correlated with the fat content in the diet.[83]

There are good reasons to be cautious about studies like these, because of the types of fat consumed. There are two convincing prospective studies, however: The Physician's Health Study and the Health Professionals Follow-up (HPFU) Study. In both studies, dietary intake was recorded regularly and not based on patients' sometimes faulty memory. The findings suggested that the risk of prostate cancer was directly related to total fat intake, but the risk was associated with animal (e.g. dairy products and meat), not vegetable, fat, and that the risk of metastatic prostate cancer was associated with dietary animal fat intake.[84]

It is important to note that prostate cancer is not the only human disease that appears to be associated with dietary animal fat intake. High-animal-fat diets have also been correlated with breast and colon cancer, heart disease and hypertension, and most cancer and heart charities recommend reduction in the amount consumed. Prostate-cancer patients and those people wishing to reduce their chances of developing the disease would be wise to reduce their intake of animal fat to an absolute minimum.[85] Many people do not realise just how much fat there is in our food now. Intensively reared animals have much more saturated fat relative to protein than in the past, when animals could exercise and were fed natural foods. For example, the amount of saturated fat in chickens has increased from 2 per cent thirty years ago to 22 per cent now.[86]

Many people are confused about the type and quantity of oils and fat they should be eating.

At a meeting on Cancer Prevention at Bethesda, USA, it was noted that the move towards lower dietary fat had failed to distinguish between unhealthy, saturated fats and healthy fats – and this mattered. Apparently, some tomato sauces available in health food stores have had olive oil removed so they could be labelled 'fat free'.[87] Also, we have been persuaded to buy spreads based on (usually altered and processed) polyunsaturated fats. Our bodies do need fats, but only in the quantities and forms which we would have consumed as hunters or gatherers. Let us try to sort out the unhealthy from the healthy forms of fat, because the right fat profile in your diet is crucial to good health.

Fats are solid at room temperature, oils are liquid. However, scientists often use the term 'fat' to include all oils and fats, whether they're solid or liquid. Chemically, fats are made up of three molecules of fatty acids and one of an alcohol called glycerol. The word 'triglycerides' is also used to describe fat – it means three ('tri') fatty acid molecules plus glycerol – triglyceride.

Fatty acids are, simply, acids found in fats. There are four major fatty acids: palmitic, stearic, oleic and linoleic. Remember, each molecule of fat contains three of these four fatty acids. It's the *combination* of these acids in the fat molecule that determines whether the fat is saturated, unsaturated, or polyunsaturated – words we've all heard a great deal in the past few years. Let me explain them.

Lipids (fats and oils) which are made from various combinations of fatty acids combined with glycerol, have long tails of carbon atoms (often fifteen to seventeen carbon atoms long) combined with hydrogen. Some fatty acids are chains of carbon atoms attached by single bonds and all their spare bonds are attached to hydrogen. They are therefore called saturated (with respect to hydrogen) because all their bonds are used up. Some have double bonds between carbon atoms and are called unsaturated. Unsaturated fatty acids can have one (monounsaturated) or many (polyunsaturated) double bonds between carbon atoms. Double bonds make fatty acids and lipids melt more easily, hence most oils are unsaturated while fats, especially animal fats, which are generally saturated, are solid at room temperature.

Saturated

Saturated fat is known to raise the level of cholesterol in your blood. The more you eat, the higher your cholesterol level, and the greater your chances of suffering a stroke or heart attack. Animal fat – hard cheese, butter and meat fat – contains lots of saturated fat. Cheese and butter contain so much saturated fat that they have been officially classified as junk food in the UK following the earlier example of Illinois in the USA.[88] A few plant fats – principally coconut and palm oil – also contain significant amounts. Among all the controversies about foods, the message to minimise saturated fat in our diet has remained unchanged for more than thirty years, despite the marketing of dairy produce and red meat as sources of CLAs now. Similarly, the advice against consuming trans-fatty acids, which can be formed during the manufacture of margarine and which can be high in many bought cakes and biscuits, remains unchanged. I avoid all margarines including those claiming to be high in polyunsaturates because they have been hydrogenated (involving passing hydrogen gas through them under pressure often in the presence of a nickel catalyst). This process can produce 'trans fat' which some nutrition experts believe are unhealthy and which has been implicated in breast cancer.[89] The Western diet typically contains large quantities of trans fatty acids (TFAs), which experimental evidence suggests impair essential fatty acid metabolism.[90] The TFAs are somewhat similar in structure and behaviour to saturated fatty acids and the WHO recommends that manufacturers reduce the levels of TFA in spreads. Since January 2006 trans fats have to be listed on products sold in the USA and they have been banned in Denmark. In the UK, action appears to be being left to large retailers. Most spreads now state the amount of trans fatty acids they contain: one organic soya spread my family uses contains only trace quantities.

Monounsaturated

Oleic fatty acid has eighteen carbon atoms and one unsaturated carbon bond. So it's called 'monounsaturated'. Ongoing research suggests that monounsaturated fat is much healthier than saturated fat. Experiments on humans show that switching from saturated to monounsaturated fat not only decreases the risk of heart disease but may also lower your blood pressure. A major source is olive oil. This contains more than 80 per cent monounsaturated fats and is naturally resistant to oxidation, which means it is relatively safe for cooking and is also less prone to rancidity than other types of unsaturated fat.

I avoid rapeseed or canola oil. Canola has been bred from old varieties of rapeseed in Canada, and is reported to contain very low levels of erucic acid suspected to have pathogenic potential in diets high in the original rapeseed oil in experimental animals.[91]

Canola oil is now the most widely consumed food oil in Canada and is approved by the US FDA.

Polyunsaturated

Linoleic fatty acid has eighteen carbon atoms and two unsaturated carbon bonds, so it's called 'polyunsaturated'. Early research indicated that polyunsaturated fats lowered total and LDL cholesterol more than monounsaturated fats. The latest research, however, finds no difference in their cholesterol-lowering ability. However, the more polyunsaturated an oil is, the more it can be damaged by heat, air and light. Most polyunsaturated oils should only be used raw because once damaged they form free radicals. Good sources of polyunsaturated fats include sunflower and corn oil.

Essential fatty acids

The two classes of essential fatty acids, omega-6 fatty acids such as linoleic acid (which, when conjugated – or linked up – forms CLAs), and omega-3 fatty acids, continue to receive considerable attention. They are both necessary for good health because they provide the catalysts for various metabolic functions (e.g. in the synthesis of prostaglandins, which are important as cell regulators and for the proper functioning of the immune system). They are called 'essential' because the body cannot make them, and they must be obtained from food sources. Most vegetable oils provide EFAs to a greater or lesser extent.

Omega-6 fatty acids (e.g. linoleic acid) are found in vegetable seeds and the oils produced from them. Good sources include oils made from safflower, sunflower, corn, soya, evening primrose, pumpkin, walnut, and wheat germ.

Omega-3 fatty acids (e.g. alpha linolenic acid) are found in oily fish such as salmon, mackerel and sardines, and also in linseed (flaxseed), borage seed and soya bean oil. In addition to being protective against cancer, evidence is mounting that they are protective against a range of other conditions including coronary heart disease and high blood pressure, arthritis, eczema and psoriasis, BPH[92] and depression. The food supplement spirulina (a microscopic algae) contains both linoleic and linolenic acids – indeed the omega-3 fatty acids in oily fish are derived from such sources.

Gamma linoleic acid is a particularly good Omega-3 fatty acid. It is enriched in organ meats such as liver (but eat only from organically reared animals) and in evening primrose oil – but do not have this in gelatine capsules (which are made from rendered animal carcasses).

Japanese researchers have shown that a deficiency of these essential fatty acids leads to an impaired ability to learn and recall information. Much new information suggests that the human brain, which contains much fatty material,[93] depends for optimal functioning on adequate supplies of omega-3 and omega-6 fatty acids and that their proportion in the diet is also important.[94]

There has been a huge change in the proportion of omega-3 to omega-6 fatty acids, especially in the Western diet.[95] With settled agriculture, which began about 10,000 years ago, people started to rely on cultivated foods, and the consumption of omega-3-rich fish and wild game declined. With the industrialisation of the food industry in the twentieth century, there was an even more dramatic shift in the proportion of omega-6 fatty acids to omega-3 fatty acids in the diet, a situation made worse by the hydrogenation of oils to make them keep longer. A typical Western diet now contains sixteen times as much omega-6 fatty acids as omega-3, whereas a century ago our diet would have contained similar amounts of each type of fatty acid. The advice is to eat more of the foods that are high in omega-3 fatty acids such as fatty fish, walnuts, flaxseed and olive oil for health.

Oils

I will no longer eat dairy produce in any guise ever and I rely mainly on first-pressed extra-virgin olive oil for everything from cooking to salad dressings. I never re-use the oil in cooking and I cook food slowly so that the oil is not damaged and the food absorbs the flavour. I avoid brands of margarine based on olive oil but which also contain dairy produce.

The only oils I use have been organically grown and extracted by cold pressing. There are three methods of extraction:

- Cold pressing. This is the traditional hydraulic pressing process where the temperature is kept low throughout and which therefore preserves temperature-sensitive vitamins. The end

product is expensive, but the oil is nutritious and tastes and smells good. It may be more expensive but you consume less!
- Screw or expeller. This process involves the use of high-pressure, which generates high temperatures, thereby destroying vitamins. Such oil is dark, strong smelling and needs further refining and deodorising – and I do not use it.
- Solvent extraction, using solvents such as benzene, hexane or heptane and lots of other processing and chemical treatment. I avoid this at all costs.

All oils should be stored in dark opaque stoppered glass bottles in dark cupboards or pantries to minimise oxidation and ideally used cold in salad dressings. I prefer to eat whole flaxseed rather than the oil. According to Ingram and others[96] it is flaxseed – but not flax oil – that is rich in anti-carcinogenic lignan precursors, and it is also excellent for avoiding constipation and hence piles and varicose veins.[97]

In many Mediterranean restaurants it is usual to have virgin olive oil flavoured with herbs to dip bread into. It is so much tastier and healthier than butter. I do this now if I have dinner parties. Usually my guests eat their bread dipped in flavoured olive oil with great relish, and I have noticed many of them have copied the idea. The Spanish, Italian and Greek people I know use olive oil with fish or tomato paste and salad for example to make sandwiches, instead of butter or processed spreads on their bread. This is not only healthier but the sandwiches and snacks are much more delicious than those most people in the UK eat.

It is particularly important to obtain fats from fresh, unpolluted sources, since many of the most health-damaging pollutants, including some powerful endocrine disrupters, are highly fat-soluble. Large quantities can accumulate in the fatty tissue of farmed fish, fresh fish downstream of sewage works and dairy fat, for example.

For the same reason I try never to use oils from plastic bottles since many of the potentially harmful chemical substances in plastics are fat soluble.

The plant called oil-seed rape, from which rapeseed oil is obtained, contains goitrogens and I avoid this in my diet and anything that contains unspecified vegetable oils since this could include such oil.

In summary, I never eat cheese, butter or margarine, nor do I eat meat or eggs from intensively farmed animals or fish. I eat a range of extra-virgin cold-pressed oils for salad dressings and use olive oil for cooking. I avoid rapeseed and canola oil.

TEN WAYS TO MODIFY YOUR FAT INTAKE

If You Used To Do This . . .	*Now Do This!*
Make your sandwiches with a thick layer of butter, then with a thick layer of peanut butter or houmous	Leave out the butter
Spread your toast with a thick layer of butter or margarine	Drizzle a little organic, cold-pressed extra-virgin olive oil over your toast instead. It tastes delicious, especially with tomato paste or savoury food
Buy oil labelled canola or unspecified 'vegetable' oil	Buy only cold-pressed extra-virgin organic olive, walnut, sesame or sunflower oils
Prepare a fondue every weekend	Keep the little forks but switch ethnic loyalties and prepare a plate of raw and steamed vegetables surrounded by a selection of Thai, Japanese and Chinese dips and sauces
Buy a cheese and pickle sandwich from your local supermarket every lunchtime	Buy a tub of their houmous instead, with a salad and a few baby pittas to dip into it
Buy crackers and snack foods without reading the labels	Read all labels for fat and hidden-dairy content! Buy fresh and dried fruit and nuts instead of fatty, salty or sugary snacks
Insist on eating popcorn while watching that film	Go ahead, but use an air-popper to make it. They make a good gift and

	require no fat. Add your favourite spices
Order the Four Cheeses pizza from your local	Try the Marguerita without the mozzarella, but request extra olives, capers, mushrooms, garlic, etc
Order the baked potato with butter, chilli con carne and cheese sauce	Order the baked potato with baked beans or houmous and a side salad
Go crazy for any dessert topped with cream	Make some fruit sauce and drizzle a little organic maple syrup over your favourite non-dairy dessert

FOOD FACTOR 5: SEASONING, FLAVOURING AND ADDITIVES

One of the most dramatic differences in our diet now compared with the end of World War II is the increase in fast and convenience foods. There are now more than 320,000 different processed foods and drinks on the market.[98] As well as preservatives to give it a long shelf life, such food frequently contains artificial flavouring and colouring agents. Eric Schlosser in *Fast Food Nation* about the problems caused by the fast-food industry in America recounts how the strawberry flavour in milkshakes sold by one outlet is prepared from more than 55 different artificial chemicals. Such chemical concoctions are used to give a consistent taste and improve the acceptability of low-cost food.

Until recently the main methods of preserving food were to add lots of salt, especially to meat and vegetables, sugar to fruit, and alcohol to a range of products. It has been said that the British, because they shipped so much food from their overseas territories, developed a particular liking for these tastes. Food naturally contains sodium so we do not need to add any to our food. Overuse of salt and sodium bicarbonate have been linked by Gerson to cancer and it continues to be implicated by some researchers in promoting certain types of cancer, including naso-pharyngeal (nose and throat) cancer.[99] Recent research by Djamgoz and his team at Imperial College, London[100] has shown that cancer cells metastasise more readily in the presence of sodium. Other common sources of sodium include monosodium glutamate, the 'extra meaty flavour' in cheap meat products and some soya sauces, and sodium sulphite used as a preservative in many wines.

On the other hand, healthy food doesn't have to be – indeed, *shouldn't* be – bland food. After a while when you cut down on salt you will find food tastes much better with more subtle flavours. Oriental people, however, consume lots of salt in soya sauce, for example, so I do not think that reducing salt intake is one of the most critical things to do in combating prostate cancer; but it is helpful to your health generally.

Many anti-cancer diet books recommend against the use of spices. Korean and Thai food and food from Hunnan and Szechuan provinces in China, however, are very heavily spiced, and the rates of prostate and breast cancer there are exceptionally low. In *The Plant Programme* many of the delicious recipes include spices, since by the time we wrote the book we were aware of the use of many spices as anti-cancer treatments in traditional Indian Ayurvedic and Chinese medicine. Turmeric, for example, one of the main ingredients of curry powder, contains curcumin, which has been shown to have powerful antioxidant and anti-cancer properties, suppressing the proliferation of cancer cells. Curcumin has even been shown to help prevent cancer cells producing their own growth factors, as they do in advanced cases of the disease. In particular, curcumin inhibits the growth of oestrogen-receptor-positive breast cancer.[101] Real saffron, made from crocus stamens and traditionally used to colour rice yellow, contains carotenoids and has anti-free-radical properties, but never eat the horribly yellow or pink food now sold as Eastern food in some shops, restaurants and supermarkets.

I grow fresh herbs such as parsley, thyme, chives, marjoram, rosemary and mint in a small patch in the garden and buy others from the supermarket. Herbs are good for you and help to make food taste delicious.

Celery seed, garlic, onions, ginger and turmeric contain substances which stimulate the activity of an important de-toxifying enzyme GST (glutathione-S-transferase), and are useful for making delicious food.[102] Rosemary, sage, oregano and thyme are also strong antioxidants,[103] and rosemary and sage have documented anti-tumour activity.[104] Ginger contains more powerful antioxidants than even vitamin E,[105] and many other herbs and spices contain substances considered to be cancer-preventive agents.[106]

TEN HEALTHY WAYS TO SPICE UP YOUR FOOD

If You Used To Do This . . .	Now Do This!
Shower everything with salt	Stop cooking with salt. Try seasoning your meal with tamari (wheat-free soya sauce) and extra herbs and spices
Spread yeast extract on your toast	Spread miso on your toast for a similar-but-different flavour and added nutrient value
Serve boiled carrots with a dollop of butter	Steam them and then toss them in a light sauté of garlic and/or freshly grated ginger with organic extra-virgin olive oil
Think white pepper is the only spice	Arrange a small collection of spices on the table including black pepper, chilli pepper flakes and Tabasco sauce. Visit your local ethnic grocer to explore a new world of spices, then experiment . . .
Use 'salad cream' and nothing else on every salad you are given	Mix finest olive oil with a herb-flavoured cider vinegar and freshly crushed garlic. Or drizzle a little freshly squeezed lemon juice and sesame or walnut oil over your salad. A splash of Tabasco will also lift the flavour
Think boiled cabbage and potatoes were only there to soak up the gravy	Steam the vegetables very lightly, and then toss them gently in a light sauté of caraway seed and chopped garlic. Season with black pepper, to taste

Think every soup needed a hefty dose of beef broth and monosodium glutamate (MSG) to be tasty	Make your soups with a strong vegetable broth including the seaweed, kombu, which has flavouring and thickening properties similar to MSG but is healthier
Think all vinegar was white or brown malt vinegar	Mix together organic cider vinegar and organically grown fresh herbs. Try tarragon, rosemary, basil or garlic. Some delicatessens sell raspberry and other delicious fruit vinegars
Think that rice was a white and fluffy but rather bland way of bulking out the good stuff	First, change your brand of rice! Buy whole-grain, basmati or wild rice then zip up the flavour this way: heat 1 teaspoon olive oil in the saucepan and sauté one teaspoon of Chinese Five Spice or Spices for CousCous. Stir in your dry rice, then add the water and follow the usual cooking routine
Think roast onions tasted of cooked water	Leave small onions whole, and slice larger ones in half. Then press two or three whole cloves into each onion and place in the baking tray with potatoes, parsnips and half the oil you would normally use. Dissolve a tablespoon of yeast extract in a little warm water and pour over the veg before roasting

FOOD FACTOR 6: CEREAL FOODS, SNACKS AND TREATS

Eating good food is one of life's great pleasures, and the Plant Programme is not a hair-shirt regime! I eat sorbets and soya ice creams and organic dark dairy-free chocolate for occasional treats. My favourite treat is fish and chips – 'the great British experience' – which I eat about once a week, although I remove all the batter unless I buy it from my local fish-and-chip shop, where they are kind enough to make it without milk. This is much better, on health grounds as well as taste, than cow burgers on white bread!

I eat masses of dried fruit of all descriptions. Prunes contain anti-cancer chemicals and figs are an excellent source of calcium. Pumpkin, sesame and sunflower seeds make delicious, nutritious snacks. I often buy a lunch box full of delicious vegetable sushi from a Korean or Japanese shop for lunch or to snack on.

Whole-grain versus refined

Most cancer-prevention diets include plenty of whole-grain cereal foods such as bread and pasta.[107] Clearly if you are intolerant of or allergic to gluten you may need to avoid food and drink containing wheat, rye or barley, although many people can tolerate some gluten-containing foods better than others (wheat contains the most gluten). Good substitutes include rice and corn, and some new scientific evidence suggests that oats may be safe.[108]

Whole grains contain a wide range of phytochemicals that reduce the risk of cancer.[109] The active phytochemicals are concentrated in the bran and the germ, so that refining wheat, for example, causes a 200- to 300-fold loss in valuable phytochemical content.[110] Tumour cells synthesise and accumulate cholesterol faster than normal cells, and one group of chemicals in whole-grain cereals (and fruit and vegetables) suppress tumour growth by limiting cholesterol synthesis.[111] Other anti-cancer substances in whole grains induce the production of the detoxifying enzyme GST.[112]

On the other hand, consuming highly processed bread and cereals that are too easily digested floods the body with sugar, stimulating it to produce high levels of IGF-I.[113] Acne may be an indicator of the over-production of IGF-I as a result of this process. (Several people following my diet have reported that their acne has disappeared, but I think that giving up dairy produce helps this too.)

Undoubtedly, consuming lots of refined cereals can be harmful. Processing wheat to make white flour for white bread and many commercial pastries removes much of the proteins, vitamins and minerals – which are then often used for animal fodder. In order to compensate, inorganic nutrients such as chalk as a source of calcium, iron and vitamins are added back. Despite adding these vitamins, such processed flour has often lost much of its vitamin B6, vitamin B5 and molybdenum; nearly all of its vitamin E, cobalt and zinc content; much of its chromium and some selenium content, too. The degradation of nutritional content is made worse by the addition of bleaches and 'improvers' such as potassium bromate, some of which have been shown to be toxic.[114] Always check the list of ingredients carefully when buying bread and ensure that it is free of chemical additives. If I had the time, I would make my own bread with freshly purchased organic wheat or other cereals, using one of the bread-making machines which are now widely available, but my life is far too busy at the moment!

Do try to buy organic wherever possible, because unfortunately much wheat is now produced mainly by monoculture methods under prairie-like conditions, with the liberal use of artificial fertilisers and pesticides.[115]

Try to eat only organic wholemeal brown bread made with stone-ground flour. I eat many other types of organically grown cereals, including porridge and oatcakes, organic whole-grain brown rice and wholemeal brown organic pasta, all widely available in health-food stores and supermarkets. Despite some recently published versions of anti-breast-cancer diets, there is nothing wrong with muesli providing it is based on organic produce and provided it is not the commercial 'muesli' made with sugar or milk-derived components. Use rice, oat or soya milk or fruit juice rather than dairy milk to moisten it. If you are staying in a hotel, use the juice from fresh-fruit salad or if there is none use the juice from the prunes which are almost always on the buffet. It is important to eat zinc-containing protein (such as meat or eggs) at least eight hours after eating food such as cereal, because cereals contains high levels of substances called phytates which can bind zinc, making it unavailable for absorption. An exception is the fibre in flaxseed, which has been shown in experiments not to bind zinc.[116]

TEN HEALTHY TREATS

If You Used To Do This . . .	Now Do This!
Tuck into a giant bag of crisps	Pour a small handful each of sesame, sunflower and pumpkin seeds into a bowl and munch them instead
Leave a trail of sweet wrappers around the place	Mix your own blend of organic dried fruits such as figs, dates, apricots, mango and raisins, and place little bowls or cartons of them in handy places: the car, your desk, near the phone . . .
Eat sweet and sticky desserts	Take an organically grown orange, slice it in half and use a grapefruit knife to slice around the segment edges. Sprinkle the sliced surface with a tiny pinch of nutmeg or cloves and a hint of maple syrup. Bake for about 15 minutes
Reward yourself with sweet and sticky desserts layered with cream	Take an organic Bramley apple, remove the core and fill it with raisins, chopped banana, cinnamon and a little maple syrup. Place it in a dish and bake for about 15 minutes. Serve with soya cream or soya ice cream
Eat whole variety packs of snack crackers	Buy rice cakes and oatcakes and arrange them on a plate with a little houmous, tofu dip, tahini or home-made salsa
Get a sweet craving at least twice a day	Soak a mixture of chopped organic dried fruit in filtered water overnight. Eat a small bowlful dressed with a little rose water and chopped pumpkin seeds

Get a serious snack attack once a day	Fight back with a piping hot baked potato filled with houmous or dairy-free baked beans. Sometimes a bean salad will do the trick
Blow out on ice cream and chocolate	Go ahead, but with soya ice cream and dairy-free dark chocolate
Eat a packet of biscuits every day	Pack your own stack of oatcakes, spread with home-made jam. Sweet, crunchy and very nutritious
Eat toast made with white bread and whatever until the whole loaf is gone	Buy only wholemeal organic loaves made with organic flour and be fussy about what you spread on them. Try tahini, barley miso, mashed banana or olive paté

FOOD FACTOR 7: SWEETENERS

Use raw cane sugar molasses, unrefined honey (preferably wild) or maple syrup as sweeteners. Refined white sugar (called 'pure, white and deadly' by Professor Yudkin) is just empty calories stripped of nutrients; I never eat it. A natural herbal substance called stevia, which has been used as a sweetener and flavour enhancer in Paraguay for centuries and is also suitable for diabetics, is now available from good health stores.

I avoid any products containing man-made sweeteners such as aspartame,[117] cyclamates, or saccharin, or refined sugar. I do so because some of these artificial sweeteners have been linked in laboratory studies to a range of diseases.[118] Artificial sweeteners are frequently found in soft drinks, over-the-counter and prescription drugs, vitamin and herbal supplements, yoghurt, confectionery, some processed cereals, sugar-free chewing-gum, some desserts, some ready-made meals, some milk-shakes, sweeteners, and some instant teas and coffees. So read all labels carefully!

Traditionally, Chinese children have eaten very few sweets. Their treats were pumpkin seeds or dried fruit.

FOOD FACTOR 8: WHAT TO DRINK

As I mentioned earlier, I drink freshly-made vegetable and fruit juices from organic produce. Clean, pure water is also fundamental for good health. Unfortunately, the only way the water companies can provide adequate supplies of water now, in areas of high population density, is to recycle it by treating or reprocessing it at sewage works. Indeed, we joke that when people drink a glass of water in the East End of London, ten people have previously drunk the same water! During treatment, the water is filtered through progressively finer material to remove particles, microbes and chemicals, and it is often mixed with other water to dilute harmful chemicals so that their concentration falls below legal requirements. Finally, chlorine is added to kill the remaining microbes.

Many medical professionals seem to be unaware of the problems associated with the use of recycled treated sewage water as the principal drinking-water supply in urban areas (*see* further under Lifestyle Factor 6 in Chapter 6) – or so it seems to me. For example, I remember a TV interview in which a senior cancer specialist from a famous London hospital accused me of putting cancer patients to unnecessary trouble in advising them to filter and boil their water before drinking it. It emerged that he had no idea that levels of natural and synthetic oestrogens (the latter from the female contraceptive pill) and other endocrine-disrupting chemicals in water from sewage-discharge systems could be so high in the UK that 100 per cent of the male fish downstream of such discharges are feminised.

Reprocessed drinking water can contain many other harmful chemicals, including benzene and cancer-causing organic chemicals, pesticides and disinfection by-products such as trihalomethanes and haloacetic acids. More rigorous limits for disinfection by-products are being legislated for in America.[119] For these and other reasons, I do not drink water straight from the tap. Some water from extraction wells has also been found to contain an amazing range of pharmaceutical residues – everything from the female contraceptive pill and HRT to Viagra, antidepressants and chemotherapy agents. Nevertheless, I continue to advise against bottled water, since some bottled waters can contain such high levels of radioactivity or nitrates that they would be illegal if they came out of the tap. This is important advice when travelling. For example, the Indian government has ordered a revision of national safety standards for drinking water after the Centre for Science and Environment in New Delhi found pesticide residues in bottled drinking water that were 36 times higher than the maximum limits set by the European Commission.[120]

I use tap water, but I filter it through charcoal into a glass jug. I have found it impossible to buy a filtration unit made completely of glass but the plastic is hard and when thoroughly washed is unlikely to release the high concentrations of phthalates associated with soft plastic. After filtering I always boil the water before drinking it to remove or further reduce harmful chemicals and to take out germs not removed by water treatment. These can occur in tap water and bottled water from shallow sources, and I always add tea or herbal teas to try to further remove pollutants (lots of organic plant matter absorbs harmful chemicals onto the surface, removing it from the liquid that you drink). This takes out or reduces many harmful chemical residues, which, if they are given the opportunity, will sorb on to something such as charcoal or organic matter instead. One recent book about fighting cancer recommends reverse osmosis to clean up tap water, but this generally involves forcing chlorinated water through plastic membranes so I prefer to keep my simple jug filter.

It is particularly important to boil water before drinking when undergoing chemotherapy because such patients are regarded as immunocompromised. Over the past fifteen years or so it has become apparent that a protozoan parasite (related to the malaria parasite) called *Cryptosporidium*, can cause severe sickness, vomiting, dehydration and diarrhoea in immunocompromised people, with symptoms which can persist indefinitely (although the gastroenteritis it causes usually clears up on its own in healthy individuals). In 1993 more than 400,000 people were affected and several people died after *Cryptosporidium* breached a water filtration plant at Milwaukee, Wisconsin. Prevention involves boiling (even boil bottled water if it is from shallow sources), and frequent and thorough hand washing and bedding changes. Infection has been reported via pets, livestock and wildlife.[121]

I never drink coffee, but I drink lots of Chinese, Japanese and Korean green tea with no milk (of course!) (if you use lemon or lime, remove the peel first unless you are using unwaxed organic fruits). Extracts of green tea have been shown to prevent cancer in experimental animals. The chemicals thought to have anti-cancer properties in green tea are polyphenols known as cathechins including epigallo-cathechin-3-gallate, an antioxidant that accounts for much of the solid materials in brewed green tea.[122] It is thought that the well-known anti-cancer activity of green tea is because it inhibits one of the most frequently over-expressed enzymes in human cancers, called urokinase.[123]

Evidence of the cancer-protecting properties of green tea continue to emerge. Recent studies have confirmed that epigallo-catechin-3-gallate has a protective role against several types of epithelial cancers, including prostate cancer.[124] Experimental studies on mice with a type of prostate cancer that mimics a progressive form of human prostate cancer showed that an infusion equivalent to six cups of green tea a day for humans significantly inhibited the development and spread of the cancer and increased overall survival. It has also been suggested that green tea is a stronger antioxidant than vitamin C[125] and helps to neutralise free radicals.

Drinking tea this way is exactly what the Chinese do. When I first worked in China, I used to wonder what the jam jars with strange looking bits in the bottom were in the front of taxis. Eventually, I realised they were jars of green tea! Chinese, Japanese and Korean green teas used to contain less pesticides than commonly produced black tea, although this may no longer be true, as they become increasingly Westernised. In China, green tea is valued for its digestive properties and for assisting circulation and regulating body temperature. Preparation of black teas, unlike green teas, involves fermentation.[126] Black tea can contain twice as much caffeine (in the form of theine) as coffee; the tannin content of black tea can also inhibit iron uptake, and brewing black tea oxidises the cathechins, according to some authors destroying any beneficial effects.[127] Interestingly, new research has shown that adding cow's milk to tea removes its health benefits. Once again the problem is casein (milk protein), which blocks the beneficial effects of catechins.[128]

I recommend drinking at least six cups a day of organic green tea certified by the Soil Association (and buy Fair Trade, which guarantees a better deal for Third World producers, whenever you can).

I also drink herbal teas, mostly peppermint or camomile with honey (many people do not like the taste of pure camomile at first). I also use fruit teas, but sparingly because some are so acid that if I drink too much they give me cystitis. Some fruit teas contain artificial chemicals of the kind used to flavour jellies and sweets (the give-away is that they are called 'fruit flavoured') and I avoid these.

Alcohol has been incriminated in prostate cancer, although, observing the quantities of rice wine and moutai (the Chinese equivalent of strong spirits) drunk by Chinese men, it is difficult to believe that it can be implicated in prostate cancer.

Oliver and others[129] found that those with prostate cancer were more likely than those without the disease (19 per cent v 26 per cent) to be heavy alcohol consumers (22 units a week or more), but the studies were carried out on Western men likely to be eating a typical Western diet.

Studies are also being carried out in Sweden to assess the effects of alcohol on IGF-I and the proteins which can inactivate IGF-binding proteins.[130]

Alcoholic beverages such as red wine can contain hidden animal-produce ingredients which it would be difficult to take account of in such studies. Also, if wine is stored in plastic-lined vats it can contain the endocrine-disrupting chemical bisphenol A (BPA).[131] According to the website of the Vegan Society,[132] many wines on sale have been fined, or cleared, using one of the following: animal blood, bone marrow, chitosan (from the hard parts of insects and crustacea such as shrimps and crabs), albumen (egg white), fish oil, gelatin (obtained by boiling animal tissues such as skin, tendons, ligaments or bones), isinglass (a fish's swim bladder), milk or milk casein (precipitated from milk). Non-animal alternatives used in wines labelled as vegan include limestone, clays and silica gel. But remember that wines labelled as vegetarian may have been fined using casein (milk protein). In the case of beer, isinglass is used especially for real ales. Keg, canned and some bottled beers are usually cleared without the use of animal substances. The production of spirits generally does not involve the use of animal substances (vodka is filtered using birchwood charcoal). The Vegan Society website[133] gives a list of good sources of vegan alcoholic beverages. I continue to drink organically produced cider, perry and beer. I avoid all diet drinks since these are likely to contain man-made sweeteners. Some ciders also contain man-made sweeteners.

I drank very little alcohol before I had cancer and I had none during treatment. I drink some alcohol now.

When I had active cancer I drank no black tea or alcohol and I never drink coffee. One of the benefits of removing these substances from my diet when I was ill was that I felt less anxious (without caffeine) and less depressed (without alcohol). Some of my fellow patients who felt the need to drown their sorrows noticeably fared badly and many were clearly depressed. You should certainly avoid alcohol during chemotherapy.

THIRST QUENCHERS: TEN DRINKS TO DELIGHT YOU

If You Used To Do This ...	Now Do This!
Start the day with a hot black one	Make it a hot yannoh instead. This is the finest cereal 'coffee' on the market. Try brewing it with 2–3 pods of cardamom and a few whole cloves
Drink strong milky tea all day long (as I used to do)	Try switching to rooibos tea, available at health-food stores. It is strong, caffeine-free and tastes good with soya milk
Drink black tea with sliced lemon	That's better, but better still try green tea or a strongly flavoured herbal tea such as nettle or dandelion
Treat yourself to a Starbuck's hot chocolate	Order it made with soya milk. When you make it yourself, try making it with carob instead. This is a chocolate-flavoured bean that is tasty and nutritious but caffeine-free
Guzzle cola all day long	Buy sarsaparilla concentrate from a health-food shop or herbalist and dilute to taste with sparkling mineral water

Swig soft drinks by the gallon	Dilute natural fruit or flower cordials, such as elderflower, with sparkling mineral water. If you have active cancer, prepare freshly made vegetable and fruit juices and down as many as you can.
Enjoy a jug of iced coffee now and then	Brew the yannoh and cardamom, above, and leave to cool. Pour a little into an ice cube tray and freeze. Blend the cooled yannoh with cold soya milk, whisk and serve with an ice cube
Lead a single-handed campaign to double the government recommendations for intake of alcohol	Switch to the types of alcohol from the vegan website and drink in moderation
Spend huge amounts on fresh juices from the chill cabinets in your supermarket	Make juices fresh with your own juicer and organic fruit and veg. Try melon, apple and celery, pear, apple and fennel, carrot and parsley, and so on
Think carrot juice was a cure for sunburn	Make your own with organic carrots. Add a quarter pint of carrot juice to a half pint of cold soya milk, stir well and serve with a straw

THE PLANT PROGRAMME

A report from the Royal College of Physicians asks doctors to pay more attention to nutritional status, something they have neglected in the past and which can cause many health problems and delay recovery. It can also increase health-care costs. Their report calls for nutrition to be tackled seriously and included in undergraduate and post-graduate training of doctors and other health-care staff.[134] Hear! Hear! – and about time too!

In the meantime, *The Plant Programme* gives full details of what to eat and what not to eat for those with prostate or other types of cancer, and provides dietary regimens for those suffering from active cancer and for those wanting to avoid recurrences of cancers. Living on processed food, as many cancer patients I see have done, is not good for health, so above all learn to cook – starting with the easy-to-follow recipes in *The Plant Programme* or *Eating for Better Health*.

CHAPTER 5 IN A NUTSHELL

- Organisations such as the WHO, the FAO, the US National Cancer Institute and the Physicians Committee for Responsible Medicine,[135] all agree that up to 40 per cent of all cancers could be prevented by diet.
- Evidence is accumulating that dietary changes such as those in the Plant Programme can also help to *treat* prostate cancer, although diet should be used to complement, not replace, conventional medical treatment.
- Vegetables and fruit are the energy foods we evolved to eat. Numerous components in vegetables and fruit, including dietary fibre, vitamins, minerals, live enzymes and various phytochemicals (i.e. plant chemicals) including those that act as anti-oxidants, contribute to a reduced risk of cancer. In contrast, animal foods lack fibre and contain saturated fat, cholesterol and animal protein as well as hormones and growth factors, all of which are associated with increased risk of cancer. There is no dispute about the health benefits of fruit and veg among mainstream scientists.
- The *Plant Programme* is based on sound science from the peer-reviewed scientific literature, and it follows the principles of diets that have been studied by teams of internationally renowned scientists. Such diets have been found to prevent not only prostate and breast cancer but other cancers such as colorectal cancer and pancreatic cancer as well as a host of other diseases.
- Many anti-cancer diets are based on junk science. Advice to eliminate all fruit, as well as vegetables such as potatoes and tomatoes, from the diet demonstrates total ignorance of the peer-reviewed scientific literature and diverts attention from the real culprit foods.
- One of the first and most essential things you can do to reduce your risk of prostate cancer is to remove **ALL** dairy products

(whether from cows, sheep, goats or any other animals) from your diet. You can replace them with soya, oat, rice or any other vegetable substitutes. The important thing is to ditch the dairy.

- Forget the anti-soya propaganda. It is not based on good science! In experiment after experiment, casein (cows' milk protein) has been shown to promote cancer, whereas soya protein has no such effect. Dairy milk contains *dangerous* growth factors *and* animal oestrogen while soya, just like other peas and beans, contains *protective* phyto-oestrogens.
- Some men express concern to me that eating the phyto-oestrogens in soya will feminise them. Man-boobs (gynaecomastia) are far more likely to reflect intake of dietary animal oestrogens or xeno-oestrogens from the environment than eating soya. In all my years of working in China and other oriental countries I did not see a single person with man-boobs there although it is hard to avoid seeing men with them in the UK or US.
- The evidence of the presence of pesticide residues in conventionally produced food continues to mount, as do the beneficial effects of eating organic food, but it should be produced to the standards of and policed by organisations such as the Soil Association.
- It is estimated that only 5 to 6 per cent of our daily calorie intake should be protein, with a maximum intake of about 10 to 11 per cent. Many people in the West consume much more. Too much protein, especially animal protein such as cheese, makes the body too acid, increasing the risk of a range of disease from cancer to osteoporosis. Instead, eat plenty of organic whole-grain cereal foods and other seeds, pulses and nuts as a source of protein.
- The risk of prostate cancer, including metastatic prostate cancer, has been linked to dietary animal-fat intake. Substitute vegetable oils. Extra-virgin cold-pressed oils are excellent for salad dressings, and use them for cooking too.
- Use herbs and spices to flavour food and cut down or cut out salt.
- Use raw cane sugar, molasses, unrefined honey (preferably wild) or maple syrup as sweeteners, rather than refined white sugar or artificial sweeteners.

- Drink freshly made vegetable and fruit juices from organic produce, lots of green tea and some herbal teas made with filtered tap water.
- Finally, remember the Plant Programme is not a hair-shirt regime! The recipes include delicious soups, smoothies, stir fries and curries – even chocolate sorbets – and they are easy to make.

6. THE LIFESTYLE FACTORS

There are important things, in addition to diet, that you can change to help cut your risk of prostate cancer. In this chapter I explain eight lifestyle factors, from strategies for coping with stress to ways of avoiding harmful substances in your environment, to help prevent and treat cancer.

LIFESTYLE FACTOR 1: VITAMINS, MINERALS, SUPPLEMENTS AND FOOD FORTIFICATION

M ost vitamins (A, B complex and folic acid, C, D, E and K) and several minerals, including selenium, zinc and iodine, are considered to protect against cancer, partly because of their antioxidant properties. Zinc, for example, helps to maintain epithelial and tissue integrity and acts as an antioxidant.[1] After iron, zinc is the next most important trace nutrient needed by our bodies,[2] and it is an active participant in maximising the effect of several other antioxidants.[3] It is involved in more than 200 enzymes in the human body and is essential for healing so it is important to have adequate zinc to help recover from surgery, radiotherapy and chemotherapy.

In men its highest concentration in the body is in the prostate gland, suggesting that zinc is particularly important for its proper functioning. Zinc is also involved in cell division, and in the way

IGF-I is controlled. Researchers at the University of Illinois, USA have shown that a complex interactive set of factors are required to ensure that IGF-I activity occurs only when conditions are right for cell growth, and they describe a discrete role for trace nutrients – especially zinc – in regulating IGF-I activity.[4] They have suggested that one of zinc's functions is to help to inactivate IGF-I. Good sources of zinc include crabs, snails and oysters (especially Atlantic oysters) or, if you are a vegan, sesame seeds (best as tahini – a delicious spread made from sesame seed), pumpkin seeds, sunflower seeds or wheat germ.

Research also indicates that selenium may play a crucial role in prostate health. In one trial, men consuming higher concentrations of selenium, 150 mcg/day, had three times less risk of prostate problems than men taking 86 mcg/day. One estimate suggests that the average intake of men in the UK is less than half that. Once again, it is best from natural sources. In addition to seeds and garlic, good sources include wholemeal bread, organic eggs, onions, broccoli and tomato, but I do not eat brazil nuts as a source of selenium for the reasons given on page 203.

A study published in the *Journal of the American Medical Association* asserts that nearly all adult Americans have dietary deficiencies in one or more vitamins and should be taking multivitamin supplements.[5] In the UK it has been suggested that in the last half of the 20th century intakes of vitamin A, iron, iodine, magnesium and potassium were lower than recommended.[6] There is little doubt that levels of essential minerals such as copper, zinc and iodine have fallen in soils and the crops grown on them, while levels of toxic elements such as cadmium have increased as a result of modern intensive agriculture.[7]

Let us look in a bit more detail at why we might have developed deficiencies and what we can do to overcome them without taking man-made vitamin and minerals, using the example of the chemical element iodine. Iodine is called a conservative element because it prefers to stay in water. This means that it is most highly concentrated in the oceans and the main dietary source of iodine is seafood. A hundred years ago fish waste and seaweed were used as fertiliser, but these have now been mostly replaced by inorganic fertilisers, especially rock phosphate, which generally has low iodine content but high levels of the toxic element cadmium. The Soil Association are careful to limit the amounts of cadmium and other toxic substances allowed in rock-phosphate fertiliser for food production, and they ban the use of sewage sludge, which can have high levels of cadmium and other heavy metals. Another reason to eat organic!

To ensure that I have enough iodine I take kelp tablets. All seaweed has high concentrations of iodine and other nutrients, but it can also concentrate pollutants. I therefore try to buy kelp from Iceland, which has a low population, uses only natural geothermal energy, and is further away from most pollutant sources than any other supplier of seaweed I know of. Taking kelp in my diet has improved my skin enormously. If I run out of tablets for any length of time my skin becomes rough, initially around my elbows and knees and the roughness gradually extends over progressively larger areas until I take kelp again, when the roughness retreats.

An extra bonus is that iodine is good for the brain.[8]

Vitamin and mineral pills and cancer

Taking foods such as kelp which have high concentrations of nutrients is helpful, but there can be many problems as a result of taking man-made vitamins and minerals for cancer patients. One of the first experimental and observational studies to show that taking vitamin pills does not help treat cancer involved beta-carotene. In a study beginning in 1985, beta-carotene was included in two large long-term chemo-prevention trials sponsored by the National Cancer Institute in the USA. Previous epidemiological studies had suggested that diets high in beta-carotene (e.g. from carrots) reduced lung cancer incidence. In the trial studies, daily doses of beta-carotene in combination with either vitamin E or vitamin A were administered for several years to tens of thousands of people thought to be at high risk of developing lung cancer. What happened? The rate of lung cancer in those taking the pills increased in both trials![9]

A recent Canadian study also showed that women who took large doses of vitamins and minerals during conventional treatment for breast cancer were more likely to relapse and die than women who did not.[10] The five-year survival rate for patients prescribed vitamin C, beta-carotene, niacin (vitamin B3), zinc, selenium and coenzyme Q10 was 72 per cent, compared with 81 per cent for the control group. Over a ten-year period, those who took large doses of vitamins and minerals were 10 per cent more likely to die. The investigators were surprised with the results, because they were expecting that the patients prescribed vitamin and mineral supplements would have a 25–30 per cent increase in survival rates.

In an editorial article in the *BMJ* in July 2002,[11] consideration of the value of daily doses of multivitamin tablets concluded that regular consumption would probably do no good unless your intake is inadequate as a result of poor diet. The article recommends only folic acid for women before and after conception (but if you eat enough green leafy vegetables – or fruits such as melon – this is unnecessary), and perhaps vitamin D in elderly people. Regarding cancer, the article refers to unexpected results that more people receiving supposedly protective supplements died than people receiving placebos.

The vice chair of the panel of US Preventive Services Task Force has also stated that there is insufficient scientific evidence to support the notion that taking vitamin supplements will prevent cancer. She pointed out that people should strive to eat the healthiest diet possible and that nutrients from supplements may not offer the same benefits that they do when consumed as part of a healthy diet.[12]

In the UK, the Food Standards Agency has suggested that many people could be damaging their health by taking vitamin and mineral supplements in doses that are too high. The agency's expert group on vitamins and minerals spent four years looking at the evidence on the potential harmful effects of taking high doses of 34 vitamins and minerals that can be bought over the counter. It found enough evidence to suggest safe upper levels for eight of them and suggested guidance on 23. It also issued statements on three minerals. Two supplements – namely beta carotene and chromium – were found to have the potential to cause cancer in some people and should be avoided by smokers and those who have been exposed to asbestos. Chromium picolinate supplements may also cause cancer and should be avoided.[13]

Other evidence against taking pills involves zinc, which, as discussed earlier, is crucial for prostate health. Men who took more than 100 mg a day of zinc supplements were found to have more than twice the risk of advanced prostate cancer. These levels are far above the recommended doses. However, in the USA, a significant number of men take zinc supplements higher than the recommended levels, partly because of their supposed benefit in preventing colds. Again the message is clear: DO NOT take man-made vitamin or mineral supplements. Have them as nature intended – as part of a good diet.[14]

Oakley has suggested that as many as 350,000 deaths from coronary heart disease could have been prevented over the last decade in the UK if the government had fortified flour with folic acid when the evidence was first published.[15] According to Reynolds, however, fortifying flour with folic acid understates the potential risks to the nervous system. Experimental studies confirm that folates cause convulsions if the blood-brain barrier is circumvented.[16] I am totally opposed to fortification of our food or water, whether by folic acid or fluoride. It is likely to be driven by some vested-interest group or other, and someone somewhere will be cashing in.

Calcium and vitamin D

Let us look in more detail at how taking mineral substances can adversely affect prostate cancer, using calcium as an example. There is much evidence that vitamin D blocks prostate and breast cancer by several mechanisms, including by interfering with the IGF-I signalling pathways, decreasing cancer-cell proliferation and increasing apoptosis.[17] Vitamin D has been reported to be antiproliferative.[18] It has been suggested that vitamin D compounds help to normalise telomerase activity (*see* Chapter 2).[19] Results from a study on prostate regression in rats provide additional support for these findings. Treatment of the rats with a vitamin-D-like substance caused a marked regression of their tumours. In addition, a significant increase in the number of apoptotic cells was observed in tissue sections from the vitamin-D-treated animals. One type of vitamin D has been shown to delay the rate of increase of serum PSA in a pilot trial involving men with early recurrent prostate cancer after primary therapy with radiation or surgery.[20] Studies of vitamin D on EGF-I and its receptor show a similar relationship, but most of the studies relate to breast cancer.[21]

Calcium, especially in the excessive amounts in dairy milk or in supplements, blocks the activity of vitamin D. Evidence of a dose-response relationship between dairy consumption and prostate cancer noted by Barnard,[22] for example, was suggested partly to reflect the deleterious effect of high-calcium foods on vitamin D balance. Colleen Doyle, director of nutrition and physical activity for the American Cancer Society in Atlanta explains: 'Calcium, especially when it is taken as a supplement, has the ability to suppress the amount of vitamin D that circulates in the blood. Vitamin D is thought to be important in suppressing the growth of prostate cells'.[23]

There is an emerging consensus. Vitamin D is present in small quantities in our food and it has been proved to reduce the incidence of prostate cancer significantly, but its ability to do this is limited by the effects of excessive calcium (and protein) in the diet. This is considered to be one of the important connections between the Western diet with its high levels of dairy and prostate cancer.[24] Dairy milk is loaded with calcium and taking large amounts of calcium, whether as supplements or otherwise, lowers blood levels of the type of circulating vitamin D which prevents cancers.[25] One cannot help wondering how much cancer is being caused by people taking too much calcium as pills or as dairy. More recently vitamin D has been shown to cut the risk of pancreatic cancer by 86 per cent.

Vitamin D forms in the skin under the influence of solar ultraviolet light, so that outdoor exercise wearing light clothing in sunny weather usually enables your body to produce all the vitamin D that it needs. Good food sources include oily fish and eggs, so only vegans living in cold climates or the housebound elderly need consider taking supplements. In the latter case I would recommend the ultra-pure versions of fish-liver oils. Always remember that too much vitamin D is toxic.

Selenium supplements

The only synthetic supplement I have taken since my first diagnosis of cancer 20 years ago is selenium. Selenium is important for thyroid function, immune function generally and as an antioxidant, but its status is often marginal to deficient in UK diets. It works best in conjunction with vitamin E, since both are antioxidants and can increase the production of antibodies by up to thirty times,[26] greatly enhancing the immune response. Although selenium is essential to health, it is required only in minute quantities. Although it is not certain at precisely what level it begins to cause adverse effects, it has been found that doses of 900 micrograms (0.9 mg) per day can make hair and nails fall out and affect the nervous system.[27]

Whole foods not pills

In general, I prefer to eat whole foods because, as I have indicated, problems often arise when we try to separate food into constituent parts. Moreover, taking too much of one or other man-made supplement, can cause a deficiency elsewhere in our diet. For example, taking the trace element molybdenum blocks copper intake. The body knows how to deal with nutrients from natural foods, but may absorb too much or too little from man-made chemical supplements.

Food such as fruit, vegetables and whole grains contain hundreds of antioxidants (and other phytochemicals) and at least some of them work together (i.e. synergistically).[28] The protective effect of a mineral-vitamin-phytochemical-rich diet is best obtained from the consumption of adequate amounts of fruit, vegetables, legumes and whole-grain produce[29] based on a good, well-balanced diet such as that in the Plant Programme. All this was confirmed by a recent report in *New Scientist*.[30] Paul Coates, who is responsible for dietary supplements in the US National Institute of Health, is quoted as saying, 'just because a certain compound in food is beneficial it does not mean that a nutraceutical (with the same chemical compound in it) is.' The article goes on to say 'the advice is simple, stick to foods such as flavanoid rich vegetables and fruit but do not take high dose supplements or fortified foods. Hence fresh or frozen cranberries are recommended rather than cranberry capsules, green tea rather than green tea extract and fresh fruit is recommended rather than vitamin C pills. This is advice every cancer patient needs to take on board, because it seems that they are prey to unscrupulous practitioners selling pills and potions at exorbitant prices, cashing in on their distress. Some people who come to see me have bags full of pills. One man with prostate cancer, who had recently been given a very bad prognosis, had more than twenty preparations he had been told to take. Some were in a lactose (milk sugar) base and some were coloured with E number substances. We agreed to junk them all and he is now doing very well. Save money by not buying unnecessary vitamins, minerals supplements and extracts and spend it instead on the best locally grown organic vegetables and fruit.

The food supplements I use

Unfortunately EU supplement laws introduced in 2005 mean that many favourites have been replaced with synthetic chemical versions manufactured by pharmaceutical companies. Fortunately the supplements I use are still available; they are not man-made synthetic substances: they are foods that are naturally enriched in trace nutrients. I continue to take kelp* to avoid iodine deficiency and also brewer's yeast,* which is a good source of many trace elements such as iron, selenium, chromium and zinc and of B vitamins. These are important if the body is to synthesise important compounds such as co-enzyme Q10, which is essential to the optimal functioning of all cell types and is also an antioxidant.

(Note that brewer's yeast will not cause candida, as some practitioners might try to persuade you. Candida infection reflects overuse of antibiotics, other medications or a diet that is too acid-generating with too much animal protein and white sugar.) I now take balanced omega-3, omega-6 vegetable oils* daily and Seven Seas ultrapure cod-liver oil,* which I store in a cool, dark place. These are all natural, not synthetic, substances. I took tablets containing selenium and vitamins A, C and E when I had active cancer. I always follow manufacturers' instructions.

If you must take man-made minerals, vitamins, supplements or any pharmaceutical products, do ensure that they are not in a lactose matrix and do not contain artificial colouring or flavours.

LIFESTYLE FACTOR 2: FOOD PACKAGING

Food packaging is very important. A recent report on the abundance of chemicals that mimic the female hormone oestrogen, from the authoritative British Institute of Environment and Health (IEH), has suggested that a group of chemicals called

---

* Follow the manufacturer's instructions and do not exceed the recommended amount – the quantity of tablets or oil depends on the brand.

phthalates seriously disrupt reproduction in animals (including damaging the testes in males). Indeed, recent studies have shown that phthalates are strongly implicated in the feminisation of baby boys. Scientific experiments suggest that certain phthalates may also cause cancer.[31] One of the main sources of phthalates identified in the report is soft plastics such as those used to wrap and cover food. The chemicals leak from the plastic into the food, and then accumulate in our body fat. Try whenever possible to buy food in good old-fashioned brown paper bags – be prepared to make a fuss if necessary. One of my friends dumps all plastics wrappings at supermarket tills, although I must say I have never dared go as far as that. If you find it impossible to buy food not pre-packed in plastic, and this is increasingly difficult, try to wash food as thoroughly as possible or in the case of vegetables peel or scrape off the surface which has been most in contact with the plastic. Unfortunately the chemicals concerned are fat soluble so it is best to avoid them if possible since they are difficult to remove by washing. This is of particular concern if you are buying oily foods such as fish. My fishmonger now wraps my fish in paper or foil.

Try to minimise consumption of water or juices sold in plastic bottles and food purchased in cans or wines stored in vats[32] lined with plastics, which can contain the endocrine-disrupting substance bisphenol A. Try to eat fresh or frozen food, and drink wines stored in oak.

LIFESTYLE FACTOR 3: COOKING

Love it or hate it, cooking is an essential part of our diet and lifestyle. In amongst all the aromas and sizzles, it has an effect on the food that can be enhancing or potentially destructive. For instance, it changes starches, proteins and some vitamins into forms that the body can absorb readily as well as releasing nutrients in some foods which are otherwise unavailable – like the amino acid tryptophan in cornmeal. Cooking of some foods is necessary to destroy toxic substances, such as those found in red beans, and cooking also makes some foods more palatable. However, cooking can destroy and leach fragile nutrients in food, although there are ways in which you can reduce this nutrient loss.

The style of cooking recommended in the Plant Programme ensures that fresh, wholesome ingredients are cooked in the healthiest way possible and served as soon as possible. Two very important rules are:

- Never use a microwave cooker, because free radicals are formed in the food
- Never use a pressure cooker, because it destroys vitamins and other important nutrients

Storing food is also important. Melons, citrus fruits and avocados are all best stored at room temperature, rather than in the fridge, and eaten ripe.

Meat

The way meat is cooked is important. My mother and all her generation of British women were taught to cook meat thoroughly, and that meant slowly. For all sorts of reasons, including preventing cancer, I will not now eat undercooked meat under any circumstances. Meat is a poor conductor of heat and if it is not cooked properly hormones in it (whether natural or introduced by man) will not be destroyed. Even if it is well-cooked, steroid hormones such as those used in the USA, may survive.

Cancer-promoting chemicals (heterocyclic amines (HCA), the most abundant of which is known as PhiP) are likely to be formed in burned meat, while cancer-promoting chemicals including hormones will remain intact in the relatively raw meat inside. I never eat meat that could contain ground-up dairy animal, such as hamburger or beef sausages. Remember, official figures show that dairy cow meat contains even more IGF-I than milk. Amounts of HCA range from very low in poached, steamed or stewed meat and fish to very high levels in grilled or barbecued meat. PhiP has been linked to prostate, breast and colon cancer.[33] High levels of HCA also occur in pan-fried meat.[34] Other toxic by-products of interaction between sugars, fats and proteins also form when food is cooked at too high a temperature.[35]

Seafood

It is important to cook seafood in a way that will preserve essential minerals such as iodine. The distinctive chemistry of iodine means that it is easily lost when processing and cooking food. (Chinese people tend to cook fish in sealed containers and use the juices to make soup. This ensures that all the iodine in the fish is consumed.)

Fried food

In the last few years there has been concern about the presence of a potentially cancer-causing chemical called acrylamide in certain foods, especially fried food, including chips and potato crisps. The levels of acrylamide in some foods are compared with the US Environmental Protection Agency (EPA) limit for this chemical in water in Table 6.1.

Research first announced by Swedish scientists in April 2002 and subsequently confirmed by studies in Norway, Switzerland, the UK and the USA shows levels of acrylamide in certain foods well above the WHO guideline values for drinking-water.[36]

Swiss researchers have also reported relatively high levels of the substance in ground roast coffee.[37]

Studies to date suggest that a minimum temperature of 120°C is needed to form acrylamide in food, although the levels increase at temperatures between 140° and 180°C. Scientists have found a

Table 6.1   Levels of acrylamide in foods, in micrograms per serving

Water, 8oz, EPA limit	0.12
Boiled potatoes, 4oz	<3
Taco shells, 3, 1.10z	1
French fries, uncooked, 3oz	5
French fries, baked, 3oz	28
Breakfast cereals, 1oz	6–7
Tortilla chips, 1oz	5
Corn chips, 1oz	11
Potato crisps, 1oz	25
French fries, 5.6–6.2oz, and potato wedges, 6.2, purchased from fast-food outlets	39–82

Data from http://www.cspinet.org/new/200206251.html

ten-fold difference between normal and overcooked chips.[38] Some scientists in North America have suggested that the substance forms at high temperature by interaction of a natural amino-acid called asparagine with certain sugars such as glucose.[39] Experts recommend a diet with plenty of fresh fruit and vegetables to help to counteract the problem.

Increased incidences of tumours have been observed in rats orally exposed to acrylamide. In the USA, levels of acrylamide are highly regulated.[40] The EPA has classified acrylamide as a probable human carcinogen,[41] and it is classified as a substance which may reasonably be anticipated to be a carcinogen by the US Department of Health.

Previously, concern about acrylamide had centred on occupational exposure (i.e. through the skin, or by inhalation of dust or vapour), during its manufacture and use by industry, and environmental exposure.[42] Acrylamide is used in the manufacture of adhesives, dyes, soil-conditioning agents, products for sewage and waste treatment, chemical grouting, the manufacture of non-iron fabrics, crude oil production, the processing of paper and pulp, and some ores and concrete.[43] Some home appliances and parts of cars and other vehicles are coated with acrylamide resin and other acrylics. Acrylamides are also contained in some cosmetics and soaps, in which they act as thickeners, in dental fixtures, hair-grooming preparations and pre-shave lotions.[44] In a report published in 1997, it was stated that no information about the natural occurrence of acrylamide was found in the readily available literature.[45]

All this information tends to suggest that acrylamide might be expected to occur at low levels in the environment in industrialised countries, from man-made sources.[46] It is a water-soluble, rather than fat-soluble, substance,[47] with a high water solubility which increases with temperature.[48]

Despite the statement by the UK Food Standards Agency[49] that frying and baking creates high levels of acrylamide in a wide range of food, the levels could partly reflect environmental pollution. When food is fried, the acrylamide will not be dissolved out into the fat and is likely to become more concentrated in the food as water is lost in cooking. On the other hand, where food is boiled, the highly soluble acrylamide is likely to be lost to the cooking water. My advice remains the same as for avoiding other harmful man-made chemicals in food and drink. Eat as organically as possible, following the methods of preparation and cooking set out in *The Plant Programme*. My advice for avoiding harmful substances generally (*see* pp. 258–75) would seem to apply to acrylamide.

Other cooking methods

I lightly steam vegetables in a stainless steel or bamboo steamer; otherwise I stir-fry lightly after first thoroughly washing and dipping vegetables in boiling water like the Chinese do. Fruit and vegetables should be eaten as raw as possible in order to preserve the vitamins and enzymes they contain. I use only organic extra-virgin olive oil to soften or gently fry vegetables. Any meat I eat is cooked slowly in the oven or under a grill and the fish I eat is just lightly grilled. I also make stewed and curried meat and fish dishes. I add no additional fat or salt to meat or fish, which I cook slowly with herbs or garlic, black pepper or other spices for flavouring. I do not own a microwave and try to avoid food cooked or heated in one. Unlike normal heating, microwaving food works by vibrating water molecules in food. This generates free radicals and I suspect would not destroy as many 'bad' chemicals as ordinary cooking (although I have been unable to find any data on this). There is no comparison between the taste of a jacket potato cooked in the traditional way and the soggy unpleasant-tasting equivalent prepared by microwaving.

Here are some general guidelines:

- If you cook with fat, don't let it become so hot that it starts to smoke. At this temperature the essential fatty acid linoleic acid is destroyed.
- Fats which have been used for cooking once should be discarded since the linoleic acid and vitamins A and C will have been lost; they may have been chemically altered and become potentially carcinogenic.
- If you boil food, steam it instead and do so for the minimum amount of time; then use the water for stock. The fragile water-soluble vitamins as well as some minerals leach into cooking water, which is why soups are so nutritious.
- Don't add bicarbonate of soda to cooking water, even if it is recommended in cookery books for cooking pulses. It destroys B vitamins, and added sodium is not good for cancer patients.

- Prepare food immediately before cooking – remember that vitamin C is destroyed once cells are damaged in vegetables – and for the same reason try not to chop them too finely. Scrubbing vegetables is better than peeling them.
- Once prepared, immerse the vegetables in boiling water straight away before stir-frying.
- Use pans with close-fitting lids and avoid using copper pans which encourage oxidation and vitamin C loss. I do not use non-stick cookware, made with fluorinated chemicals or orange or other highly coloured cookware. I use stainless steel pans and bamboo baskets for steaming.
- Once food is cooked, eat it straight away. Keeping it warm will result in further nutrient loss, which is why eating out too frequently may be less healthy for you.
- Never dehydrate food between plastic sheets.
- Do not store unripe fruit and vegetables in the fridge or vital vitamins will fail to build up. Melons, citrus fruits and avocados are all best stored at room temperature and eaten ripe.

Living dangerously

An amazing number of people I see who have cancer do not cook at all. They simply buy pre-prepared meals from supermarkets and reheat or microwave them. I have no scientific data to prove my theory, but I think this really is living dangerously. The meals in the Plant Programme are all healthy and nutritious and many are very easy to make. Start with a simple soup or curry.

LIFESTYLE FACTOR 4: DEALING WITH STRESS

The stress of coping with cancer

The word 'cancer' is terrifying to most people, and in *Your Life in Your Hands* I described the horror I felt at discovering I had breast cancer. But remember that new medicines have been developed that effectively relieve most of the worst symptoms of cancer, including pain and nausea – including that caused by treatment. Modern treatments for prostate cancer are effective and are given with an increasingly significant chance for a positive response.[50]

In an article entitled 'ABC of psychological medicine: Cancer',[51] White and Macleod point out that cancer is the most feared of diseases and causes considerable psychological distress, including depression and anxiety, in patients and their families, and even in health professionals who care for them. A diagnosis of cancer can precipitate feelings similar to bereavement (it is worth noting that a recent study showed that people who profess stronger spiritual beliefs seem to resolve grief more rapidly than people with no spiritual beliefs[52]). Severe and persistent depressive disorder is up to four times more common in cancer patients than in the general population, and occurs in 10–20 per cent of people affected by the disease. Feeling of loss may be reaction to perceived loss, for example of sexual potency in the case of prostate cancer, the role in family or society, or impending loss of life. Anxiety can manifest itself as apprehension, uncontrollable worry, restlessness, panic attacks, and avoidance of people and of reminders of cancer. Patients may overestimate the risks associated with treatment and the likelihood of a poor outcome. Anxiety may also exacerbate or heighten perceptions of physical symptoms that patients can interpret as cancer symptoms, and post-traumatic-stress symptoms occasionally follow diagnosis or treatment that the patient has found particularly frightening. Certain cancers and treatments are associated with specific fears. For example, patients may develop phobias and conditioned vomiting in relation to treatments such as chemotherapy.[53]

Distress is more likely to occur at specific points in a patient's experience of cancer. These include:[54]

- *Diagnosis*, when doctors should explain that feelings such as shock, anger, disbelief and distress are normal.
- *During treatment*, especially at times when treatment appears to be failing.
- *At the end of treatment*, because of the fear that the cancer might recur.
- *After treatment*, because of fear of recurrence and misinterpretation of symptoms (such as believing that pain associated with a muscle strain represents a recurrence of cancer).
- *Recurrence*. Most patients report recurrence of cancer as more distressing than receiving the initial diagnosis.

The principles of treatment[55] to help such patients involve:

- A clearly identified principal therapist to coordinate care.
- Sympathetic interest and concern.
- Effective symptomatic relief.
- Understanding the patient's concerns and needs.
- Collaborative planning of continuing care.
- Good information and advice.
- Involvement of the patient in treatment decisions.
- Involvement of family and friends.
- Early recognition and treatment of psychological complications.
- Clear arrangements to deal with urgent problems.

Let me turn now to some of the things that I found helpful and those I did not.

The idea that cancer could be cured by thinking positively had always seemed ill-founded to me. One of the particular problems with the 'think positive' approach is that people who do not get better often feel guilty that they are not trying hard enough, and this is sometimes reinforced by well-meaning friends. In the book *You Can Heal Your Life* by Louise Hay, there is a list of diseases and their probable causes. In the case of cancer, the probable cause is given as 'deep hurt, long-standing resentment, deep secret or grief eating away at the self; carrying hatreds; what's the use'. The advice is to develop a new thought pattern as follows: 'I lovingly forgive and release all of the past. I choose to fill my world with joy. I love and approve of myself.' This may be admirable as a general attitude to life, but when it comes to preventing cancer I prefer a more rational approach, based on science.

It has also been claimed that there is a particular personality type that is likely to be affected by breast cancer. Much has been written about the 'cancer personality' especially by Lawrence LeShan, an American psychotherapist. According to LeShan, the typical personality had an emotionally deprived youth, followed by a period of fulfilment in an intense relationship or all-involving work, followed by the loss of that relationship or work at which time the cancer occurs. The other main characteristic is the person's inability to express anger, particularly in their own defence; such a person is often described by others as being like a saint. LeShan believed that this pattern fitted 76 per cent of his patients. This is certainly not a description of me or my life and I cannot think of anyone else I know who has had breast cancer that fits this description!

All carefully controlled research indicates that this theory is wrong. The concept is unhelpful, and again tends to lead to feelings of guilt. As indicated earlier, the problem is one of chemistry and is rooted in the Western diet. The book *Wild Swans* by Jung Chang provides a vivid example of the high levels of stress that Chinese women have suffered in the past, yet they retained low rates of breast cancer except when they have changed to a Western diet.

A recent systematic review of the influence of psychological coping on survival and recurrence in people with cancer[56] supports the view that positive thinking is not key to fighting cancer. It found that most of the studies that investigated fighting spirit or feelings of helplessness or hopelessness found no significant associations with survival or recurrence. The authors conclude that people with cancer should not feel pressured into adopting particular coping styles.

Also some people feel guilt that their cancer is some form of punishment. I certainly felt that, but as I now say in all the many lectures I give cancer is not brought about by a wrathful God. Almost all cancers and certainly prostate cancer have far more rational explanations, as discussed in this book.

Because stress has been implicated as an important factor in cancer generally, people can become worried and hence more stressed by problems so that a vicious circle is set up. Over the last fourteen years I have faced up to some extremely stressful situations in my family life and at work, and yet my cancer has not returned – because fundamentally it was a problem caused by harmful chemicals from my food and the environment causing problems in my body. Now my diet and lifestyle are sound, I cope much better with stress.

Helping yourself cope

However, for your health and general well-being it is helpful to reduce the stress and distress in your life as much as possible and scientific evidence that stress has physiological effects suggests that it is worthwhile working on methods of reducing sources of stress. The chemical changes in the body caused by stress would need a book in themselves. Hormones from the adrenal gland as part of the body's 'fight or flight' mechanism increase the amount of blood sugar available, boost the heart rate and slow down digestive function to enable us to run or fight. Too much for too long, however, can affect the immune system. As mentioned earlier, prolactin levels increase as a result of stress. Other damaging hormones, growth factors and biochemicals that increase under chronic stress include cortisol, noradrenaline, growth hormones, thyroxin testosterone and oestrogen.[57]

When humans are confronted with an important loss or change in their lifestyle – such as a diagnosis of cancer – their emotions are likely to follow a pattern which is well known to counsellors and others trained to help with our emotional well-being. Initially, denial, shock, numbness and grief may be experienced, followed by resistance, gradual acceptance and depression before beginning to let go of the old reality and adjust to the new one. People differ in the intensity of their emotions and the time taken for each part of the cycle. Indeed, faced with a diagnosis of cancer some people simply give up hope and never leave the 'trough of despair'. This can be a particularly serious problem with prostate cancer, I suspect, because of fear of impotence and incontinence. Some people remain in denial, and I receive much correspondence from people intending to refuse conventional medical treatment and simply follow my programme. I always advise against such a course of action in the strongest possible terms.

In my case, when confronted with problems I tend to move to the 'what can be done about it' stage very quickly and of course one of the frustrations with being confronted with a diagnosis of prostate (or breast) cancer is that according to orthodox medicine the answer is, 'nothing'. If you have heart disease you can follow a diet and exercise plan, if you have an infectious illness you can take tablets and rest, but with prostate cancer you are told there is nothing you can do.

I totally disagree with this and with doctors who advise that you simply accept your fate because it will bring peace. On the contrary, you must be empowered to help yourself and, as I have explained, there is a lot you can do to help yourself with crucially important changes in diet and lifestyle. The diet itself, in addition to helping you fight cancer directly, will help your state of mental and emotional well-being by providing greatly improved nutrition.

Several complementary and alternative-medicine treatments have been suggested to improve the well-being of patients with cancer. These include: mind-body programmes for stress; acupuncture or acupressure for nausea; tai chi and other gentle exercise techniques to improve strength; therapeutic massage and relaxation techniques to reduce stress; and herbal medicines for depression and anxiety.[58] Certainly talking therapies can be very helpful.

Dealing with the stress of cancer

Let us look at some of the particular problems associated with coping with prostate cancer, such as incontinence and loss of sexual potency.

Concerns about sexuality are often of very great concern to men with prostate cancer and it is important to discuss worries with partners as well as the patients, because they are affected as well. Partners are usually concerned about how to express their love during and after treatment. Suggestions that may help a man cope better include involving his partner as soon as possible after treatment, openly communicating feelings, needs, and wants, and seeking the support of others.[59] Some marriages and family relationships break down following the wife and mother suffering from breast cancer, and I have heard of many such cases. However, I cannot think of a single case where this has happened with any of the prostate-cancer sufferers who correspond with me or who I talk to.

I shall now try to share with you some of the coping strategies I developed with the help of a wonderful psychotherapist whose help was made available to me by Charing Cross Hospital. It was difficult for me to agree to see her initially because of fear evoked by my childhood memories of the appalling treatment my father had received at the hands of psychiatrists, combined with difficult experiences with my first husband, also a psychiatrist. When I expressed my reservations to her, she quickly reassured me, and promised me that, as a psychotherapist, she would not under any circumstances suggest the use of ECT or drugs.

With her help I was able to come to terms with the loss of my breast. Also she helped me to address and come to terms with problems in my life and personality and reactions. I learned that unresolved feelings of fear, anger and guilt are especially damaging, negative emotions. With her help, I revisited, reinterpreted and finally dealt with events in my past and memories which generated negative emotions. In some cases I wrote to or telephoned people I had not spoken to for years to try to heal unpleasant situations and reduce my emotional baggage. But in some situations this was not possible and the only way to come to terms with the past was to develop a new perspective.

With help, we can do the same with even the most distressing situations. I found psychotherapy helpful even over the few months I worked with my doctor. According to MIND, the mental health charity, psychotherapy may last for several years and is particularly helpful in understanding, and coming to terms with, past events.

With my psychotherapist's help I learned two other coping strategies which I found particularly helpful in dealing with cancer. The first is cognitive therapy. Part of being a creative thinker, which I need to be as an innovative scientist, is that I develop large 'worry castles' from one or two odd bricks. In dealing with cancer it is particularly easy to develop frightening scenarios for the future. Cognitive therapy teaches you to trace the building of the worry castle backwards and stop at the facts. You can then develop a more sensible, rational, less frightening vision. Again according to MIND, cognitive therapy is about learning to think and behave in positive ways. It is a type of behavioural therapy which is helpful in overcoming negative thinking. If you think this would be helpful, ensure that you consult an expert in cognitive therapy, since most GPs have had little training in this field.[60] My psychotherapist also taught me how to be more assertive without being aggressive, which helps one to avoid situations where one is affected by negative emotions. For example, if you calmly but clearly state your concerns or dislikes, many situations that lead to negative emotions can be avoided. There are many excellent books on cognitive therapy and assertive behaviour which are well worth reading.

I have to say that I found counselling of the type based on trying to release pent-up emotions far less helpful than the psychotherapy sessions. The analogy I would use about my counselling sessions is that of a pond in which emotions had settled to the bottom and the water had cleared, and every week I was encouraged to put in a large stick and stir it around until I became upset. Counsellors are trained never to give reassurances and I found that by repeating answers to 'how do you feel about that' or 'what is your worst fear' I was giving my brain only negative feedback and reinforcing my fears. Others I know have found counselling very helpful – it just did not work well for me. Also I tried self-help and support groups but found these made me feel that I was 'wallowing in cancer'. Again, others I know have found attending such groups helpful.

The person I found most helpful was a lady called Peggy Heason who is a hypnotherapist. I found sessions with her extremely helpful. Also, having brought up her children and grandchildren through difficult situations she has so much common sense and she was prepared to reassure me where she could. But above all she was always there for me. She cared for me but she was not so emotionally involved as my own family so she was better able to help me. If you have cancer or any other serious problems in your life, my advice is to find yourself a Peggy Heason.

Basic methods of reducing stress

The basis of most techniques to reduce stress and tension start with relaxation. First, turn off the telephone, doorbell etc. so you will not be interrupted. Then turn off the light or draw the curtains and lie flat (I do this without a pillow – at most use only one) and make sure you are warm and comfortable. Then systematically relax each part of your body beginning with your toes, then your feet, your lower legs, gradually progressing up through the body. Repeat until you feel totally relaxed. This way you relax each bit of you from toe to top. There are several good relaxation tapes based on these methods but Peggy Heason's was the one that I found the best. At the same time I used diaphragm breathing which is very relaxing. When we are anxious we tend to take lots of shallow breaths by breathing using only the ribcage. Diaphragm breathing is a technique to ensure you are using your full lung capacity by using the large muscle called the diaphragm at the base of the lung cavity to suck in and expel air. You simply place your hands on your abdomen and make sure that they go up and down as you breathe in and out. Used with imagery you can accompany your relaxation by imagining yourself walking through a beautiful calm garden listening to the birdsong or walking along a beautiful beach with waves gently crashing on the sand. It is possible to buy tapes to guide you through imagery and relaxation but do listen to them first. I found some voices on tapes that I bought incredibly irritating. It is important to find ones that you enjoy and find helpful, because you will probably use them many times. Many such tapes are readily available from health and new-age shops. Some include affirmations (quiet verbal instructions) and subliminal messages to your body.

I also learned meditation which I still use, and despite being such a simple method, it clears worries out of the mind and allows deep relaxation. I chose the word crystal, and I repeat it continuously in my mind and visualise the crystal sparkling. After a time one feels truly relaxed. I found meditation difficult at first because I am normally a busy-busy sort of person but the technique really does clear my mind and helps me in my work, especially in solving problems. I now find yoga helpful as well. There is a great deal of evidence of the effectiveness of such techniques in reducing stress and the physical symptoms that this creates in the body: for example, several of the methods lower blood pressure.

Another technique sometimes used for cancer patients is visualisation, a technique made famous by the Simontons in the USA. This involves imagining your body killing the cancer, removing the debris and finally visualising situations where you are well and whole again. This is how one of the visions begins: 'Your white blood cells are fish swimming in and eating up the greyish cancer cells. Project this image as if it were on a screen that you're viewing in your mind's eye. When you have that image very clearly then become one of the fish and lead the rest of the pack into the attack. Feel yourself as the fish eating. At the end of each visualisation, imagine yourself engaging in activities you would pursue if you were healthy. Picture yourself at the healthiest time in your life and create images of the present, feeling just that way.' I found visualisation techniques unhelpful but others feel better for using them.

Working with family and friends

What I learned was how important it is that you understand how distressed your family is, if your relationships are to survive cancer. They will all react differently. They are having to come to terms with their own distress, fears and anxieties about your illness as well as helping and supporting you. They have different personalities with different capabilities and methods of coping. I soon learned not to dump my fears, feelings and anxieties onto my family – they were too close and too frightened and upset already and as a family we could quickly enter damaging downward-spiralling emotional situations.

I learned instead to rely on others who cared about me but who were not so close that their fears became amplified and spiralled out of control. I found my women friends, my vicar, my former doctor and Peggy Heason whom I have already mentioned, the best equipped to help me. They knew me well enough to care about me and give me support but there was not the intense emotion that there is in the family. A group of my women friends, all professionals with busy lives, each gave some of their time to take me to hospital and stay with me during radiotherapy and chemotherapy treatments. Somehow they worked together as an efficient team, each giving the help and the time they could spare to provide me with a wonderful cocoon of total care. When they asked me how they could help I managed to shed my typically British reserve and independence and tell them.

Working with your friends is a two-way process and can be so helpful. If you want to do something for a friend with cancer, ask them sincerely how you can help and show that you mean it. All sorts of practical things – doing some shopping, going with them for treatment, means so much at such times.

Some friends simply cannot cope. This is a common experience for cancer patients. Try to understand that these people do care about you; they just do not know how to cope themselves. Do not allow yourself to become bitter. Let them back into your life when they feel able to cope.

Working through

The level of fatigue after cancer treatment is the largest factor in predicting a return to work. Nearly two thirds (64 per cent) of cancer survivors in a study of 235 patients were back at work within 18 months. The duration of sick leave depended on diagnosis, treatment, age, physical complaints and workload.[61]

During my illness, I found it helpful to keep working and I took the minimum of sick leave: for example, four days twice a month when I was on chemotherapy (two days for treatment and the following days to recover from the nausea). This gave me a sense of purpose and took my mind off my problems. Many other friends and colleagues with cancer or with partners with cancer have also found the routine of going to work helpful in coping with the disease. Of course, this depends on the type of work you do, the working environment and your personality, and it requires a supportive boss and colleagues. Friends and colleagues showered me with flowers, messages and cards, and they telephoned me a lot – this type of support can be very important in maintaining morale, although other cancer sufferers prefer just to be left alone.

The right and wrong way

I think that the best way of coping emotionally can be summed up by quoting a friend and former colleague Dr Chris Evans whose wife, Norma, sadly died of cancer in 1995, 'I learnt during the four years that Norma was ill that we all react differently. There is no right or wrong way. There are people out there who can help and people who are going through the same thing. These people can suggest a range of coping strategies but friendship, openness and love are at the heart of most.'

THE BIG DOS AND DON'TS

- Do not believe the old adage 'cancer equals death'. Today, many cancers are curable; others can be controlled for long periods during which new treatments may become available.
- Do not believe that you caused your cancer. There is no evidence linking specific personalities, emotional states or painful life events to the development of cancer.
- Do rely on strategies that helped you solve problems in the past, such as gathering information, talking to others and finding ways to feel in control. Seek help if they don't work.
- Do not feel guilty if you can't keep a 'positive' attitude all the time. Low periods will occur, no matter how good you are at coping. There is no evidence that these periods have a negative effect on your health. If they become too frequent or severe, though, seek help.

- Do use support and self-help groups if they make you feel better. Leave any that make you feel worse. A list of support groups and other such resources you can call on are listed at the end of the book. I have recently launched a website with my friend Laura Jones that helps people find the latest information about anti-cancer diets and lifestyles. It also has a forum that enables people to offer help and support to each other, which has many contributions about prostate cancer. The address is www.cancersupportinternational.com.

- Do not be embarrassed to seek counsel from a mental-health professional. It is a sign of strength, not weakness, and it may help you to tolerate your symptoms and treatments better. I recommend against pills for anxiety wherever possible. I am still suffering the after-effects of such treatment after nearly fourteen years (see further under sleeplessness). My book about this dreadful experience written with psychologist Janet Stephenson will be published shortly.[62]

- Do use any methods that aid you in gaining control over your emotions, such as meditation and relaxation.

- Do find a doctor of whom you can ask questions and with whom you feel mutual respect and trust. Insist on being a partner with him or her in your treatment. Ask what side effects to expect and be prepared for them. Anticipating problems often makes them easier to handle if they occur.

- Do not keep your worries to yourself. If the person closest to you can cope, involve them. If they find it difficult you may need to involve a group of friends so each can give you some support. If all else fails, phone the Samaritans and talk to them of your fears. Ask a close friend to accompany you to visits to the doctor when treatments are to be discussed. Research shows that you often don't hear or absorb information when you are very anxious: a second person will help you to interpret what was said.

- Do explore spiritual and religious beliefs and practices that may have helped you in the past. They may comfort you and even help you find meaning in the experience of illness.

- Do not abandon your treatment in favour of an alternative method, especially those which make no sense and are irrational. But do change your diet and lifestyle in the ways described here to help you to overcome your disease and withstand treatment.[63]

LIFESTYLE FACTOR 5: SLEEPLESSNESS AND FATIGUE

One of the common problems of cancer sufferers is that of sleeplessness. Almost fourteen years on, I am still affected by this problem. In my case, it was probably made worse by the strong tranquillisers I was prescribed to make me sleep when it was thought that I was terminally ill.[64]

Alternative techniques for helping people to sleep include herbal substances, but I have found these to be ineffective.

Methods I have found to be helpful include the use of acupressure cones, which can be bought from high-street chemists and applied to the acupuncture sleep points on the wrists as shown in the accompanying leaflets. One tip is to buy travel bands instead, since, unlike the cones, they can be re-used many times. They work on the same principle as the cones, but are intended for use on different acupuncture points on the wrists, to prevent nausea. I use them with the studs placed on the sleep pressure points, which saves money and reduces using yet more plastic.

I listen to self-hypnosis tapes, available widely in bookstores and health food shops. I also find it calming to have a bowl of organic porridge with a little soya milk before going to bed (though this may not be suitable for those with a gluten allergy); oats were the traditional treatment for hyperactivity in children and are still used by herbalists to help overcome benzodiazepine and valium addiction, alcoholism and some other types of drug addiction.[65]

LIFESTYLE FACTOR 6: AVOIDING HARMFUL SUBSTANCES IN YOUR ENVIRONMENT

Cancer cells are relatively big, and when they spread they usually get trapped in the first network of capillaries (the very fine blood vessels that take blood to and from all the tissues in our bodies) that they encounter downstream of their origin. The first highly vascularised organ encountered by blood leaving most organs in our bodies is the lung, except in the case of the intestine from which the blood supply goes to the liver first. Thus the organs to protect from secondary tumours are the lungs and liver. Protecting the pelvic bones and other bones is particularly important in the case of prostate cancer.

The effects of exposure to harmful chemicals depends on the dose, the duration, how and when you are exposed and the presence of other chemicals. The main task of the lungs is to exchange 'old blood' containing carbon dioxide created by body processes for 'new blood' invigorated with fresh oxygen. They can cope with some dust, particles and bad chemicals but if you overwhelm them with harmful chemicals (for example from tobacco smoke or if you live in a city environment where the air usually contains high levels of car, aeroplane and other exhausts containing benzene, a potent cancer-causing agent, as well as many other cancer-causing agents) they are far more likely to become diseased with primary lung cancer. Also, they are far less likely to be able to fight against invading cancer cells trying to establish secondary tumours.

The liver is an amazing organ, responsible for eliminating poisonous chemicals from the body, including those produced by the body's own metabolism, as well as manufacturing all sorts of important enzymes and other chemicals essential for the body to function. The liver detoxifies the system and produces anti-cancer chemicals. My strategy was, and continues to be, to have as many good nutritious substances as possible to help my liver to help me and to keep it as unburdened as possible with pollutants in my food, applied to my skin or inhaled.

One of the main sources of pollutants to try to eliminate is tobacco smoke. It is estimated that smoking tobacco causes approximately 30 per cent of all cancers in the USA alone. Smoking tobacco not only causes cancer in the lungs but is also implicated in many other types of cancer.

One study, which focused on men younger than age 65, calculated that, even after taking account of ethnicity and prostate cancer in close relatives, the risk of prostate cancer increases by 40 per cent when men smoke. The effects are worse in heavy smokers who have smoked for a long time. For example, smoking two packs a day for 20 years was found to double a man's risk of aggressive prostate cancer – but if he had given up smoking for ten years before 40 years of age, he was no more likely to develop prostate cancer than if he had never smoked.[66]

Oliver and others[67] found, in contrast, that men with prostate cancer were more likely to report a lifetime history of non-smoking, while other studies have also no association, either positive or negative, between smoking and prostate cancer.[68] Oliver and others conclude that the effects of smoking on prostate cancer are unclear when studied in isolation from other factors.[69] I find it hard to believe that smoking is such a key factor in prostate-cancer risk, since many Chinese men smoke so heavily and prostate cancer rates in China are so low. On the other hand, cigarettes contain a lot of cadmium, which is a carcinogen and seems to make testosterone more dangerous in its effects on the prostate gland.[70] It is also an endocrine-disrupter and is particularly damaging to bones,[71] which need to be specially protected in prostate cancer. Other authors have also indicated that there is a positive association between smoking history and IGF-I level.[72]

I think it sensible to try not to smoke, and to avoid passive smoking. If people ask you if you mind if they smoke in your presence, just say 'yes'. If you smoke and are addicted to nicotine and find it difficult to give up, you can reduce your risks by having nicotine as patches or by chewing nicotine-impregnated gum – it is the tar in tobacco which contains the powerful cancer-causing agents, not the nicotine.

I am now going to tell you about some other damaging chemicals in the environment before advising you on how to cut your exposure to them. The concentration of many of them, especially the endocrine-disrupting chemicals, can actually be measured by their effects on cancer cell cultures. Many are persistent and fat soluble and bioaccumulate up the food chain, becoming especially concentrated in milk and oily fish.

CANCER HAZARD: POLYCYCLIC AROMATIC HYDROCARBONS (PAHs)

Because so many combustion processes favour production of PAHs, they can be abundant in the environment from sources such as engine exhausts, cigarette smoke, grilled food, and coal and wood smoke. Coal tars and petroleum residues such as road and roofing asphalt and many con-taminated land sites such as old gas works also have high levels of PAHs.

They deserve special attention because as well as acting as endocrine-disrupting chemicals (EDCs, see p. 264) some of them cause cancer in other ways. They have particularly sinister chemical properties in the body, because as the liver tries to eliminate them their oxidised metabolites can react chemically and become permanently inserted into the structure of DNA, introducing mistakes into it. It is this property that makes some of the PAHs so carcinogenic.

The complicated name of this group of chemicals refers to the fact that they comprise more than one ring of carbon atoms. Benzene is the basic single ring structure of six carbon atoms, each with one hydrogen atom attached. It is itself a very powerful carcinogen. PAHs are built up from this basic unit. Some PAHs, including benzo(a)pyrene, the molecules of which comprise an arrangement of five benzene rings and which is concentrated in tobacco smoke, are well known to be the precursors of cancer-causing metabolites.

There are special regulations for the use of benzene in laboratories, in order to meet Health and Safety requirements, so it always strikes me as strange that we are allowed to be exposed to this dangerous chemical every time we fill our cars with petrol or walk down the street and breathe in car exhaust fumes.[73] Typical tests on exhaust fumes from cars show that they emit about 10 mg of benzene for every kilometre travelled.[74]

CANCER HAZARD: DIOXINS

The major source of dioxin in the environment (95 per cent) used to come from incinerators burning chlorinated wastes. Dioxin is formed as an unintentional by-product of many other industrial processes involving chlorine, such as chemical and pesticide manufacturing, pulp and paper bleaching, and the production of Polyvinyl Chloride (PVC) plastics. Dioxin is the primary toxic component of Agent Orange, and was one of the main contaminants at Love Canal, New York. It was the cause of the evacuation at Seveso, Italy, and the Bhopal disaster in India.

Dioxin is a general term that describes a group of hundreds of chemicals that are highly persistent in the environment. The most toxic compound is 2,3,7,8-tetra-chlorodibenzo-p-dioxin or TCDD. The name dioxin is also used for the family of structurally and chemically related polychlorinated dibenzo-para-dioxins (PCDDs), polychlorinated dibenzofurans (PCDFs) and certain polychlorinated biphenyls

(PCBs). Some 419 types of dioxin-related compounds have been identified but only about 30 are considered to have significant toxicity, with TCDD being the most toxic.[75]

TCDD dioxin is, in fact, one of the most toxic chemicals known. According to the September 1994 report of the US Environmental Protection Agency (EPA), not only does there appear to be no 'safe' level of exposure to dioxin, but levels of dioxin and dioxin-like chemicals have been found in the general US population that are 'at or near levels associated with adverse health effects'. The EPA report confirmed that dioxin is a cancer hazard to people; that exposure to dioxin can also cause severe reproductive and developmental problems (at levels 100 times lower than those associated with its cancer-causing effects); and that it can cause immune system damage and interfere with regulatory hormones so that it is an EDC.

Chronic exposure of animals to dioxins has resulted in several types of cancer. The IARC (International Agency for Research on Cancer) announced in February 1997 that the most potent dioxin, 2,3,7,8-TCDD, is now considered a Class 1 carcinogen.

Dioxin is fat-soluble and bioaccumulates up the food chain; it is found mainly (97.5 per cent) in meat and dairy products.[76] The North American intake based on a total exposure of 119 pg (picograms)/day is as follows: dairy products and milk, 34 per cent; beef 32 per cent; chicken 11 per cent; pork 11 per cent; fish 7 per cent and eggs 3 per cent. Milk in the UK also contains dioxins and PCBs.[77]

Extensive stores of waste industrial oils with high levels of dioxins exist throughout the world. Long-term storage of this material may result in releases into the environment and the contamination of human and animal food supplies. Dioxins are not easily disposed of, and incineration at temperatures above 850°C remains the best available method, with temperatures above 1,000°C required for large amounts. Further information on dioxin is available on several websites, including those of the WWF, the WHO and the US EPA.

CANCER HAZARD: POLYCHLORINATED
BIPHENYLS (PCBs)

The abbreviation PCB refers to polychlorinated biphenyls, a family of man-made chemicals that contains 209 individual compounds of varying toxicity. Commercial formulations of PCBs enter the environment as mixtures consisting of a variety of PCBs and impurities. They have very high chemical, thermal and biological stability and low vapour pressure, and are good electrical insulators and fire retardants. Between the 1930s and 1970s these properties led to their widespread use as coolant-insulation fluids in transformers and capacitors; for the impregnation of cotton and asbestos; as plasticisers; and as additives to some epoxy paints. The same properties that made the extraordinarily stable PCBs so useful also contributed to their widespread dispersion and accumulation in the environment. The manufacture of PCBs was discontinued in the US and their uses and disposal were strictly controlled after 1976.

It has been estimated that since 1929 a total of 1.2 million tons of PCBs have been manufactured,[78] of which 31 per cent (370,000 tons) has so far escaped into the environment. However, 780,000 tons of PCBs are still in use in transformers and capacitors or have been sent to landfills. Thus the amount that could potentially be released into the environment is approximately twice that already released.

PCBs enter the body through contaminated food and air and through skin contact. They are particularly enriched in fatty food, including milk.[79] Fish have been implicated, but a survey of fish products reported in 1997 indicated that fish-liver oils contained higher concentrations of PCBs and dioxins than fish-body oils, so fish is safer than fish oils – though it is now possible to buy purified oils with greatly reduced levels.[80] Exposure from drinking water is minimal.

It is known that nearly everyone has PCBs in their bodies, including infants who drink breast milk containing PCBs.[81] Animal experiments have shown that some PCB mixtures produce adverse health effects, including liver damage, skin irritations, reproductive and development effects and cancer. Some PCBs cause mutations in cells and they are endocrine disrupters (*see* p. 264).

While the risk of PCBs in producing cancer in humans cannot be clearly defined, the available evidence provides a basis for concern.

The FDA specifies PCB concentration limits of 0.2 to 3 parts per million (milligrams PCB per kilogram of food) in infant foods, eggs, milk (in milk fat), and poultry (fat). The American EPA guideline for drinking water ranges from 0.005 to 0.5 micrograms of PCBs per litre of water, which is associated with the risk of a person developing cancer of between one in 10,000,000 and one in 100,000.

In Britain, levels of PCBs in soils peaked in the late 1960s but have now fallen to 1940s levels, and between 1982 and 1992 the estimated UK dietary intake of PCBs declined significantly.[82] Disposal of PCBs from discarded electrical equipment and other sources remains a problem.

CANCER HAZARD: ENDOCRINE DISRUPTING CHEMICALS (EDCs)

One of the ways in which many pollutants are now implicated in causing cancer is in the way they have been shown to mimic hormones or otherwise disrupt the endocrine system, so they are called endocrine disrupting chemicals (EDCs). Because prostate cancer, along with testicular cancer, is considered to be a hormone-dependent cancer, EDCs are of particular significance to its prevention and treatment.

Since the term 'endocrine disruptor' was first introduced by Theo Colborn in 1993, EDCs have received a great deal of attention; the media often describe them as 'gender benders'. Following Colborn's work it was realised that a lot of man-made chemicals that are manufactured in large quantities and to which we are exposed in consumer items and through the environment might be implicated in many health problems including cancer.

EDCs are defined by the UK Environment Agency as 'naturally occurring or synthetic substances that interfere with the functioning of hormone systems resulting in unnatural responses'.[83] They cause problems, including by (1) mimicking the natural hormone and producing a similar response by the cell, (2) binding to cell receptors and preventing a normal response and (3) interfering with the way natural hormones and receptors behave. Perhaps of most concern is the evidence that EDCs or their breakdown products can directly damage DNA to alter the cell cycle, affect repair processes, or interfere with cell-to-cell signalling – all processes implicated in the initiation of cancer.

Concern about this group of chemicals has mushroomed since 2000. The concern reflects: (1) the discovery that a range of widely used man-made chemicals, including substances used in detergents, herbicides, pesticides, plastics, the female contraceptive pill, hormone replacement pills and by-products of other industrial and waste-disposal processes, to which we are exposed daily, can act as EDCs[84] (127 pesticides have recently been suggested to be EDCs[85]); (2) hypothetical links to an increase in disorders of reproductive development and function in the human male and in some species of wildlife;[86] and (3) the striking coincidence between human exposure to these chemicals and the increase in prevalence of a range of hormone-dependent human reproductive cancers (prostate, breast, endometrial, testicular and ovarian). Some of the substances have been used for a considerable length of time in household and personal-care products and even in the manufacture of children's toys and teething rings. One particularly powerful EDC, NPE, has been used in the formulation of many herbicides and insecticides used to spray on food crops. Bisphenol A (BPA), an oestrogenic EDC, can leach from the plastics used to line tin cans and even from some types of composite dental fillings.[87] Countries around the world are phasing out the use of many of these substances of concern.[88]

In addition to oestrogen-mimicking substances, EDCs include chemicals that are thought to block oestrogen, mimic or block testosterone and other androgens (male hormones) and possibly also mimic or block thyroid hormones. Most people now have body burdens of EDCs similar to those that cause abnormalities in other vertebrates.[89] Proving a causal link between EDCs and cancer is difficult for many reasons, including the multifactorial nature of the disease and differences in the duration and intensity of exposure. Despite these difficulties, evidence is accumulating from laboratory animal, wildlife and human studies that exposure to EDCs can promote hormone-dependant cancers.[90] Case-control studies, for example, have found that breast cancer risk is increased in women with high body burdens of organochlorine pesticides.[91] Organochlorines have also been shown to alter tumour-suppressor genes *in vitro*, promoting the growth of prostate-cancer cells as well as breast-cancer and ovarian-cancer cells.[92]

There are now many sources of information on EDCs. For example, a new database (REDIPED), launched in 2002 by the Department for Environment, Food and Rural Affairs in the UK, provides information on 79 confirmed or suspected EDCs.

Recent advances in molecular biology demonstrate that the hormones used by vertebrates all have a similar structure.[93] Because EDCs are related to hormones, an infinitesimal quantity can have a significant effect.[94] Indeed, recent evidence suggests that extremely low doses of EDCs can have effects as damaging as higher doses.[95] Male frogs suffer from conditions such as undescended testes and even hermaphrodism when exposed early in their development to tiny doses(1–2 parts per billion) of a commonly used herbicide called atrazine. Some persistent EDCs can accumulate in the body and be passed from one generation to the next.

Some researchers have suggested that xeno-oestrogens are unlikely to cause harm because we are already exposed to phyto-oestrogens. Humans and their pre-human ancestors have been eating phyto-oestrogens for millions of years, however, whereas most xeno-oestrogens have been around for, at the most, a few decades. Moreover bioaccumulative persistent xeno-oestrogens and other endocrine disrupters accumulate in body tissues to much higher levels than phyto-oestrogens.[96] All of the epidemiological and other research I have read suggests that phyto-oestrogens are protective while xeno-oestrogens are potentially very harmful.

HARMFUL SUBSTANCES AND PROSTATE CANCER
Several studies indicate an increased risk of prostate cancer associated with exposure of farmers and pesticide applicators to pesticides. One study showed that several organo-chlorine

pesticides, a pyrethroid and a fungicide all caused proliferation of human prostate cancer, and considerable evidence links exposure to endocrine-disrupting chemicals in the environment, especially where exposure occurs on foetuses and baby boys. BPA has been shown to cause enlargement of the prostate in laboratory animals exposed as foetuses to low levels of this substance. Cadmium and arsenic have been linked to prostate cancer; the evidence is particularly strong for cadmium. High risks have also been found in those exposed to metallic dusts, metal-working fluids, PAHs and liquid-fuel combustion products.[97]

SOME OTHER HAZARDOUS ENVIRONMENTAL CHEMICALS

The occurrence of pharmaceuticals in the environment and the extent to which they pose a risk to the environment and humankind has also received considerable attention since the early 1990s. An initial risk assessment for the UK,[98] of more than sixty compounds thought to account for more than half of the known tonnage of pharmaceutical consumption, suggested that the substances of most concern were paracetamol/acetminophen, aspirin and dextropropoxyphene (pain killers), fluoxetine (antidepressant), oxytetracycline (antibiotic), propranolol (for heart disease and migraine), aminotriptyline (for neuralgia) and thioridazine (for adult schizophrenia).

Recently the United States Geological Survey carried out the first nation-wide reconnaissance of the occurrence of pharmaceuticals, hormones and other organic contaminants in water.[99] The most frequently detected compounds were coprostanol (faecal steroid), cholesterol (plant and animal steroid), N,N-diethyltoluamide (insect repellent), caffeine (stimulant), triclosan (disinfectant), tri(2-chloroethyl)phosphate (fire retardant) and 4-nonylphenol (detergent breakdown product). More than one of the contaminants was commonly detected in samples, and there were as many as 38 in some samples. Little is known about the potential interactive effects that occur from such complex mixtures and their breakdown products and their overall effect on human health and the environment.

Other monitoring programmes in Europe and the Americas have detected pain-killers, cholesterol regulators, antiseptics, chemotherapy agents, antibiotics and hormones in water.[100] One of the problems is that conventional sewage-treatment technologies vary greatly in their ability to remove drug residues and, in some instances, have even been shown to increase the bioactivity of the pharmaceutical residues.[101] Activated carbon filtration, which is used by some states in the USA, continues to be one of the most effective known methods of removing drug and other contaminant residues from drinking water. Please see the section on Food Factor 8 'What to Drink' in Chapter 5, to reduce your risk of taking in harmful substances through your drinking water.

HARMFUL GASEOUS SUBSTANCES
Brominated flame retardants (BFRs), widely used for fire proofing everything from televisions and computers to carpets and curtains, are now known to be persistent, bioaccumulating and toxic – and have been detected in human breast-milk samples![102] Harmful gaseous substances are increasingly of concern in buildings and vehicles. The Hamburg Environment Institute has analysed gaseous emissions from household and office appliances such as computer mice and mobile phones.[103] They have also tested carpets and wallpaper. Their study identified a hundred compounds emitted from the products tested, including carcinogens and EDCs. Volatile organic compounds can reach particularly high levels in new cars.[104] A useful leaflet entitled *Volatile organic compounds (including formaldehyde) in the home* has been posted on the website of the UK Institute for Environment and Health.[105]

The problem of synthetic chemicals in food, air and water has not been helped by the fact that many doctors take little or no interest in the environment and they often do not know much about the chemicals used in industry, agriculture or even in the home environment, or their effects. For example, an article in the October 1999 issue of the *BMJ* implied that crop yields would go on increasing, but there was no mention of the input of chemicals that this would require.[106] Nor was there any mention of the pesticides and other chemicals that have been used in order to achieve the increase in yield in the past. I have served on committees and attended many meetings concerned with the environment and health. Usually all the environmentalists sit through the presentations given by medical specialists. However, the doctors used to leave before any of the papers on the environment were presented (we now mix the papers in sessions to prevent this happening). Thank goodness for doctors such as Professor A J McMichael at the London School of Health and Tropical Hygiene, author of the book *Planetary Overload*,[107] who has developed a broader vision of the causes of ill health related to the environment – including as a result of industrialisation of agriculture – and pollution.

According to a report entitled 'Chemicals in the European Environment: Low Doses, High Stakes', published by the European Environment Agency (EEA) and the United Nations Environment Programme (UNEP) in 1999, there are now many thousands of (man-made) chemicals on the market, and little is known about their fate or their impact on people or the environment. Monitoring of some of these substances is required by law in the US and Europe, but only a few. Moreover, since much of the monitoring involves analysis of water samples and the compounds of concern are generally not water-soluble, the monitoring schemes are likely to underestimate their true impact and presence in the environment. The Royal Commission on Environmental Pollution's Report 24 'Chemicals in products: safeguarding the environment and human health' takes this further and states that 'ignorance outweighs knowledge at every stage in our understanding of synthetic chemicals'. Recently Professor Sir Richard Peto, co-author with Doll of the now notorious 1981 paper that discussed risk from pesticides, pronounced in an article in the *Independent* newspaper that links between chemicals in the environment and breast cancer are 'rubbish'. Mmm! What did the Royal Commission say about ignorance and chemicals?

Some chemicals, such as pesticides, are released into the environment deliberately. Other releases have been an unfortunate side effect of the use of substances by the manufacturing industry. In addition, harmful organic chemicals have accumulated in the environment because of energy generation, especially the combustion of fossil fuels. Some chemical releases have caused major incidents, for example the release of dioxins at Love Canal in Niagara Falls, New York and Seveso, Italy – but contamination is usually a more insidious process.

As discussed in Chapter 4, dairy milk contains testosterone, oestrogen and progesterone. These chemicals can cause severe biological damage, even very low levels. One illustration of this was the problem caused by the effects of a chemical called tributyl tin (TBT) on dog whelks on Britain's south coast. The chemical was developed for use in paint to coat the underside of ships to prevent 'fouling' or the growth of creatures such as barnacles that increase friction and thus slow down ships and boats. The levels of TBT in water were only about five parts in a millionth of a million of seawater and were barely detectable. Nevertheless, in the 1980s, over a wide area of Britain's south coast where minute traces of the chemical occurred, female dog whelks died when their egg tubes became blocked by their own eggs because they had developed male organs which had overgrown their female organs. It is difficult to comprehend that such an infinitesimal amount of a substance could, in the open sea, have such a profound effect: but it did. Unfortunately, the chemical is still licensed for use in larger ships including those used by the British Navy. Interestingly, TBT's mode of action is thought to be by blocking the conversion of testosterone to oestrogen in organisms because it inhibits aromatase. Aromatase inhibitors are now being widely prescribed for breast cancer, and I have yet to meet an oncologist who has heard of the damage caused by TBT.

Let me quickly summarise how I and many other earth and environmental scientists see the situation.

Life on Earth has evolved in a complex interrelationship with the environment for at least 3,500 million years. Modern man, whose body chemistry has developed over that period of biological evolution, has appeared in the last ten-thousandth of the planet's history (equivalent to the last ten seconds on the 24-hour clock). In the past fifty years or so (much less than a fraction of a second on the 24-hour clock) we have set about dramatically changing the types and proportions of chemical molecules in the environment.

In particular, we have reconfigured organic chemicals, which were the basis of all life, into new 'organic' substances to use in industry and industrialised agriculture. Some of the new 'organic' substances, which range from plastics to pesticides, their by-products or their metabolites are the antithesis of life. The genes that code for the molecules that make up our hormone systems that help control our bodies such as testosterone and oestrogen evolved as long as 550 million years ago.[108] Some of the new chemicals and their by-products are implicated in causing cancer. Chemicals which disrupt the endocrine system whereby chemical messengers or hormones control our physiological function are of particular concern in hormone-dependent cancers such as those of the prostate.

Making sense of it all – the practicalities

Here is some practical advice to cut down your individual exposure to such chemicals and that of society more generally, although it is impossible to do this completely. Indeed, many of the chemicals of concern are distributed across the globe and are even found in the blubber of seals and other creatures at the polar regions.

My advice is to have as few man-made chemicals in your life as possible. Never use perfumed soap, aftershave, deodorant or similar products. Most women I know find highly perfumed men a joke! I recently read the label on some expensive shower gel marketed by a prestigious company, to find that it actually listed phthalates – one of the main groups of endocrine disrupters implicated in the feminisation of fish – among the chemicals it contained. Moreover, research by Professor John Sumpter of Brunel University, London, now suggests that parabens could be an EDC (see p. 264).[109] With cosmetics, as with all other products, read the label, and remember: the simpler and more old-fashioned the better. As a 1960s teenager, I cannot be without my make-up, but I buy hypoallergenic products which are unperfumed and generally contain less damaging chemicals.

I do not add chemicals other than simple salts such as Epsom salts to my bath water. Even familiar man-made chemicals are often eventually shown to cause problems. A report in the magazine *Nature* suggests that a commonly used anti-bacterial agent, Triclosan, may work by causing mutations in bacteria.[110] Triclosan is used in many antibacterial soaps, lotions, mouthwash, toothpaste, plastic toys, socks and cutting boards. I prefer to use good, old-fashioned simple soap which will bind with dirt, fat-soluble chemicals and 'germs' and wash them away.

I do not use chemicals to stay young artificially. Some doctors in America and at some London clinics are reportedly providing their patients with human growth hormone to prevent ageing! A study published in the *BMJ* in 1998 reported that high natural levels of this hormone could lead to premature death from cancer. Growth hormones available to athletes and body builders must also be of concern.

Many other cancer-causing agents have been identified, mainly as a result of occupational exposure to high levels of particular chemical substances – by, for example, factory workers, painters and decorators, and hairdressers. Some of the most dangerous chemicals implicated include benzene (used in the manufacture of some furniture and rubber and emitted from some types of fresh paint and car exhausts); formaldehyde (often used as a preservative for example on fabrics in new cars, clothes and furnishing and in some cosmetics and shampoos) and hair dyes.[111] It has been shown that golf-course superintendents in the USA have increased mortality from prostate cancer, non-Hodgkin's lymphoma and cancer of the brain. The increase in these diseases was related to their exposure to pesticides.[112]

Avoid dark-coloured hair dyes, some of which contain chemicals suggested to cause cancer when applied directly to the scalp. Anyway, men with grey hair usually look much more distinguished than those with dyed hair. I do not know why, but most women I know think men with dyed hair ridiculous (although it's OK for us women to dye our hair!). Discuss with your hairdresser any chemicals they use on your hair and ensure that they have checked the information on their carcinogenicity.

One of the alternative therapies I question as a treatment for cancer is aromatherapy, especially if you are undergoing chemotherapy. Your liver already has a massive job to do to clear out all the unwanted chemicals and dead cells and other debris from the treatment without having to deal with other powerful chemicals. The skin is the body's largest organ and a proportion of many of the things we put on it are absorbed into the bloodstream.

In aromatherapy a carrier oil such as almond oil (thought not to be absorbed by the skin) is used as a base and an essential oil which normally evaporates (and has molecules that can pass through the skin) is added to achieve particular effects. Some of the oils absorbed through the skin are concentrated extracts of powerful chemicals. Many people wrongly believe that because the essential oils used in aromatherapy are extracted from plants and flowers they cannot be harmful, despite being delivered in high concentrations through the skin. In nature they are at low concentrations as part of a total fruit, flower or leaf. Many of the 'essential' oils have never been tested scientifically for their side effects, but medical research has shown that camphor, hyssop and sage oils can have such serious side effects as causing fits. Limonene – the lemon-smelling aromatherapy oil – is known to be capable of causing kidney damage. Basil oil, which is said to lift mood, and tarragon oil also contain a chemical called estrogole which causes cancer in rodents. Dr Sharon Hopkiss of the Department of Pharmacology and Toxicology at St Mary's Hospital Medical School in London has been quoted as saying that many oils used in aromatherapy are extremely potent natural agents.

Remember that the characteristic smell of a new car reflects the fact that it is emitting nasty chemicals such as plasticisers and brominated flame retardents. If you have a new car, make sure it is well ventilated when you use it. The only car I drive is an old Land Rover of 1973 vintage with an engine converted to use lead-free petrol. If anything goes wrong we simply buy a new part and put it in. Any volatile organic chemicals used in manufacture or sprayed on its interior will long since have evaporated. Even so, I try to use it as little as possible and to travel by public transport. The chemicals emitted by cars, even when well tuned and running optimally, include many hazardous substances such as benzene (*see* John Pearson's book *The Air Quality Challenge*).

If you paint your house or have it painted, ensure it is well ventilated (some of the oil-based paints used in Britain are now banned in Scandinavia). Remember that new furniture, curtains and upholstery can be important sources of toxic chemical fumes, including BFRs. Vinyl chlorides (PVCs) should also be avoided as much as possible. In an article in *The Times* of 11 November 1999 by Martin Fletcher, it was reported that the European Commission had called for an emergency ban on soft PVC toys, including rattles and dummies which babies suck, because they contained dangerous chemicals – phthalates again.

Be careful of gardening chemicals. If some plant in your garden is going to die, so be it. Feed it with composted household waste to help it survive but I minimise any use of chemicals around the house or in the garden. My garden has lots of different wild bird species, butterflies, ladybirds, toads and hedgehogs. The degree of biodiversity in my garden compared to those of many friends who use chemicals says a great deal about the damage our use of chemicals does to the animals, so why do we think that we will be unaffected? We have already discussed problems associated with pesticides implicated in reproductive cancers generally. To avoid irresponsible use of chemicals in the environment, I never buy or give cut flowers. It is much better to give a garden plant. In my garden, Susan's rose, Eileen's buddleia and Georgina's astilbe bloom, reminding me of them every year. Many organophosphates, well known to be damaging to the central nervous system, are now known to be EDCs. Aside from sheep dip and shampoos to kill headlice, many familiar products are based on these substances, including many insecticides, sprays and treatments for lice or fleas on pets including flea collars. Avoid all such products, and never use aerosol sprays for hair, deodorants, cleaning, gardening or any other purpose because of the increased risk of inhaling man-made chemicals. Evidence has recently emerged of the high levels of EDCs that we can be exposed to in cabin air when flying.[113]

Pesticides are also widely used in some leisure industries. Golf courses, for example, are often kept looking perfect as a result of using large quantities of killer chemicals including herbicides, insecticides and rodenticides to kill moles. Try to persuade any facilities you use that you would prefer less visual perfection in return for less use of toxic chemicals.

Use wood, glass, ceramics and natural mineral materials in the home, stainless steel, enamel or toughened glass for cooking, and aluminium foil to wrap food. Whenever possible, use natural materials for clothing and furnishing, with as few plastics or man-made fibres or other chemicals in your life as possible. Always wash and thoroughly rinse new clothes before wearing them to remove preservatives. Minimise the use of detergents and ensure they are thoroughly rinsed from crockery and clothes before use. Ideally, use the ecofriendly varieties. You might find it strange that someone who has spent her professional career working as a geochemist should try so hard to avoid chemicals in everyday life. Like many of my colleagues, I have a healthy respect for what chemicals can do to biological processes and so try to minimise my exposure.

If you have good, nutritious food and reduce exposure to pollutants, you will find your skin and general appearance improves without the need to add polluting man-made chemicals to your body or the environment. We can all reduce our personal risk from hazardous chemicals, and by doing so we help the environment generally, with cleaner air, water and soils and hence more wholesome food. To most natural scientists this is all just common sense.

So, whenever you read or hear a new advertisement for a new 'personal care' product, man-made fabric or garden spray, for example, think very carefully whether you really need it. Almost certainly you do not. People who avoid such products are frequently portrayed as odd especially by those wishing to sell us products that we do not need in order to make money. No one looking at me, spending time with me or visiting my home would think I was a crank. Unless pointed out to them they probably would not notice anything is missing or different. Indeed, people comment on how normal I am (presumably despite being a scientist)!

There is additional information on hazardous chemicals at www.cancersupportinternational.com.

LIFESTYLE FACTOR 7: EXERCISE

Outdoor exercise in daylight, which increases levels of a particularly beneficial form of vitamin D, may be helpful against prostate cancer, and other forms of gentle exercise, especially some types of yoga or tai chi, may be helpful in coping with stress and building strength.

LIFESTYLE FACTOR 8: SEXUAL ACTIVITY

Prostate cancer affects a gland that is under the control of male hormones, suggesting the possibility of a relationship between the disease and the levels of male hormones in the blood and sexual activity. Evidence for this includes findings that patients with prostate cancer have an increased likelihood of having had a sexually transmitted disease, to have had more sexual partners and possibly to have a greater libido than men without prostate cancer. This study, 20 years ago, involved only a small number of people, but more evidence emerged in 2001 confirming the possible link between sex and prostate cancer, linking numbers of partners and lack of condom use with an increased risk of prostate cancer. Circulating levels of the male hormone testosterone have been measured in patients with prostate cancer and compared with levels in patients with normal prostates and those with BPH. Recent evidence suggests slightly higher levels of testosterone in prostate-cancer patients than in healthy men.[114]

Personally, from the many men I know affected by prostate cancer I think it most unlikely that promiscuity is a factor, unless a viral infection is involved and they have just been unlucky, as in the case of cervical cancer in women – though documenting the sexual behaviour of others is notoriously difficult! There is also contrary evidence that a higher risk of prostate cancer is associated with a lack of sexual activity. One study reported that men who ejaculated most in their twenties, thirties and forties had about a third less prostate cancer risk than men in the lowest category of ejaculation. In the absence of a sexual partner, masturbation was recommended.[115]

I suspect that if sexual activity influences prostate health at all it is a relatively minor factor compared with diet and other lifestyle factors such as exposure to harmful chemicals.

AWAY FROM HOME

All of the factors described in Chapters 5 and 6 are easy to control in your own surroundings. I travel a lot internationally and here are a few tips to help you maintain the Plant Programme while on your travels.

1. When travelling, allow plenty of time for every aspect of the journey. Do not allow yourself to become stressed or upset by delays. If flying, try to fly at night to cut your exposure to cosmic radiation.

2. Count out the number of kelp, brewer's yeast and red clover tablets to cover your entire time away, prepare small bottles of your oils and take a small pot of dried soya milk (normally sold in cans for babies and infants). Take herbal tea bags and enough fruit to see you through until you can find a local supply.

3. When flying, ensure you order a vegan meal and check that the travel agent uses the code VGML, as other codes can include dairy. Drink lots of boiled water flavoured with your own herbal tea bags to avoid dehydration. Drink beer to make you sleepy.

4. Travel only on 'No Smoking' flights or in 'No Smoking' train compartments.

5. When you arrive at your destination, locate the nearest fruit and vegetable stall or shop and buy fresh supplies daily. In many countries these must be washed in boiling water before eating. This is really a brief immersion (use the hotel sink) similar to the blanching process used in cooking.

6. Before you travel, look up key words in a dictionary and jot them down in the language of the country you will be visiting. For example, in France 'soya' is 'soja': having a small number of ready-translated words to hand is very helpful. Ask your hotel where to buy the items you need using the written version if necessary. There will usually be a supermarket near your hotel where you can buy supplies, including beer, and thus avoid using the hotel's expensive minibar.

7. Research the local cuisine and check which dishes you will be able to eat without problem or fuss.

8. Tell everyone you are terribly allergic to dairy produce and insist that you have none at all. (I have found this is most difficult in France.) If all else fails you can remove the cheese, or scrape off the yoghurt or cream etc. – I do so ostentatiously!

9. Be inventive in avoiding dairy produce. For example, at the breakfast buffet use prune or other fruit juice to moisten your cereal.

10. If you have trouble sleeping in a different time zone, camomile is soothing and beer usually makes me sleepy.

CHAPTER 6 IN A NUTSHELL

- Scientific evidence shows there can be many problems as a result of taking man-made vitamins and minerals for cancer patients. Instead use supplements, naturally enriched in trace nutrients such as kelp and brewer's yeast but most importantly have a healthy diet.

- Harmful chemicals can leak from plastic wrappings into the food, and then accumulate in our body fat. Try whenever possible to buy food in good old-fashioned brown paper bags.

- Learn to cook and prepare healthy nutritious meals such as those in *The Plant Programme* or *Eating for Better Health*.

- It is helpful to reduce stress as much as possible because scientific evidence indicates that it can have physiological effects. Methods of reducing stress include meditation, relaxation and visualisation and in some cases cancer patients require professional help from a counsellor or psychologist.

- Try not to punish yourself. Some people feel that their cancer is some form of punishment but cancer is not brought about by a wrathful God. Almost all cancers and certainly prostate cancer have far more rational explanations, as discussed in this book.

- The problem of chemicals in consumer products and as contaminants in food, air and water is not helped by the fact that many doctors take little or no interest in such chemicals or their effects. So learn how to cut down your exposure for yourself.

- Outdoor exercise in daylight increases levels of a beneficial form of vitamin D that helps protect against prostate cancer; other forms of gentle exercise, such as yoga or tai chi, may be helpful in coping with stress.

- If sexual activity influences prostate health it seems likely to be a relatively minor factor compared with diet and other lifestyle factors such as exposure to harmful chemicals.

7. WHY ARE OUR LIVES IN OUR OWN HANDS? TEN SIMPLE GUIDELINES

I am convinced that our lives really are in our own hands. Much of the advice given to us, even from some government sources and charities, cannot be regarded as reliable, because of the overwhelming influence of vested-interest groups such as the food and pharmaceutical industries. We must, therefore, rely on ourselves and our own efforts in safeguarding our health, and try to distinguish objective, unbiased information based on good science from data biased by commercial or political interests. This chapter gives some advice on how to do this and concludes with ten simple guidelines.

As I wrote in the first edition of *Your Life in Your Hands*, much of the scientific evidence presented here has been widely known for decades by scientists around the world, so why have we, the public, not been told? Let us look first at dietary factors.

According to Campbell, scientists know an enormous amount about the links between nutrition and health but the real science has been buried beneath a clutter of junk science, fad diets and food industry propaganda. Many elements of the Western diet, such as the high levels of saturated fats and cholesterol in dairy products and meats, have been known to cause disease for decades. In 1961 the results of the seminal Framingham study in the USA showed clearly that cardiovascular disease did not reflect the heart wearing out, as previously thought; it reflected instead high intakes of animal fats in the diet.[1] (These findings have been confirmed time and time again, and it has even been shown that heart disease can be reversed using diet alone.[2]) Yet this has not been clearly communicated to the public, who, instead of being helped to change their diet and lifestyle, have been treated with a succession of pills and potions, many with unfortunate side effects.

In presenting the results of the China study, which I discussed in Chapter 3, Campbell and Junshi showed that even small intakes of food of animal origin are associated with significant increases in chronic degenerative diseases, including several types of cancer.[3] These findings are confirmed by all the research results into prostate cancer, breast cancer and osteoporosis that I have studied over the last fourteen years and published in a series of books.[4] Campbell and Junshi noted that in the West, reduction in fat consumption was being achieved by using lower-fat foods e.g. low-fat dairy foods, while their central fruit-vegetable-cereal recommendation appeared to have received little attention. Concerned by this distortion of their important message, the scientists speculated that pressure from food-industry lobbying groups influenced both the media (and hence the public) and also policymakers.

According to an article entitled 'Food industry obfuscates healthy eating message'[5] this practice continues to the present day. The article describes how food giants are still going to enormous lengths to obfuscate US government messages on healthy eating. To counteract this problem, one US-based organisation is now sponsoring 'Clean Science in Regulation' to explore how to establish a proper relationship between an independent scientific community and the business community. The centre wants to prevent regulated industries from attacking and discrediting valid scientific information, and to examine bias in the membership of advisory committees and conflicts of interest in the sponsorship of scientific studies. Dr Marion Nestle of the Department of Food and Nutrition Studies, New York University, sums up the situation: 'Food is big business, $1.3 trillion ... and the food industry will do everything to make sure that no regulatory agency and no nutritionist ever suggests eating less . . . and what [we] should eat less of'.

Recently the food industry in the USA has been accused of generating a 'toxic food environment',[6] dominated as it is by animal products, refined cereals and chemical concoctions that bear little resemblance to natural food.[7] Americans are increasingly sick, despite having the highest per capita spending on health care of any country in the world. An amazing two thirds are overweight and over 15 million have diabetes, and America has the highest rate of prostate cancer in the world.

Let us look in more detail at the role of the food industry in marketing food that is damaging to health, using the dairy industry as an example.

DAIRY IN THE DOCK

As discussed in Chapter 4 and *Eating for Better Health*, in addition to the overwhelming evidence that dairy products are implicated in prostate, testicular, breast and ovarian cancer and osteoporosis, dairy is associated with a very wide range of diseases, including serious infectious illness. Industrialisation of the dairy industry has made matters worse. Cows are kept in large industrialised units, in which they are fed concentrates rather being allowed to graze naturally, and they continue to be milked when they are pregnant. To quote from the *Sunday Times*, 'In reality, the modern high-yield dairy cow is a pitiful ramshackle embodiment of market-driven exploitation. The new UK model, so help us, is the American Holstein battery cow. A shed-housed fermentation vat on legs, teats dragging on the ground, it's a sight to frighten children'.[8] The article includes a photograph of 'a large-uddered milker, one of the grotesque products of the modern dairy industry'. The article goes on to point out that farmers have not been able to resist the genetic promise (of developing such creatures) – a 2 per cent compound increase in milk yield annually.

In the UK, the industry has been immensely damaging to our economy, including tourism, as a result of BSE, which was mainly a disease of dairy, not beef, cows, the foot-and-mouth crisis of 2001, and more recently bovine tuberculosis. Milk makes up 14 per cent of EU agricultural output and the annual turnover in the dairy-processing sector is about 117 billion euros.[9] Yet it continues to be heavily subsidised under the European Common Agricultural Policy. In fact, the EU's support for dairy farmers amounts to around £11 billion per year, which works out as about £1.40 per day for each cow. Put another way, the average EU cow now receives more than the income of half the world's population. Dairy is big business, with the total value of milk production in the UK estimated at £2.7 billion, 3 times the value of the production of fresh vegetables.[10]

Concerns about marketing cows' milk to replace breast feeding have been around for many years. The late Dr Benjamin Spock, in *Baby and Child Care* (the United States' best selling book, other than the Bible, over the past fifty years), after recommending that no one consume cows' milk and cataloguing a host of ills associated with milk consumption (heart disease, cancer, obesity, antibiotic residue, iron deficiency, asthma, ear infections, skin conditions, stomach aches, bloating and diarrhoea*), concludes: 'In nature, animals do not drink milk after infancy, and that is the normal pattern for humans, too ... Children stay in better calcium balance when their protein comes from plant sources.' Dr Spock recommends human mother's milk for baby humans.[11]

Dr Spock's book has been hugely influential. A great deal of his advice has been followed conscientiously by parents in America and all round the world. Why has his simple advice on milk not been followed equally conscientiously? And why has it taken about fifty years since Dr Spock's book was published for the UK Department of Health to endorse the resolution passed at the World Health Assembly in May 2001 that babies should be exclusively breast fed for the first six months of life?[12]

One of the reasons action has taken so long is perhaps illustrated by the example of the recent prosecution of SMA Nutrition, part of Wyeth, one of the world's biggest manufacturers of infant formula milk. This company was fined and ordered to pay legal costs after being convicted of six separate breaches of illegal advertising direct to consumers. In what is thought to be the first case of its kind, the judge described the company's breaches as 'cynical and deliberate ...'[13]

---

* Other scientists link type 1 diabetes to the consumption of cows' milk by babies and infants, especially genetically susceptible children.

The insidious ways that milk has been marketed to us are outlined by Butler.[14] She describes, for example, how school milk has been central to the promotion of dairy, most recently through the School Milk Project (TSMP) funded by the Milk Development Council. Dr Peter Atkins of Durham University has reviewed the motivation behind the introduction of cows' milk in schools early in the twentieth century. He concludes that the nutritional benefits were debatable, possibly even negative where dairy replaced other foods, but the dairy industry did well for itself creating new markets at a time of depression.[15] Free school milk continued until 1971 when Margaret Thatcher withdrew school milk on economic grounds. The emotional argument that followed and the nickname 'Thatcher, Thatcher milk snatcher' is a warning to anyone acting against the interests of the powerful dairy industry lobby.

I have certainly come under strong personal attack for my anti-dairy advice. For example, 'Jane Plant's statements are truly unfortunate. A study describing a single case history, particularly when it is the author's own, is scientifically unacceptable and lacks any objectivity', says Gregory D. Miller, PhD, FACN, vice president of nutrition research for (guess who!) the US National Dairy Council. He continues 'There is no scientific evidence . . .'[16] those of us in the UK know how little statements beginning 'There is no scientific evidence . . .' mean after the problems with BSE and new variant CJD that we have experienced.[17] What the US National Dairy Council website attacking *Your Life in Your Hands* totally fails to mention is that it contains more than 600 references, mostly from the peer-reviewed literature, medical textbooks and websites such as those of the WHO. I have become accustomed to such arm-waving attacks which are deliberately misleading. As an experienced scientist, I am quite prepared to listen to specific facts that are wrong and to change my book accordingly. In the seven years since it was first published I have received no such comments.

As well as attacks on my work, there have been several attempts to buy me off. The latest, amazingly in the presence of my lawyer, was an offer by a probiotics (or yoghurt) company mediated by the head of a well-known cancer charity to persuade me that 'probiotics were not such a bad food after all'. In return for changing my position I would be given funding for my new website. Of course I was not prepared to accept such an offer and we left, indeed we swept out of the meeting immediately.

But back to the attacks, the study most frequently quoted against my books and in favour of the health benefits of dairy products is the Harvard Nurses' Health Study (HNHS), which purported to show the benefits of dairy products.

Dr RM Kradjian, Chief of the Breast Surgery Division, Seton Medical Center, California, in his book *Save Yourself from Breast Cancer*,[18] has much to say about the Harvard study in relation to breast cancer. In Appendix 1 of his book, he strongly criticises the methodology of the study, documenting several serious flaws in the scientific methodology. He concludes:

> When one carefully dissects this report, it is revealed as a very peculiar piece of work. The problem is that very few physicians, American women, or members of the press seem to have read the article in close detail; nor did more than a handful apparently read the twelve pages of remarkable supplementary material. They were apparently comforted by the names – Harvard, National Institutes of Health, and the American Cancer Society – and looked no further.

He himself discourages all use of cows' milk and all other dairy products. He notes that human beings are the only mammals on earth that continue to drink milk after weaning. 'Despite the fact that milk drinking is widespread among Westernised people, it is a truly bizarre habit.' Appendix 2 of his book is entitled 'Research Funding: an incentive for bias'. The first question is 'Who sponsored the Harvard Nurses' breast cancer study?'

> At issue is the funding of university studies and university researchers by interested food-industry groups. Such funding could clearly result in pressure on those investigators to deliver conclusions that are acceptable to the sponsors, should the investigators hope to continue receiving funds from those sponsors.

Much of the following section of the Appendix describes how he repeatedly contacted the Freedom of Information Office at the (US) National Institute of Health, but was unable to obtain an answer to the simple question 'Is the food industry involved in the funding of the Harvard Nurses' Health Study?' After a year of persistent probing, he had received 'only a verbal acknowledgement from one of the authors that the dairy industry is involved in "some part of the study"'.

There are several other papers that purport to show that there is no relationship between dairy and cancer or, worse, that dairy is protective. All the ones that I have read were funded by the dairy lobby. A recent example, funded by the UK dairy industry, a paper by Patricia G Moorman and Paul D Terry entitled 'Consumption of Dairy Produce and the Risk of Breast Cancer', has been used to send out the message, through a host of magazines, that dairy is not linked to cancer. Some of the many flaws in the paper are discussed on the website www.cancersupportinternational.com.

In *Your Life in Your Hands* I warned about the consequences of the privatisation of science. The *Sunday Times* article I quoted above in relation to the dairy industry makes the same point:[19]

> Of course, commercial science will look to where it's paid. 'CLA research was actually got going by the American meat and dairy industry', says Dr Campbell [Dr T. Colin Campbell, one of the most eminent dietary epidemiologists in the world], 'and it's very depressing when people start looking into little components of this and that. Let's face it, if dairy products contained all the good things that fruit and vegetables do, we'd be tired of hearing about them by now.'

In the UK, until recently, one of our main cancer-treatment centres defended consuming dairy produce. The leaflet 'After Treatment', produced by the Royal Marsden Hospital and issued to a breast-cancer sufferer in 2002, dismissed dietary therapy and claimed that there was no scientific evidence to support exclusion of dairy products from the diet. Clearly the authors of the leaflet have not read the extensive scientific reviews such as those by Outwater and others[20] and the European Commission[21] or the more recent review by Yu and Rohan[22] or the many, many other scientific references cited in my books.

Many people find it difficult to reconcile the advice given by me and others such as Kradjian with the conflicting advice given by their own doctors, nurses and dieticians. I thought this was mainly just the conservatism of the profession, but according to one source,[23]

> The **dairy industry** has a powerful hold on the nutrition industry in this country [the USA]; it **pays huge numbers of dieticians, doctors, and researchers to push dairy**, spending more than $300 million annually, just at the national level, to retain a market for its products. **The dairy industry has infiltrated schools, bought off sports stars, celebrities, and politicians, pushing all the while an agenda based on profit, rather than public health** [my bold].

My book with Gill Tidey on osteoporosis came under fierce attack in a review published in Science in Parliament.[24] Here is an extract from our response[25] which I think sums up the situation.

> Our osteoporosis book is based on more than 450 references mainly from peer-reviewed sources and includes seven dietary and eight lifestyle factors so we are always suspicious when someone seizes on the non-dairy message. In the case of the lead reviewer of our book, Susan A New, her university website indicates that her PhD was funded by a 'nutritional consultative panel UK dairy industry scholarship'. Our response also notes New's consistent track record in raising significant research income. Moreover in 2001 she was awarded the silver medal of the (UK) Nutrition Society, where a senior officer recently confirmed that their funding was from publications, grants and fees for membership – and their membership includes mainly representatives of the food, feed and pharmaceutical industries.

R.M. Kradjian, head of the breast surgery division, Seton Medical Centre Calfornia,[26] draws attention to the problem of science funded by vested interest. He states, 'the issue is clear. Much of our highly varied, desired and profitable food supply has been found to be dangerous. The people who furnish this food and who are enriched by its sale do not want you to know this. They have generously contributed to scientists who have supported and are willing to continue to support their products.'

In their response[27] to our criticism of their biased review, New and her co-author stated 'We entirely refute Plant and Tidey's inference that our views have been influenced by any political conflict of interest, which we have always disclosed.' Unfortunately, there was no such disclosure in their review of our book on osteoporosis!

In contrast to the findings of scientists in receipt of funding and honours from the dairy industry, leading non-aligned nutritional scientists generally agree that osteoporosis is linked to high dairy consumption (Chapter 4). To quote John Robbins, author of *Diet for a New America*,

> The National Dairy Council has spent tens of millions of dollars to make us think that osteoporosis can be prevented by drinking more milk and eating more dairy products. But the only research that even begins to suggest that the consumption of dairy products might be helpful has been paid for by the National Dairy Council itself.[28]

Let me finish this section with some extracts from reviews of *Your Life in Your Hands* posted on the Amazon.com website. One reviewer, a physician, writes: 'This book is a must read for any breast cancer activist and any health care professional who treats breast cancer in women. It is surprising that the book has not gotten more publicity and attention. I suspect the American dairy industry may have had something to do with that.'

A second writes: 'No wonder the dairy industry hates this book. Others have said this book is as important as Rachel Carson's "Silent Spring". I agree.'

Cheese is junk food: official

In the UK there are some signs of improvement in the information given to the public, especially from the FSA under its new director Dame Deidre Hutton. New labelling of foods according to the amount of saturated fat, salt and sugar they contain mean that several dairy products will be given a red traffic-light symbol to warn of the high levels of saturated fat they contain. Also, since they are now formally classed as junk food, they will not be allowed to be advertised on television at times when children might be watching. So there have been some successes against the dairy lobby.

The Empire fights back and drops the D word

A recent article noting the growing anti-dairy lobby, especially in the UK, described how the industry intended to fight back with the help of a supermarket chain.[29] Certainly, there seem to be endless dairy advertisements, and cheese and cream are extensively used in TV cooking programmes despite their designation as junk foods. Even so-called quality newspapers such as *The Times* have recently produced biased, poorly researched articles[30] assuring us that dairy is safe based on information from the official-sounding British Nutrition Federation – which is in fact funded by the Dairy Council, Dairy Crest, Kraft Foods and Nestle UK.[31] Dairy is now sold as functional food often with no mention that it contains dairy. For example yoghurt has been renamed 'probiotics' and no one mentions milk or dairy in any of the advertisements promoting the stuff. Even *ICON*, the magazine aimed at telling cancer sufferers the latest research findings about cancer, carries advertisements for probiotics without mentioning the D word.[32]

FRUITFUL ORGANIC ARGUMENTS AND THE POISON WITHIN

It is unfortunate that the Food Standards Agency in the past and the Advertising Standards Agency did not pursue the claims of the Dairy Council with the same vigour that they applied against organic food producers.

Why, for example was the UK Dairy Council allowed to make claims that 'A natural fat [CLAs] found in milk, cheese, yoghurts and butter may soon prove to contain anti-cancer properties', when, as the *Sunday Times* article (*see* p. 285) points out, 'the proportion of CLAs is only 1 in 120 parts of saturated fat; ergo, to come by a significant amount of CLAs, you'd have to eat artery-choking amounts of the fat stuff'?[33]

In Chapter 5 I have argued that one of the best ways of limiting the ingestion of toxic man-made substances is by eating organically grown food, ideally produced locally to the standards of the Soil Association.

FALSE CLAIMS[34]
Last year [2001], in an attempt to clamp down on false and misleading claims, the Advertising Standards Authority (ASA) issued guidelines for advertisers on claims about organic food. This was prompted by several complaints received by the ASA about organic claims made by well-known names, including Tesco and the Soil Association. The new guidelines state that:

- Advertisers can't claim that organic food is 'safer' or 'healthier' than conventional food, unless they have convincing evidence that this is the case.
- Organic food can't be described as 'environmentally friendly' or 'sustainable', as all managed food production systems cause some environmental damage.
- Claims that organic food uses no chemicals, pesticides or artificial additives can only be made if this is the case.

The following is an edited extract of an article in *Which?* magazine,[35] discussing the advantages of organically produced food:

One of the most common reasons our shoppers gave for choosing organic food was to avoid pesticides. Organic standards allow the use of some approved pesticides but these are mostly from natural sources. There's little data on pesticide residue levels in organic food, but the government's pesticide residue monitoring programme (see *Which?*, September 2001, p24) includes a limited number of organic samples, and residues are rarely found in those tested ... Processing can significantly reduce the levels of residues. Washing and peeling alone has been shown to reduce levels by 50 to 90 per cent in apples, carrots and potatoes. Cooking and other types of processing involving heat can reduce levels further ...

Also, by restricting the use of artificial fertilisers and pesticides, organic farmers and agricultural workers reduce the risk of harmful health effects to themselves as well as the risk of environmental damage associated with more intensive pesticide use.

Organic food can contain food additives (E numbers) and processing aids, but the list is more restricted – around 35 additives are approved, compared with hundreds in conventional food. Artificial sweeteners are banned and only natural flavourings and colourings are allowed ...

In spite of all the evidence to the contrary, the UK government took action, mainly through the Food Standards Agency, to argue that there are no health benefits to eating organically produced foods. The following is an edited extract from another article in *Which?*[36]

The health benefits of eating fruit and vegetables are clear. The government wants us to eat at least five portions a day. To encourage this the Department of Health has introduced the National School Fruit Scheme, with the aim that, by 2004, all schoolchildren aged four to six will be receiving a piece of free fruit daily.

But fruit and vegetables tested still contain pesticide residues. Although most residues fall within legal safety levels, figures show 72 per cent of apples and 81 per cent of pears have residues. And, in December [2001] it was reported that 61 per cent of grapes and 63 per cent of kiwi fruit contained toxic chemicals. Exposure to pesticides may be linked to increasing cancer rates and other health problems – young children, in particular, may be more vulnerable ...

With these concerns, you'd expect the current and long-standing advice to wash and peel fruit as 'a sensible additional precaution when preparing fruit for small children' to be emphasised or improved. Instead, the FSA wants to ditch the advice because its 'misinterpretation' could imply that 'only organic fruit should be supplied to the National School Fruit Scheme' – according to a leaked memo ...

Which? thought that the FSA approach wasn't good enough and asked the government to be more transparent about its motives.

According to an article in the *Daily Mail*, John Krebs, the former head of the FSA, was particularly sceptical about the value of organic food, and under his direction the Agency faced claims that it was biased against organic agriculture. Since Dame Deirdre Hutton took over, the FSA has funded a lecture by Lord Melchett on behalf of the Soil Association about the benefits of organic food, introduced a simple but effective traffic-light system to indicate food containing high levels of fat, salt or sugar, and classified cheese and other dairy products such as Greek yoghurt as junk food. The FSA website on organic farming and food now states: 'Organic farming is a holistic approach to food production, making use of crop rotation, environmental management and good animal husbandry to control pests and diseases. Processed organic foods use ingredients that are produced organically and organically produced ingredients must make up at least 95% of the food. There are only a limited number of additives used in organic food production. Some key aspects of organic farming are:

1. restricted use of artificial fertilisers or pesticides.
2. emphasis on animal welfare, and prevention of ill health, including stocking densities, free range, choice of suitable breeds.
3. use of conventional veterinary medicines is focussed on treating sick animals.
4. emphasis on soil health and maintaining this through application of manure, compost and crop rotation.'

My faith in the FSA has increased greatly since Dame Deirdre took over.

But what can possibly be wrong with the organic farming movement. All their stated aims seem to make so much sense. Who could possibly oppose such a movement at a time when there is so much talk of sustainability? Once again one has to look at who stands to lose out if we all buy organic. Who has a vested interest in portraying all those of us who back the organic movement as emotional unscientific crackpots? Could it be the pesticide industry – an industry worth millions of dollars a year in the USA alone? Might it be that this industry also tries to subvert the truth and to influence some scientists to act on its behalf?

On 8 December 2006 many scientists were shocked to read an email that claimed that, since the late 1970s, Professor Sir Richard Doll had been in receipt of large sums of money from pesticide manufacturers. The mail and the various newspaper articles that appeared at the time included a copy of a letter sent to Sir Richard by George Roush, director of Monsanto's medicine and environmental health department, on 29 April 1986 that read as follows

> Dear Sir Richard
> This letter is for the purpose of extending your Consulting Agreement with Monsanto Company dated May 10 1979. The consulting agreement is hereby extended for an additional one-year period beginning June 1 1986 and ending May 31, 1987.
> During the one year period of this extension your consulting fee shall be $1,500 per day. All other terms and conditions of the Consulting Agreement of May 10 1979 shall remain in effect during this extension period.
> If the foregoing meets with your understanding and approval please so indicate by executing this letter in duplicate and returning one of the signed duplicates to us.
> Yours etc

It has been suggested that Doll donated the money he received to Green College Oxford. Nevertheless, it would have been wise to declare such a serious conflict of interest, especially in the much-quoted paper entitled 'The causes of cancer' published in 1981, only two years after Doll's Monsanto consultancy began. In the paper, pesticides and other chemicals in the environment were said to be responsible for only 1–2 per cent of cancers. Recent re-examination of the Doll and Peto study suggests that it was seriously flawed and that it totally underestimated the numbers of cancers that could be prevented by better regulation of chemicals in the environment. A review of environmental and occupational causes of cancer published in 2005[37] states that it is difficult to estimate the impact of Doll and Peto's views especially by those who argue that cleaning up the environment is not going to make much difference to cancer rates. They go on to trace how the Doll and Peto study influenced other scientists, governments and cancer organisations to put relatively little emphasis on pollution compared to tobacco smoking and other personal lifestyle choices. This approach, they suggest, is still hampering the USA from implementing a comprehensive policy on chemicals regulation such as that being introduced in the European Union from 2007 known as REACH.

Of course I would not accuse Sir Richard of dishonesty nor even of bias, but it is worth pondering what would have happened if he had investigated links between pesticides and cancer with the same vigour and intensity that, as a young man, he had brought to bear on investigating the links between tobacco and smoking. It is also worth pondering how many cancers might have been prevented had chemicals been better regulated earlier.

As discussed in Chapters 4 and 5, there are increasing numbers of studies that now link cancer to endocrine-disrupting chemicals – which include many pesticide formulations. For more information on links between cancer and harmful substances in the environment you might wish to visit www.cancersupportinternational.com.

TECHNOLOGICAL MEDICINE

A doctor friend of mine describes the UK's National Health Service as the 'National Illness Service'. He is right to do so. In my own subject of environmental chemistry the whole approach would be regarded as an outdated 'end-of-pipe' solution. This approach is now discredited in favour of using a full-life-cycle analysis to avoid problems at all stages, from raw-material extraction, refining and manufacturing to end-of-life disposal of products and beneficial after-use of land.[38] In medicine, such an approach would involve placing far more emphasis on prevention, where prevention means giving people clear, truthful, readily understandable information about healthy diet and lifestyle, and becoming involved in limiting the use of cancer-causing chemicals especially in food production.

Doctors and nutrition

Very few of my friends who are medical professionals seem to know much about food chemistry, and I have often seen consultants and junior doctors at busy hospitals eating junk food themselves. The fact that many doctors do not eat healthy diets suggests they do not know the importance of good nutrition. Moreover, most doctors seem unaware of the links between the food we consume, the chemicals in our environment, and prostate (and breast) cancer. Instead, much of their knowledge is based on the literature they are bombarded with about new drugs and procedures. I think it is unrealistic to expect clinical doctors to root out all of the scientific literature on prostate cancer, but surely doctors' training could be improved. My son is now a doctor, and so I am aware how full the curriculum is, but far more proper science and far less sociology would be my prescription for producing better doctors.

Many people express concern about how little doctors know about nutrition. Why do some recommend their patients not to take soya? Do they not know that, in common with other peas and beans, it contains phyto-oestrogens which are protective against cancer? Why do many doctors fail to advise against consuming dairy, which is packed with dangerous growth factors and animal hormones such as oestrogen up to a thousand times more powerful than phyto-oestrogens? Why do many doctors recommend dairy and calcium supplements, when leading researchers at Harvard showed more than 20 years ago that such concentrated sources of calcium suppress a form of vitamin D that is vital for the immune system to protect against cancer and to protect our bones against osteoporosis? I am afraid that the answer is ignorance of the scientific literature.

Doctors and cancer prevention

Unfortunately in conventional medicine, 'prevention' seems to equate to 'early detection' – a battery of screening tests, a considerable proportion of which involve using ionising radiation or the injection of potentially harmful chemicals.[39]

According to Professor Waxman, from whose book *The Prostate Cancer Book*[40] I have quoted extensively in Chapter 1, there are three forms of cancer research:

- laboratory research to establish the molecular basis for disease from the study and analysis of cells and tumour samples,
- pharmaceutical research, carried out by the pharmaceutical industry to develop new treatments for cancer, and
- clinical research.

But what about epidemiology, diet, nutrition, lifestyle, environmental pollutants and other hazards? In other words, what about a genuine attempt by the medical profession to *prevent* prostate and other cancers – and not by the introduction of yet more screening methods?

Moreover, with improved survival rates for cancer, especially prostate cancer and breast cancer, and increased interest in the extent to which diet and complementary and alternative therapies improve outcomes, surprisingly little is known about the effects of such factors on cancer survival. Instead of emotional outbursts from some UK doctors against the use of such methods to complement conventional medical treatment of cancer would it not be better to devise some scientific studies to compare outcomes? Fortunately this has begun for breast cancer with about six studies being carried out in the USA.[41]

A report from the Health Development Agency (the NHS body responsible for promoting more healthy lifestyles) entitled *Where's the Research on Preventing and Reducing Ill Health*, states that only 0.4 per cent of studies into such issues as smoking, heart disease and cancer looked at prevention rather than cure.[42] Chaturvedi points out that medical students aim for a lucrative private practice; those opting for studies in prevention are considered academically unsound.[43]

The UK National Cancer Research Institute has produced a detailed breakdown of spending on cancer research. It estimates that more than £250 million from 15 leading charities and government organisations goes towards cancer research in the UK every year,[44] most being spent on the most lethal cancers, including prostate and breast cancer. The study showed that the biggest proportion of spending (41 per cent) goes on basic biological research, followed by research into treatment (22 per cent), while only 16 per cent is spent on researching causes. Research into prevention, care of patients, and survival attracts the least funding. The whole approach merely serves to generate yet more jobs and money in the pharmaceutical, medical-equipment and medical industries that are industrial medicine today.

Evidence-based medicine

The industrialisation of medicine increasingly depends on costly drugs and other invasive and often unpleasant treatments, for which 'Evidence-based medicine' is one of the main planks.

Writing in the *BMJ*,[45] Richard Smith discussed evidence-based medicine as a means of answering 'One of medicine's most important – and simplest – questions: "Does a treatment work?"' This is certainly a problem for prostate-cancer sufferers. He continued:

> It has now become almost the only 'gold standard' way of testing different treatments to be sure that you are comparing the same sorts of patients at the same time; that is to 'randomise' the patients to one treatment or another. To exclude 'bias' (which might, for example, lead a doctor to put all the sicker patients into one arm of the trial) neither the doctor nor the patient should know who has got the active treatment, making the trial 'double blind'.
>
> **Because the benefit from most medical treatments is so small and so hard to detect,** you need very many patients in the trial. Although 'double blind randomised trials' are considered the best way of determining whether a treatment works, **many of them have been poorly conducted and have given misleading results.**[46] [my bold]

The problems of recruitment of appropriate patients to randomised trials have been raised by Corrie, Shaw and Harris.[47] They found that even when a trial was available, eligibility criteria excluded over half of patients. Other serious problems of carrying out meaningful double-blind randomised trials have been described by Wald and Morris.[48] Moreover, results may vary according to the source of funding for the trial (see below). Nevertheless it is data from such trials that often dictate treatment.

Screening for cancer is extremely lucrative but potentially problematical, often involving ionising radiation or the use of high powered electromagnetic fields or potentially harmful chemicals. In an editorial in the *BMJ*,[49] Richard Smith wrote:

> The problems (of scans) lie in medicine's difficulties in defining normality, the devil of 'false positives', and our limited understanding of the natural history of disease. The commonest way of defining normal is that the measure lies within two standard deviations of the mean. So in a set of measurements from a normal population 5 per cent will be

classed as 'abnormal'. The whole body scan will produce hundreds of measurements. So you have almost no chance of emerging as normal . . .

Let us look in more detail at some of the other drivers of end-of-pipe technological medicine.

PHARMACEUTICALS – SOME PROBLEMS

The pharmaceutical industry is very profitable (US drug sales grew 12 per cent in 2002, to $220 billion[50]), and hence very powerful. An article entitled 'Drug companies maintain "astounding" profits',[51] states that pharmaceuticals ranked as the most profitable sector in the US annual 'Fortune 500' ranking of America's top industries, released in May 2002. Of course, there is nothing wrong with profitability itself – only with the abuse of the power that profits can bestow.

The *BMJ*, from which I have quoted extensively in this book, now asks all contributors to sign a declaration of conflicts of interests, including funding sources and competing interests. This has allowed the association between such interests and the author's conclusions to be investigated.[52] Financial competing interests are defined as funding by for-profit organisations and other competing interests such as personal, academic or political. The results showed that authors' conclusions were significantly more positive towards the experimental intervention in trials funded by for-profit organisations alone than in trials without competing interests or in trials funded by both profit and non-profit organisations. The association between financial competing interests and authors' conclusions was not explained by the quality of the methods used, the statistical power, the type of experimental intervention, involving pharmaceuticals or non-pharmaceutical approaches or medical speciality. The authors concluded that in cases where financial competing interests had been declared, randomised clinical trials significantly favour experimental interventions. In a poll conducted by the *BMJ* on its website (bmj.com), 96 per cent of the 1479 people who voted would like to see all financial relationships between doctors and drug companies conducted with transparent contracts that are disclosed to patients.[53]

In the US, too, researchers have claimed that most randomised trials of new treatments published in leading medical journals are reported in a potentially misleading way, with statistics designed to make the results more positive than if other statistical tests were used.[54]

The problem seems to have become much worse, at least in the US. Industry supported 62 per cent of biomedical research in the US in 2000, almost double the proportion in 1980; during the same period, government support declined. About a quarter of academic investigators have affiliations to industry that could influence research and publication, according to a review in the *Journal of the American Medical Association*.[55]

Concern about links between the pharmaceutical industry and experts were also raised in a study carried out by researchers in Toronto. They claim that most guidelines on clinical practice are written by experts with undisclosed links to the pharmaceutical industry. In a survey of nearly two hundred authors of 44 clinical guidelines, 87 per cent of respondents admitted to financial links with one or more pharmaceutical companies,[56] and one new American company called Time-Concepts LLC is offering doctors $50 (£34) each time they listen to a short sales pitch from a drug company representative.[57]

Another increasing concern is the direct marketing of pharmaceuticals to patients, including via the internet. According to a recent article in the *BMJ*, a fifth of Americans contact their doctor as a result of direct-to-consumer drug advertising.[58]

The drug companies have expressed the wish to inform patients,[59] and the chief executive of the Association of British Pharmaceutical Industries states: 'My feeling, from the pharmaceutical industry, is because we are the providers of medicines that people get from the health service, we should not be excluded from [giving information to patients], provided we do it in an objective way.' He denied suggestions that this might stoke demand for certain drugs.

Fortunately (in my view) moves to allow drug manufacturers to advertise directly to particular groups of patients have been rejected by European Union health ministers.[60]

In the UK, the General Medical Council has issued new guidance on the standards expected for research carried out in the National Health Service, universities and the private sector,[61] while the US government[62] has joined the American Medical Association and the drug industry in efforts to control drug-company handouts to the medical profession – but the recommendations are voluntary.

DOCTORS AND PHARMACEUTICAL COMPANIES

The real problem of the relationship between doctors and pharmaceutical companies has been summed up by Lechin as follows:

> The practice of Medicine is divided into two camps of doctors engaged in combating disease: scientists and clinicians. The former acquires knowledge about physiology, pathophysiology, pharmacology, neurochemistry, neuroendocrinology, immunology, genetics, biochemistry and many other disciplines. Unfortunately these doctors do not practice medicine.
>
> Conversely many physicians or clinical practitioners possess only superficial knowledge of the above disciplines and so are limited to rudimentary and simplistic diagnostic and therapeutic procedures for suppressing symptoms. They do their best although sadly it is seldom enough.

He concludes that 'while doctors are trained as technicians but not scientists, the pharmaceutical industry but not doctors prescribe treatments to patients.' Also too many doctors are essentially professional human biologists, when we need doctors who understand far more chemistry if they are to work as equals with the pharmaceutical companies rather than simply acting as their agents.

THE CANCER INDUSTRY

A book entitled *Breast cancer: an environmental disease*, published by Unison, Breast (Cancer) UK and the Women's Environmental Network in 2005 referred to the 'cancer industry'. This was said to be 'a generic term for the ever expanding industry which has grown up around the disease'. The book went on, 'It is a vast industry incorporating all services, products, materials and technologies for the orthodox management of the disease.

'Given its
- traditional preoccupation with control and management of the disease,
- current preoccupation with new therapies (drug and gene) to meet future demands,
- huge research and financial investment in therapies for a burgeoning future market, and
- awareness that profits for society from primary prevention represent a loss of industry profits,

there would appear to be little hope for the primary prevention of breast cancer becoming a priority for the cancer industry.'

Interestingly, the book states that cancer charities work in close association with the cancer industry and that primary prevention is not their aim; and it specifically mentions Breakthrough in this respect. In conclusion, the report states, 'A thriving industry with a guaranteed future, "cancer" is a growth industry in every sense of the word.' It would be particularly unlikely that this particular industry would champion a cause that has the potential to undermine its very existence.

CHARITIES, PATIENT ASSOCIATIONS AND RESEARCH

There is also concern about links between pharmaceutical companies and patient organisations and charities.

Writing in the *BMJ* on the subject of industry funding of patients' support groups, Paola Mosconi wrote that declaration of competing interests is rare in Italian breast cancer associations. The following is an edited version:[63]

Herxheimer reported and commented on relationships between pharmaceutical companies and consumers' and patients' associations.[64] This is a 'hot' topic: the debate on transparency of fund raising for voluntary health associations is far from being resolved, and consumers' umbrella associations have an increasingly important role in discussing health at a European level.

In Italy, at least among the 100 breast-cancer associations belonging to the Italian forum of Europa Donna, transparency of fund raising is rarely discussed and few data are available. Using a standardised self-administered question-naire on the characteristics of breast cancer associations, information on the sponsorship of 67 of them indicated that although most of the funds come from individual donations, one third received funds from pharmaceutical companies.

In the same survey it was found that only five breast-cancer associations had been open and transparent about sponsorship by pharmaceutical companies.

These data confirm the concern expressed by Herxheimer and by Hirst[65] on the independence of consumers' and patients' associations and support the need for more open-ness and transparency about funding from the pharmaceuti-cal industry and other vested interest groups for organisations participating in the debate on public health. It should be a requirement that such conflicts of interest are clearly stated on the home page of the websites of all charities and patient organisations.

Another article in the *BMJ*[66] tells 'How HRT studies have got drug firms rallying the troops':

In 2002 the powerful New York based Society for Women's Health Research, whose 'sole mission is to improve the health of women through research', held a celebrity gala . . . entirely underwritten by Wyeth. In a *Washington Monthly* article entitled 'Hot Flash, Cold Cash,' journalist Alicia Mundy reported that only a few days after the gala the company donated a quarter of a million dollars to the society.

Several weeks later, in July 2002, [negative findings about HRT were made public after the huge US Women's Health Initiative (WHI) study was prematurely halted on grounds of safety[67]] Wyeth was in a tailspin. They found support from the society . . . [which, as Mundy observed,] 'seemingly took the side of its donors – and of Wyeth in particular.' As they fervently downplayed the negative findings of the WHI study and urged women not to abandon their HRT, the society's staff failed to disclose their substantial links to Wyeth and other drug companies.

Another investigation in the USA discovered that three key organisations, the United Seniors Association, the Seniors Coalition, and the 60s Plus Association, have all received substantial contributions in recent years from the drug industry: 'When the pharmaceutical industry speaks these days, many Americans may not be able to recognise its voice. That's because the industry often uses "front groups" that work to advance its agenda under the veil of other interests.'[68]

Let us look at what some charities have said about recent reports linking diet to cancer. In November 2006, scientific researchers in the USA published the results of their findings into the links between red meat and breast cancer, based on studies of the diets of 90,000 women.[69] It was found that women who ate more than one and a half servings of red meat a day had a risk of hormone (oestrogen and progesterone) receptor positive cancer almost twice that of those who ate three or fewer servings a week. It was suggested that this was caused by hormone residues from growth hormones used on cattle in the US or the presence of heterocyclic amines created during cooking of red meat. In *Your Life in Your Hands* in 2000 I predicted that these would be avoidable risk factors for breast cancer. Dr Cho, in summarising the importance of his teams' findings, stated 'Given that most of the risk factors for breast cancer are not easily modifiable these findings have potential public health implications in preventing breast cancer.' So what did the breast cancer charities say? Sarah Rawlings of Breakthrough Breast Cancer is quoted as saying 'Very little is known about diet and breast cancer risk because we eat a variety of foods and separating out the effect of an individual food is difficult.' What nonsense! Of course trained scientists such as Dr Cho know how to process and interpret data in relation to confounding factors and as for 'very little is known about diet and cancer' one is tempted to ask if Rawlings reads? Maria Leadbetter of Breast Cancer Care's response was equally helpful and informative! She stated 'The benefits of eating a healthy and varied diet are well established and the biggest risk factors for breast cancer remain gender and age.'

Another report released in January 2007 showing that premenopausal women who ate more than 30 g fibre from foods such as wholemeal bread and fruit and vegetables in the diet had a risk of breast cancer half that of women who ate less than 20 g a day. There was again a rather muddled, lukewarm response from Breakthrough Breast Cancer. In contrast Cancer Research UK was quite positive. They stated, 'It further highlights the importance of eating a healthy diet for reducing the risk of cancer.' Of course, I am delighted with the results of such studies, confirming as they do all my findings based on analysing the scientific literature and first published in *Your Life in Your Hands* in 2000. It is interesting to recall how I was attacked by Breakthrough at the time. Their then chief executive, Delyth Morgan, attacked my findings in interview after interview. I wondered at the time what Breakthrough's agenda was and I still wonder what it is! I have generally found prostate-cancer charities to be much more enlightened and helpful, and more willing to advise their members on diet and lifestyle. Many now advise against eating dairy.

I have been asked countless times since *Your Life in Your Hands* was first published about donations to cancer charities. I recommend that any charitable donations should be given to highly reputable charities. The research charity I would choose is Cancer Research UK, which is headed by a distinguished doctor and although it errs on the conservative side of issues can, I think, be trusted. I have started a new charity, Cancer Pprevent, aimed at the primary prevention of cancer by identifying and communicating avoidable risks. The charity is part of Imperial College Trust and is headed by a distinguished cancer biologist, Professor Mustafa Djamgoz, Dr Voulvoulis, who is an expert in endocrine-disrupting substances, and me.

I also commend the charities concerned with caring, such as Macmillan Cancer Relief, Marie Curie Cancer Care and the various hospices. Before giving any donations to cancer charities, do consider what proportion of their funds are devoted to administration, or the acquisition of capital assets such as buildings, the merchandising of consumer goods, and what proportion is actually spent on cancer prevention and/or care. Cancer Pprevent has the best profile in terms of expenditure on administration and buildings relative to money spent on research, but it is still new and poorly funded. Personally I would not give a penny to Breakthrough Breast Cancer.

MEDIA AND ADVERTISING

The *BMJ* in an attack on media spin distorting the outcomes of medical studies, entitled 'The operation was a success (but the patient died)'[70] pointed out that the previous week one simple health message had dominated the US media: radical prostate surgery for prostate cancer saves lives. The media were reporting the results of a Swedish trial,[71] yet the trial showed no such thing. The trial concluded that although radical surgery did reduce death from *prostate cancer*, there was no significant difference between surgery and watchful waiting in terms of overall survival (because of death from other causes). A companion study found that the surgery also failed to improve the men's quality of life.

According to another *BMJ* article, positive reporting bias may occur for several reasons. Beyond the seemingly universal desire to believe in cures, which may underlie some of the bias in such media reports, are corporate interests, the author suggests. Journalists seeking experts for comments often turn to seemingly credible and disinterested groups, such as professional associations, non-profit health groups, and patient organisations. The article goes on to say that many journalists do not realise, or fail to report, that many groups receive substantial funding from vested interests. Hospitals in North America, facing brutal competition, have, the article suggests, started buying contracts with television stations to feature them 'in news reports'. A poll of three hundred news directors found that 43 per cent felt that such payments create pressures to exert improper influence. Dr Ivan Oransky, who teaches medical journalism at New York University, believes that the sort of investigative reporting that is standard in political coverage is lacking in medical and science reporting, with too many journalists reporting researchers' assertions uncritically.[72]

A recent development in America is the sponsored news programme, and it may be queried whether these are a new form of paid front for the pharmaceutical industry.[73] What many viewers of these news-magazine-style programmes may not realise is that healthcare companies, including pharmaceutical and biotechnology companies, are paying directly for videos and suggesting the topics to be covered, according to a report in the *New York Times*. That article named a number of senior American broadcasters as having worked for a company funded by pharmaceutical giants to make video material. The celebrity journalists were reportedly paid up to $100,000 for one day's work, broadcast as news on public television stations across the country.

In the UK recently the media have led highly charged emotional campaigns for certain drugs to be made available to sufferers of diseases such as breast cancer and Alzheimer's disease in advance of, or in some cases in spite of, the recommendations of NICE, the National Institute of Clinical Excellence, the body established to provide evidence-based advice to the NHS. In 2005 there was a particularly emotional campaign for breast-cancer sufferers to be prescribed Herceptin (trastuzumab).[74] The drug is a monoclonal antibody that acts on the HER2(erbB2) receptor which is over-expressed in about 30 per cent of early-stage breast cancers. Herceptin costs about 70 thousand dollars for a full course of treatment and debate has centred on whether the drug should be provided to all patients with HER2 metastatic cancer or only some, given that about 70 per cent of patients do not respond to treatment and cancer resistance develops rapidly in virtually all patients. Moreover, the drug is associated with heart problems in up to 7 per cent of patients and these increase when the drug is combined with certain types of chemotherapy.[75] I heard none of these complications, which call for fine clinical judgements, in media reports at the time. They simply gave the impression that by denying patients the drug we were committing them to death. Recent discussions on the BBC suggest that they are more aware of ways in which sufferers can be manipulated now.

That pharmaceutical companies devise clever ways to market their products is hardly surprising, but journalists and others should be more sceptical. They should always ask the key questions, 'Who is funding you or your research?' In an article by George Monbiot in the *Guardian* in February 2006 he stated that 'academics and the media have failed dismally to ask the crucial question of scientists' claims: Who is paying you.' He cited the example of Professor David Warburton of Reading University working for an organisation called ARISE that described itself as 'a worldwide association of eminent scientists who act as independent consultants, but which obtained more than 90 per cent of its funding from the tobacco industry.' He describes how Warburton in an uncontested interview on the Today Programme extolled the calming properties of cigarettes and poured scorn on public health messages, and was unchallenged by any of the UK press except for one article in the *Guardian*.

In general, it has been said, newspapers underreport randomised trials, emphasise bad news from observational studies, and ignore research from developing countries.[76]

WHERE DOES THE FAULT LIE?

Instead of trying to prevent disease (based on good dietary advice), we continue to treat disease with pills and potions, surgery or other expensive invasive methods to suppress symptoms. The communication of problems in our diet and lifestyle that affect our health is typically done poorly – or not at all – and usually without proper, clear advice on how to change our behaviour.

In the first edition of *Your Life in Your Hands* I asked why. I raised concerns about wealth creation being more highly regarded than quality of life, and the lack of an adequate knowledge of science in Parliament and the civil service, especially after the privatisation of much science in the late 1970s and 1980s, but I had no idea how serious the problems were. The situation is particularly serious I believe, for prostate cancer, which is such an unpleasant disease for men. The whole approach to chronic illness avoids antagonising special-interest groups, and it maintains the material wealth of (and jobs in) sectors such as farming, agrochemicals, the food industry, pharmaceutical research and the manufacture of medicines and medical equipment. But would it not be better to communicate facts as they are known, clearly and simply so that people can make their own choices and prevent disease? Would it not be better to create jobs in sectors working for the well-being of society and the environment, for example, in growing wholesome, nutritious organically produced food, with medical professionals being concerned more with health education, disease prevention and monitoring than dishing out pills?

My answer to the question of 'whose fault is the prostate and breast cancer epidemic?' is that it is all our faults – especially the relatively well-educated people in society. It remains my view that we are the ones who must make and communicate the changes that will reduce both our personal and societal risk of suffering from these diseases. We must use our spending power to show that some foods are unhealthy and they should not be produced.

The research for this book impressed upon me strongly what an unpleasant disease prostate cancer is. Not only that, but the decisions about whether to opt for watchful waiting or for one of the other treatment options – all of which may have unpleasant physical and emotional side effects – is far from easy. How much wiser it would be to concentrate on prevention rather than risk the need of a 'cure' or the anxiety and risks of watchful waiting. And yet society continues to emphasise the search for cures. The point is well made by a story attributed to Joseph Malins (1895) about a dangerous cliff and the debate whether to erect a fence at the top of the cliff, to prevent people falling off, or keep an ambulance down in the valley:

A collection was made to accumulate aid
and the dwellers in highway and alley,
gave dollars and cents, to provide . . . not a fence,
but an ambulance down in the valley.

'For the cliff is all right if you're careful', they said,
'and if folks ever slip and are dropping,
it isn't the slipping and dropping that hurts,
it's the shock down below when they're stopping.'

So for many a year, as these mishaps occur,
quick forth do the rescuers sally,
to pick up the victims who fall from the cliff
with the ambulance down in the valley.

Then one made a plea: 'It's a marvel to me
that you'd give so much greater attention
to repairing results than to curing the cause;
why, you'd much better aim at prevention.

'For the mischief of course should be stopped at its source.
Come, neighbours and friends, let us rally:
it makes far better sense to rely on a fence
than an ambulance down in the valley.'

'He's wrong in his head', the majority said.
'He would end all our earnest endeavour.
He's the kind who would shirk this responsible work,
But we will support it for ever.'[77]

OUR LIVES IN OUR HANDS

In this book I have given information to reduce individual risk of prostate cancer, but the only long-term, final and lasting answer to these scourges of our Western lifestyle is to *change* that lifestyle. There is no point expecting politicians, the medical profession or the media to help, given the powerful lobbies that influence them. But we can change our own lifestyles and show with our buying power that we don't want dairy produce, or harmful chemicals in our lives but that we do want locally grown organically produced food. In the UK this is already beginning to happen as dairy farms give way to more beneficial uses of land and the market for organic food keeps on expanding.

We have to develop greater awareness of, and sensitivity to, the impact of our lifestyle choices on our own health, that of our fellow beings, and that of our planetary home. Let me quote from Professor McMichael from the London School of Tropical Hygiene and Health and Dr Powles of Cambridge University; their paper in the *BMJ* states:[78]

> Population size and the material intensity of our economies are now so great that, at the global level, we are disrupting some of the biosphere's life support systems.
>
> Recent attempts at 'full cost accounting' estimate that the demands of the current world population already exceed global carrying capacity by approximately a third.

What they are saying is this: if we are to survive as a healthy species, we must change our values and emphasis from materialism to other measures of well-being. We need increasingly to put more value on good food, education, the arts, beautiful unspoilt environments populated by diverse species, friendships, social interaction and health – and less value on 'things'.

Looking back, I realise that I have changed my diet and lifestyle from that of a middle-class, ambitious career-minded Western woman to a woman with a more traditional Eastern diet, lifestyle and values. So here are some simple, practical guidelines that you can follow to help you to cut your risk of prostate cancer and probably many other non-communicable or degenerative diseases, and improve the health of all of us and our home planet, Earth, at the same time.

TOWARDS A HAPPY ENDING

I am delighted that in the seven years since *Your Life in Your Hands* was first published so many people have told me how helpful they have found it, and that no credible science has been published to persuade me to change one word of my advice to prostate-cancer and breast-cancer sufferers. I hope that this new edition of *Prostate Cancer: Understand, Prevent and Overcome* will be used widely to help men to reduce their risk of suffering from the disease. For those already suffering from prostate cancer, I hope it will provide help and empowerment to work with your medical professionals to overcome your illness.

Knowledge is power. In this book I have tried to empower all men and their partners to deal with prostate cancer, individually and as a society, by trying to share with them the knowledge that I have gained on the subject of prostate and breast cancer as a scientist and as a five-times cancer sufferer.

Let us all try to spread the word. 'Public opinion when it is truly aroused, can be unstoppable.' John Humphrys, *The Great Food Gamble*, Hodder and Stoughton, 2001.

TEN SIMPLE GUIDELINES

1. Make good food ingredients your top priority when it comes to spending money. Keep as closely as you can to the diet and lifestyle recommendations set out in this book and in *The Plant Programme*, and wherever and whenever possible be prepared to pay extra for organically grown food produced as naturally as possible, ideally to the standards of the Soil Association, or grow your own. This sends the clearest possible message to government and the food industry.
2. Eat only those foods which human adults have evolved to eat. Most crucially, leave out dairy produce, which is designed for baby calves, goats or lambs. Also refuse to eat food depleted of nutrients or otherwise altered by food processing, including

food which contains artificial chemical additives such as colouring and flavouring agents, preservatives and emulsifiers or food which has been chemically altered, for example fats which have been hydrogenated. Refuse to be bamboozled by marketing and advertising, look for the 'weasel words' and separate them in your mind from the underlying facts. Be suspicious – check labels and demand information. Make eating good nutritious meals based on wholesome nutritional ingredients your top priority when it comes to your time.

3. Try to be less materialistic. Buy fewer new cars or clothes – don't be a fashion victim. In fact, try to cut down on buying *things* generally.

4. Be concerned and take action to improve the environment for everybody. There are many chemicals being introduced that we can do nothing about as individuals. Collectively, we can reduce the impact of chemicals on the environment by reducing our use of materials such as fragrances for personal or home use, perfumed deodorants and aftershaves, soft plastics, detergents, cleaning products, house and garden chemicals, and man-made fibres. Remember how in the past we were sold 'wonder' chemicals such as DDT and PCBs which have turned out to cause serious problems to the health of man, animals and the environment and which are still with us. What chemicals are we using today that scientists will have a similar view of in the future? Press for more research into the environment, nutrition and human health, with more medical research on epidemiology aimed at prevention.

5. Try to understand some basic science. Usually it is your money that scientists are spending, directly or indirectly, and you need to understand what they are doing. Always ask who funds them and their work and what conflicts of interest they have. Ensure that scientists contribute more to the public understanding of science by asking questions. If you do not understand the answer, do not be embarrassed to repeat your question until you get a satisfactory answer. If a scientist cannot explain their work properly it is their problem, not yours. It is essential that a well-informed body of opinion exists if science is to be directed for the benefit of humankind rather than lead to our downfall. Books that will 'fire you up' are *Silent Spring* by Rachel Carson, *Our Stolen Futures* by

Colborn, Dumanski and Myers and *Planetary Overload* by A J McMichael. If you want to become more involved as lay members of the boards of scientific organisations, write in and offer your services.

6. Learn to understand your basic anatomy and, depending on your age, discuss with your doctor whether you should have regular PSA tests and other examinations (*see* Chapter 1).

7. If you are diagnosed with prostate cancer – use all the tools at your disposal to fight back. For your orthodox treatment ensure that you are treated at a centre of excellence which uses a specialist cancer team led by a surgeon, radiotherapist and chemotherapist. Work with your doctors and be an involved and constructive participant in overcoming your illness, not a passive victim.

8. Follow my diet and the lifestyle recommendations aimed at avoiding man-made chemicals as closely as possible. This includes minimising the use of prescriptions available from doctors and pills from pharmacists. If you are prescribed or recommended drugs, demand to know precisely how they work and what the side effects are. Take them only if you are satisfied with the explanation and convinced there is no alternative. If your physician cannot explain how the drugs work and give examples of their successes and failures, be sceptical.

9. Use methods such as meditation, hypnotherapy and visualisation and yoga to cope with any emotional distress to develop the most positive approach possible. But do not rely on positive thinking alone. It is changing your body chemistry by changing your diet and lifestyle that is the crucial thing to do. Talk to your friends and family members and allow their help and support into your life, but if they find difficulty in coping, understand that they are distressed. Forgive them and allow them back into your life as soon as they feel able to return.

10. Prostate cancer is NOT an automatic death sentence. Remember the experience of the men whose stories I recounted in Chapter 1 – as well as my own experience with breast cancer – and read the success stories at www.cancersupportinterna tional.com

Keep reminding yourself that it is possible to overcome even advanced cancer. I know because I did it.

TO FIND OUT MORE ABOUT PROSTATE CANCER

1. BOOKS

The Prostate Cancer Book by Jonathan Waxman, published by
   Vermillion.
Prostate Problems by Jane Smith and Dr David Gillatt, published
   by Hodder and Stoughton.
The China Study by T.C. Campbell and T.M. Campbell,
   published by BenBella Books.

2. BOOKLETS FROM THE US NATIONAL CANCER INSTITUTE*

Booklet About Prostate Cancer
'What You Need to Know about Prostate Cancer'

Booklet About Prostate Changes
'Understanding Prostate Changes: A Health Guide for All Men'

Booklets About Cancer Treatment
'Understanding Treatment Choices for Prostate Cancer: Know
   Your Options'

---

* http://www.nci.nih.gov/cancerinfo/wyntk/prostate.

'Chemotherapy and You: A Guide to Self-Help During Treatment'
'Helping Yourself During Chemotherapy: 4 Steps for Patients'
'Radiation Therapy and You: A Guide to Self-Help During
   Treatment'
'Pain Control: A Guide for People with Cancer and Their
   Families'
'Get Relief From Cancer Pain'

Booklets About Living With Cancer
'Taking Time: Support for People With Cancer and the People
   Who Care About Them'
'Facing Forward: Life After Cancer Treatment'
'When Cancer Recurs: Meeting the Challenge'
'Advanced Cancer: Living Each Day'

3. USEFUL WEBSITES

The Prostate Cancer Charity (UK): http://www.prostate-
   cancer.org.uk
The National Cancer Institute (US): http://www.nci.nih.gov/
   cancerinfo/wyntk/prostate and http://cancer.gov
The National Comprehensive Cancer Network, in partnership
   with the American Cancer Society (US): http://www.nccn.org/
   patient_gls/_english/_prostate/
PSA Rising (US): http://www.psa-rising.com
Cancer Support International (UK): http://
   www.cancersupportinternational.com

4. FIND OUT ABOUT LOCAL PROSTATE-CANCER SUPPORT GROUPS

5. FIND OUT ABOUT CENTRES THAT PROVIDE DIETARY ADVICE, SUPPORT COUNSELLING AND TRAINING IN RELAXATION AND OTHER COPING TECHNIQUES, SUCH AS THE BRISTOL CANCER HELP CENTRE (helpline 0117 980 9505, http://www.bristolcancerhelp.org)

And THE POSITIVE ACTION ON CANCER CHARITY
(telephone 01373 455 255, http://www.pacproject.co.uk; offering
a free counselling service to cancer patients and their families)

NOTES

WELCOME

1. Plant, Jane, 2000. *Your Life in Your Hands*. Virgin Books. Subsequent editions contain all of the first edition, unchanged, together with additional sections updating each chapter.
2. Plant, Jane and Tidey, Gill, 2002. *The Plant Programme*. Paperback edition. Virgin Books; Plant, Jane and Tidey, Gill, 2005. *Eating for Better Health*. Virgin Books.
3. Kradjian, Robert D., 1994. *Save Yourself from Breast Cancer*. Berkley Publishing.
4. Plant, Jane and Tidey, Gill, 2003. *Understanding, Preventing and Overcoming Osteoporosis*. Virgin Books.
5. Medical Report: Prostate Cancer. ICON, 2002, 1(5), 8–10.
6. Waxman, Jonathan, 2001. *The Prostate Cancer Book*. London: Vermillion.

1. PROBLEMS WITH THE PROSTATE?

1. Plant, Jane, 2000. *Your Life in Your Hands*. Virgin Books. Subsequent editions contain all of the first edition, unchanged, together with additional sections updating each chapter.
2. Plant, Jane A. and Moore, P.J., 1979. Geochemical mapping and interpretation in Britain. *Phil Trans Roy Soc, London*, B288, 95–112.
3. Plant, Jane A., Smith, D., Smith, B. and Williams, L., 2000. Environmental Geochemistry at the Global Scale. Geological Society Special Issue.
4. Finkelman, R.B., Belkin, H.E., Centena, J.E. and Zheng, B., 2003. Geological Epidemiology: Coal Combustion from China. In *Geology and Health – closing the gap*. Skinner, H.C.W. and Berger, A.R. (eds). Oxford University Press.

5. Eaton, Lynn, 2003. World cancer rates set to double by 2020. *British Medical Journal*, 326, 728.
6. Peto, R. and others, 2000. Smoking, Smoking Cessation and Lung Cancer in the UK since 1950. *BMJ*, 321, 323–9.
7. Raleigh, V.S., 1999. World Population and Health in Transition. *BMJ*, 319, 981B4.
8. Packham, D.E., 1999. Impacts of Commercialisation and Privatisation on Capabilities for Scientific Advice, Oracles or Scapegoats? IPMS Conference notes, October. See also: Packham, David and Tasker, Mary, 1997. Industry and the academy – a Faustian contract. *Industry and Higher Education*, April, 85–90.
9. Waxman, Jonathan, 2001. *The Prostate Cancer Book*. London: Vermillion.
10. http://www.nci.nih.gov/cancerinfo/wyntk/prostate
11. Waxman, Jonathan, 2001. *The Prostate Cancer Book*. London: Vermillion.
12. Clapp, R.W., Howe, G.K. and Jacobs, M.M., 2005. Environmental and occupational causes of cancer. www.sustainableproduction.org
13. http://info.cancerresearchuk.org/cancerandresearch/cancers/prostate
14. Waxman, Jonathan, 2001. *Op. cit.*
15. Plant, Jane and Tidey, Gill, 2002. *The Plant Programme*. Paperback edition. Virgin Books.
16. Coulter, Angela, 2002. Patients' views of the good doctor. *BMJ*, 325, 668–669.
17. Coulter, Angela, 2002. Patients' views of the good doctor. *BMJ*, 325, 668–669.
18. Donaldson, Liam, 2003. Expert patients usher in a new era of opportunity for the NHS. *BMJ*, 326, 1279–1280.
19. Plant, Jane and Tidey, Gill, 2003. *Understanding, Preventing and Overcoming Osteoporosis*. Virgin Books; Plant, Jane and Tidey, Gill, 2005. *Eating for Better Health*. Virgin Books.
20. Wilkins, David, 2003. Patient's response to the research. *BMJ*, 326, 1313.
21. Waern, M. and five others, 2002. Burden of illness and suicide in elderly people: case control study. *BMJ*, 324, 1355–1357.
22. Stone, Mike, 2003. What patients want from their doctors. *BMJ*, 326, 1294.
23. Berry, D.C., Michas, I.C., Gillie, T. and Forster M., 1997. What do patients want to know about their medicines, and what do doctors want to tell them? A comparative study. *Psychol Health*, 12, 467–480; Berry, D.C., Knapp, P. and Raynor, D.K., 2002. Provision of information about drug side effects to patients. *Lancet*, 359, 853–854.
24. Waxman, Jonathan, 2001. *The Prostate Cancer Book*. London: Vermillion.
25. http://www.nccn.org/patient_gls/_english/_prostate/
26. Gask, Linda and Usherwood, Tim, 2002. ABC of psychological medicine: The consultation. *BMJ*, 324, 1567.
27. Herxheimer, Andrew and Ziebland, Sue, 2003. DIPEx: fresh insights for medical practice. *Journal of the Royal Society of Medicine*, 95, 5, 209–210.
28. Cox, Peter and Brusseau, Peggy, 1992. *Superliving A Beginner's Guide to Medspeak*, Vermillion.; Rule, Ashley, 2003. Shocking Language. *BMJ*, 327, 422.
29. Watts, Geoff, 2003. Second coming for patient power. *BMJ*, 326, 520.

30. Plant, Jane, 2007. *Your Life in Your Hands*, Fourth edition. Virgin Books. pp. 246–248.
31. Medical Report: Prostate Cancer. *ICON*, 2002, 1 (5), 8–10.
32. Medical Report: Prostate Cancer. *ICON*, 2002, 1 (5), 8–10; Waxman, Jonathan, 2001. *The Prostate Cancer Book*. London: Vermillion.
33. Waxman, Jonathan, 2001. *The Prostate Cancer Book*. London: Vermillion.
34. Medical Report: Prostate Cancer. *ICON*, 2002, 1 (5), 8–10.
35. Waxman, Jonathan, 2001. *The Prostate Cancer Book*. London: Vermillion.
36. Waxman, Jonathan, 2001. *The Prostate Cancer Book*. London: Vermillion.
37. http://www.nci.nih.gov/cancerinfo/wyntk/prostate
38. Medical Report: Prostate Cancer. *ICON*, 2002, 1 (5), 8–10.
39. Wilt, Timothy J., 2002. Treatment options for benign prostatic hyperplasia. *BMJ*, 324, 1047–1048.
40. Kirby, R.S. and seven others, 2003. Efficacy and tolerability of doxazosin and finasteride, alone and in combination, in treatment of symptomatic benign prostatic hyperplasia: the Prospective European Doxazosin and Combination Therapy (PREDICT) trial. *Urology*, 61 (1), 119–126.
41. Lee, E, 2002. Comparison of tamulosin and finasteride for lower urinary tract symptoms associated with benign prostatic hyperplasia in Korean patients. *J Int Med Res*, 30 (6), 584–590.
42. Wilt, Timothy J, 2002. Treatment options for benign prostatic hyperplasia. *BMJ*, 324, 1047–1048.
43. Brookes, Sara T., Donovan, Jenny L., Peters, Tim J., Abrams, Paul and Neal, David E., 2002. Sexual dysfunction in men after treatment for lower urinary tract symptoms: evidence from randomised controlled trial. *BMJ*, 324, 1059–1061.
44. Waxman, Jonathan, 2001. *The Prostate Cancer Book*. London: Vermillion; Medical Report: Prostate Cancer. *ICON*, 2002, 1 (5), 8–10.
45. Medical Report: Prostate Cancer. *ICON*, 2002, 1 (5), 8–10.
46. http://www.nccn.org/patient_gls/_english/_prostate/
47. Waxman, Jonathan, 2001. *The Prostate Cancer Book*. London: Vermillion.
48. Medical Report: Prostate Cancer. *ICON*, 2002, 1 (5), 8–10.
49. http://www.cancer.med.umich.edu/prostcan/
50. http://www.nccn.org/patient_gls/_english/_prostate/
51. Waxman, Jonathan, 2001. *The Prostate Cancer Book*. London: Vermillion.
52. http://www.cancer.med.umich.edu/prostcan/
53. http://www.cancer.org/docroot/NWS/content/NWS_1_1x_Prostate_screening_Test_Results_Vary_Over_Time.asp
54. http://www.nlm.nih.gov/medlineplus/news/fullstory_13465.html
55. http://www.nccn.org/patient_gls/_english/_prostate/
56. *JAMA*, 289, 2695–2700.
57. Stuttaford, Thomas, 2003. Cancer: the four tests. *The Times (T2)*, 24 October 2003.
58. Chapple, A. and five others, 2002. Why men with prostate cancer want wider access to prostate specific antigen testing: qualitative study. *BMJ*, 325, 737–739.
59. Chapple, A. and five others, 2002. Why men with prostate cancer want wider access to prostate specific antigen testing: qualitative study. *BMJ*, 325, 737–739.

60. Chapple, A. and five others, 2002. Is 'watchful waiting' a real choice for men with prostate cancer? A qualitative study. *BJU (Urol Int)*, 90, 257–264.
61. *Journal of the National Cancer Institute*, 1 October 2003, reported in *The Times (T2)*, 7 October 2003.
62. Donovan, J.L., Frankel, S.J., Neal, D.E. and Hamdy, F.C., 1999. Dilemmas in treating early prostate cancer: the evidence and a questionnaire survey of consultant urologists in the United Kingdom. *BMJ*, 318, 299–300.
63. Duckworth, Martin J., 2002. Right to choose is important. *BMJ*, 324, 1392.
64. Josefson, Deborah, 2002. PSA screening leads to overdiagnosis, study says. *BMJ*, 325, 61.
65. Lu-Yao, Grace, Albertsen, Peter C., Stanford, Janet L., Stukel, Therese A., Walker-Corkery, Elizabeth S. and Barry, Michael J., 2002. Natural experiment examining impact of aggressive screening and treatment on prostate cancer mortality in two fixed cohorts from Seattle area and Connecticut. *BMJ*, 325, 740–743.
66. http://www.cancer.med.umich.edu/prostcan/
67. *Urology*, 2003, 61, 1177–1180; http://www.nlm.nih.gov/medlineplus/news/fullstory_13258.html
68. Medical Report: Prostate Cancer. *ICON*, 2002, 1 (5), 8–10.
69. Perron, Linda, Moore, Lynne, Bairati, Isabelle, Bernard, Paul-Marie and Meyer, Francois, 2002. PSA screening and prostate cancer mortality. *Canadian Medical Association Journal*, 166 (5), 586–591.
70. http://www.cancer.med.umich.edu/prostcan/
71. Thompson, Ian, Leach, Robin J., Pollock, Brad H. and Naylor, Susan L., 2003. Prostate cancer and prostate-specific antigen: the more we know, the less we understand. *Journal of the National Cancer Institute*, 95, 1027–1028.
72. Yamey, Gavin and Wilkes, Michael, 2002. The PSA storm. *BMJ*, 324, 431.
73. Cramer, Scott D. and 13 others, 2003. Association between genetic polymorphisms in the prostate-specific antigen gene promoter and serum prostate-specific antigen levels. *Journal of the National Cancer Institute*, 95, 1044–1053.
74. http://www.post-gazette.com/healthscience/20030716prostatehea1.asp
75. http://www.post-gazette.com/healthscience/20030716prostatehea1.asp
76. http://www.nlm.nih.gov/medlineplus/news/fullstory_13363.html
77. http://www.nccn.org/patient_gls/_english/_prostate/
78. http://www.nccn.org/patient_gls/_english/_prostate/
79. Gottlieb, Scott, 2003. Prostate specific antigen test must be repeated before biopsy. *BMJ*, 326, 1231.
80. *JAMA*, 289, 2695–2700.
81. http://www.nccn.org/patient_gls/_english/_prostate/
82. Waxman, Jonathan, 2001. *The Prostate Cancer Book*. London: Vermillion.
83. *Canadian Medical Association Journal*, 2002, 166, 1399–1406.
84. http://www.nccn.org/patient_gls/_english/_prostate/
85. Medical Report: Prostate Cancer. *ICON*, 2002, 1 (5), 8–10. Waxman, Jonathan, 2001. *The Prostate Cancer Book*. London: Vermillion.
86. http://www.cancer.med.umich.edu/prostcan/
87. http://www.nccn.org/patient_gls/_english/_prostate/
88. http://www.nccn.org/patient_gls/_english/_prostate/3_stages.htm

89. http://www.prostatelab.com/grading.htm
90. http://www.prostatelab.com/grading.htm
91. http://www.cancer.med.umich.edu/prostcan/
92. http://www.nccn.org/patient_gls/_english/_prostate/
93. *Cancer*, 2002, 94, 3135-3141.
94. Spurgeon, David, 2002. Scientists develop more sensitive grading system for prostate cancer. *BMJ*, 324, 1476.
95. http://www.nccn.org/patient_gls/_english/_prostate/
96. http://www.nccn.org/patient_gls/_english/_prostate/
97. Waxman, Jonathan, 2001. *The Prostate Cancer Book*. London: Vermillion.
98. Medical Report: Prostate Cancer. *ICON*, 2002, 1 (5), 8-10.
99. Waxman, Jonathan, 2001. *The Prostate Cancer Book*. London: Vermillion.
100. http://www.nccn.org/patient_gls/_english/_prostate/
101. http://www.nccn.org/patient_gls/_english/_prostate/
102. http://www.nccn.org/patient_gls/_english/_prostate/
103. Spurgeon, David, 2003. Advanced scanning techniques help doctors stage prostate cancer. *BMJ*, 326, 1418.
104. *New England Journal of Medicine*, 2003, 348, 2491-2499.
105. http://www.nccn.org/patient_gls/_english/_prostate/
106. http://www.cancer.org
107. Stuttaford, Thomas, 2003. Cancer: the four tests. *The Times (T2)*, 24 October 2003.
108. Stuttaford, Thomas, 2003. Cancer: the four tests. *The Times (T2)*, 24 October 2003.
109. http://www.nccn.org/patient_gls/_english/_prostate/
110. Waxman, Jonathan, 2001. *The Prostate Cancer Book*. London: Vermillion.
111. Waxman, Jonathan, 2001. *The Prostate Cancer Book*. London: Vermillion.
112. http://www.fgcu.edu/chp/deadlytomen/info.html
113. Kirwan, C.C, Nath, E., Byrne, G.J. and McCollum, C.N., 2003. Prophylaxis for venous thromboembolism during treatment for cancer: questionnaire survey. *BMJ*, 327, 597-598.
114. Waxman, Jonathan, 2001. *The Prostate Cancer Book*. London: Vermillion.
115. Waxman, Jonathan, 2001. *The Prostate Cancer Book*. London: Vermillion.
116. Waxman, Jonathan, 2001. *The Prostate Cancer Book*. London: Vermillion.
117. http://info.cancerresearchuk.org/cancerstats/types/prostate/survival/
118. Medical Report: Prostate Cancer. *ICON*, 2002, 1 (5), 8-10.
119. http://www.nccn.org/patient_gls/_english/_prostate/
120. Gottlieb, Scott, 2002. Watchful waiting as good as surgery for prostate cancer. *BMJ*, 325, 613; Lenzer, Jeanne, 2002. The operation was a success (but the patient died). *BMJ*, 325, 664.
121. Medical Report: Prostate Cancer. *ICON*, 2002, 1 (5), 8-10.
122. Waxman, Jonathan, 2001. *The Prostate Cancer Book*. London: Vermillion.
123. http://www.shot.demon.co.uk
124. Waxman, Jonathan, 2001. *The Prostate Cancer Book*. London: Vermillion.
125. http://www.nccn.org/patient_gls/_english/_prostate/
126. Ask the nurses. *ICON*, 2002, 1 (3, September 2002), 7.
127. *The Times*, 28 November 2006.

128. UK National Radiological Protection Board, http://www.nrpb.org/radiation-topics/risks/exposure.htm
129. Shiralkar, A. and five others, 2003. Doctor's knowledge of radiation exposure: questionnaire study. *BMJ*, 327, 371–372.
130. Medical Report: Prostate Cancer. *ICON*, 2002, 1 (5), 8–10.
131. Waxman, Jonathan, 2001. *The Prostate Cancer Book*. London: Vermillion.
132. http://www.nccn.org/patient_gls/_english/_prostate/
133. http://www.cancer.med.umich.edu/prostcan/
134. Waxman, Jonathan, 2001. *The Prostate Cancer Book*. London: Vermillion.
135. Waxman, Jonathan, 2001. *The Prostate Cancer Book*. London: Vermillion.
136. Waxman, Jonathan, 2001. *The Prostate Cancer Book*. London: Vermillion.
137. Waxman, Jonathan, 2001. *The Prostate Cancer Book*. London: Vermillion.
138. http://www.nccn.org/patient_gls/_english/_prostate/
139. http://www.nccn.org/patient_gls/_english/_prostate/
140. Waxman, Jonathan, 2001. *The Prostate Cancer Book*. London: Vermillion.
141. http://www.nccn.org/patient_gls/_english/_prostate/
142. http://www.cancer.med.umich.edu/prostcan/
143. Waxman, Jonathan, 2001. *The Prostate Cancer Book*. London: Vermillion.
144. Waxman, Jonathan, 2001. *The Prostate Cancer Book*. London: Vermillion.
145. http://www.nccn.org/patient_gls/_english/_prostate/
146. Alternative Therapy, British Medical Association, 1986.
147. *New Scientist*, 27 August 1987.
148. Vickers, A. and Zollman, C., 1999. ABC of complementary medicine: Acupuncture. *BMJ*, 9 October, 973–976.
149. Medical Report: Prostate Cancer. *ICON*, 2002, 1 (5), 8–10; http://www.nccn.org/patient_gls/_english/_prostate/
150. Waxman, Jonathan, 2001. *The Prostate Cancer Book*. London: Vermillion.
151. Waxman, Jonathan, 2001. *The Prostate Cancer Book*. London: Vermillion.
152. http://www.nccn.org/patient_gls/_english/_prostate/
153. The best way to live with cancer. *The Times*, 11 September 2003.
154. Ross, J.R. and five others, 2003. Systematic review of role of bisphosphonates on skeletal morbidity in metastatic cancer. *BMJ*, 327, 469.
155. Waxman, Jonathan, 2001. *The Prostate Cancer Book*. London: Vermillion.
156. Plant, Jane and Tidey, Gill, 2003. *Understanding, Preventing and Overcoming Osteoporosis*. Virgin Books.
157. Chapple, A. and Ziebland, S., 2002. 'I take the piss out of life, because it's the only way to get through it': what jokes do for men with testicular cancer [Abstract]. In: BSA Medical Sociology Group Annual Conference, 27–29 September 2002. Durham: BSA, 2002.
158. See, for example, section on cytotoxic (cell poisoning) drugs in the British National Formulary, 1998.
159. Josefson, Deborah, 2002. Doctors warned to be wary of new drugs. *BMJ*, 324, 1113.
160. Garattini, Silvio and Bertele, Vittorio, 2002. Efficacy, safety, and cost of new anticancer drugs. *BMJ*, 325, 269–271.
161. http://www.nccn.org/patient_gls/_english/_prostate/
162. http://www.nccn.org/patient_gls/_english/_prostate/
163. http://www.cancer.gov/

164. Modified after: Chemotherapy and You: A Guide to Self-Help During Cancer Treatment. Information about what to expect during chemotherapy and what patients can do to take care of themselves during and after treatment. *NIH Publication* −99–1136; http://www.cancer.gov/cancerinfo/ chemotherapy-and-you (There are, however, other recommendations in this booklet with which I do not agree.)
165. http://grants1.nih.gov/grants/guide/rfa-files/RFA-DK-01-008.html
166. Suicide cells. *The Times (T2)*, 10 October 2003.
167. http://www.news.harvard.edu/gazette/2001/05.10/gleevec.html
168. Pagan Westphal, Sylvia, 2003. Behind the mask. *New Scientist*, 19 July 2003.
169. Drug companies delve deep to advance the battle against cancer. *The Times*, 27 October 2003.
170. Waxman, Jonathan, 2001. *The Prostate Cancer Book*. London: Vermillion.
171. Waxman, Jonathan, 2001. *The Prostate Cancer Book*. London: Vermillion; http://www.nccn.org/patient_gls/_english/_prostate/
172. Coulter, Angela, 2003. Killing the goose that laid the golden egg. *BMJ*, 326, 1280.
173. Coulter, Angela, 2003. Killing the goose that laid the golden egg. *BMJ*, 326, 1280.
174. Ernst, E., 2003. Herbal medicines put into context. *BMJ*, 327, 881–882.
175. Waxman, Jonathan, 2001. *The Prostate Cancer Book*. London: Vermillion.
176. Dyer, Owen, 2003. Aspirin could be used to prevent cancer. *BMJ*, 326, 565.
177. Flower, Rod, 2003. What are all the things that aspirin does? *BMJ*, 327, 572–573.
178. UK limits use of aspirin by under 16s. *BMJ*, 2002, 324, 1294.
179. Bartram, Thomas, 1998. *Bartram's Encyclopedia of Herbal Medicine*. London: Robinson; http://www.prostatepointers.org/cmyers/pf0696.html
180. Astralagus. *ICON*, 2002, 1 (3), 23.
181. Medical Report: Prostate Cancer. *ICON*, 2002, 1 (5), 8–10.
182. De La Taille, A. and five others, 1999. Effects of a phytotherapeutic agent, PC-SPES, on prostate cancer: a preliminary investigation on human cell lines and patients. *Br J Urol Int*, 84, 845–850.
183. Ernst, Edzard (editor), 2001. *The Desktop Guide to Complementary and Alternative Medicine: an evidence-based approach*. Mosby.
184. Waxman, Jonathan, 2001. *The Prostate Cancer Book*. London: Vermillion.
185. Bartram, Thomas, 1998. *Bartram's Encyclopedia of Herbal Medicine*. London: Robinson.
186. Medical Report: Prostate Cancer. *ICON*, 2002, 1 (5), 8–10.
187. Campbell, T.C. and Campbell, T.M., 2006. *The China Study*. BenBella Books.
188. http://www.nci.nih.gov/cancerinfo/wyntk/prostate
189. Medical Report: Prostate Cancer. *ICON*, 2002, 1 (5), 8–10.
190. Greenwald, Peter, 2002. Cancer chemoprevention. *BMJ*, 324, 714–718.

2. CELLS BEHAVING BADLY

1. http://bioscience.igh.cnrs.fr/2001/v6/d/hansen/2.asp
2. Clarke, M.F. and Becker, M.W., 2006. Stem cells: the real culprits in cancer? *Scientific American*, July 2006, 53–59.

3. Study reveals how growth factors affect human stem cells. www.hhmi.org/news/melton.html
4. Weinberg, Robert A., 1996. How Cancer Arises. *Scientific American*, Special Issue, What you need to know about Cancer, September, 275, 3, 62–70.
5. Woolf, Neville, 1998. *Pathology, Basic and Systemic*. W.B. Saunders Publishing Co. Chapter 28, p. 274, Figure 28-3.
6. Davey Smith, George, Gunnell, David and Holly, Jeff, 2000. Cancer and insulin-like growth factor-I. *BMJ*, 321, 847–848; Holly, J.M.P., Gunnell, D.J., Davey Smith, G., 1999. Growth hormone, IGF-I and cancer. Less intervention to avoid cancer? More intervention to prevent cancer? *J Endocrinol*, 162, 321–330.
7. http://www.intouchlive.com/cancergenetics/onco.htm
8. Oliver, S.E., Gunnell, D.G., Donovan, J. and others, 2004. Screen-detected prostate cancer and the insulin-like growth factor axis: Results of a population-based case-control study. *International Journal of Cancer*, 108, 887–892.
9. Reuters, 4 August 1999.
10. Ludwig, T., Fisher, P., Ganesan, S. and Efstratiadis, 2001. Tumorigenesis in mice carrying a truncating BRCA1 mutation. *Genes and Development*, 15 (10), 1188–1193; Xu, X., Wagner, K.U., Larson, D., Weaver, Z., Li, C., Ried, T., Hennighausen, L., Wynshaw-Boris, A. and Deng, C.X., 1999. Conditional mutation of BRCA1 in mammary epithelial cells results in blunted ductal morphogenesis and tumour formation. *Nature Genetics*, 22 (1), 37–43; Paull, T.T., Cortez, D., Bowers, B., Elledge, S.J. and Gellert, M., 2001. Direct DNA binding by BRCA1. *Proceedings of the National Acadamy of Sciences of the USA*, 98 (11), 6086–6091.
11. Jensen, R.A., Thompson, M.E., Jetton, T.L., Szabo, CI., van der Meer, R., Helou, B., Tronick, S., King, M-C., Page, D.L. and Holt, J.T., 1996. BRCA1 is secreted and exhibits properties of a granin. *Nature Genetics*, 12, 303–308; http://www.mc.vanderbilt.edu/cancer/research/roster/jensen.html
12. Waxman, Jonathan, 2001. *The Prostate Cancer Book*. London: Vermillion.
13. http://www.cancer.med.umich.edu/prostcan/
14. http://www.mercola.com/2002/apr/27/sv40.htm
15. Waxman, Jonathan, 2001. *The Prostate Cancer Book*. London: Vermillion.
16. Murray, R.K., Granner, D.K., Mayes, P.A. and Rodwell, V.W., 1990. *Harper's Biochemistry*. Appleton and Lange Norwalk, CT, p. 653.
17. Weinberg, Robert A., 1996. How Cancer Arises. *Scientific American*, Special Issue, What you need to know about Cancer, September, 275, 3, 62–70.
18. Clarke, M.F. and Becker, M.W., 2006. Stem Cells: The Real Culprits in Cancer? *Scientific America*, July 2006, 53–59.
19. Jain, R.K., 1994. Barriers to Drug Delivery in Solid Tumours. *Scientific American*, July, 271(1), pp. 58–65.
20. Davey Smith, George, Gunnell, David and Holly, Jeff, 2000. Cancer and insulin-like growth factor-I. *BMJ*, 321, 847–8.
21. Lichtenstein, P, Holm, N.V., Verkasalo, P.K., Iliadou, A., Kaprio, J., Koskenvuo, M. and others, 2000. Environmental and heritable factors in the causation of cancer – analyses of cohorts of twins from Sweden, Denmark, and Finland. *N Engl J Med*, 343, 78–85.

22. Hursting, S.D., Slaga, T.J., Fischer, S.M., DiGiovanni, J. and Phtang, J.M., 1999. Mechanism-based cancer prevention approaches: targets, examples, and the use of transgenic mice. *Journal of the National Cancer Institute*, 35, 2031–2038.

23. Newby, J.A. and Howard, V.C., 2006. Environmental influences in cancer aetiology. *Journal of Nutritional and Environmental Medicine*, 2006, 1–59.

24. Cheeseman, K.H. and Slater, T.F., 1993. *Free Radicals in Medicine*. Churchill Livingston.

25. Cheeseman, K.H. and Slater, T.F., 1993. *Free Radicals in Medicine*. Churchill Livingston.

26. Holly, J.M.P., Gunnell, D.J. and Davey Smith, G., 1999. Growth hormone, IGF-I and cancer. Less intervention to avoid cancer? More intervention to prevent cancer? *J Endocrinol*, 162, 321–330.

27. Gann, P.H., Hennekens, C.H., Ma, J., Longcope, C. and Stampfer, M.J., 1996. Prospective study of sex hormone levels and risk of prostate cancer. *Journal of the National Cancer Institute*, 88, 1118–1126.

28. Waxman, Jonathan, 2001. *The Prostate Cancer Book*. London: Vermillion.

29. http://grants1.nih.gov/grants/guide/rfa-files/RFA-DK-01-008.html

30. http://grants1.nih.gov/grants/guide/rfa-files/RFA-DK-01-008.html

31. Miller, W.R. and Sharpe, R.M., 1998. Environmental oestrogens and human reproductive cancers. *Endocrine-Related Cancer*, 5, 69–96.

32. Miller, W.R. and Sharpe, R.M., 1998. Environmental oestrogens and human reproductive cancers. *Endocrine-Related Cancer*, 5, 69–96.

33. Yu, H. and Rohan, T., 2002. Role of the insulin-like growth factor family in cancer development and progression. *J Natl Cancer Inst*, 92, 1472–1489.

34. Rose, Steven, with Mileusnic, Radmila. 1999. *The Chemistry of Life*. Fourth (revised) edition. Penguin Books.

35. Voet, Donald and Voet, Judith, 1995. *Biochemistry*. Second edition. John Wiley & Sons, Inc.

36. Outwater, J.L., Nicholson, A. and Barnard, N., 1997. Dairy products and breast cancer: the IGF-1, estrogen, and bGH hypothesis. *Medical Hypotheses*, 48, 453–461.

37. Oliver, S.E., Gunnell, D.G., Donovan, J. and others, 2004. Screen-detected prostate cancer and the insulin-like growth factor axis: Results of a population-based case-control study. *International Journal of Cancer*, 108, 887–892.

38. Gunnell, D, L, and 10 others, 2003. Are diet – prostate-cancer associations mediated by the IGF axis? A cross-sectional analysis of diet, IGF-I and IGFBP-3 in healthy middle-aged men. *British Journal of Cancer*, 88, 1682–1686.

39. Yu, H. and Rohan, T., 2002. Role of the insulin-like growth factor family in cancer development and progression. *J Natl Cancer Inst*, 92, 1472–1489.

40. Yu, H. and Rohan, T., 2002. Role of the insulin-like growth factor family in cancer development and progression. *J Natl Cancer Inst*, 92, 1472–1489.

41. Loeb, L.A., 1991. Mutator phenotype may be required for multistage carcinogenesis. *Cancer Research*, 51, 3075–3079.

42. Barres, B.A., Hart, I.K., Coles, H.S.R., Burne, J.F., Voyvodic, J.T., Richardson, W.D. and Raff, M.C., 1992. Cell death and control of cell survival in

the oligodendrocyte lineage. *Cell*, 70, 31–46; Harrington, E.A., Bennett, M.R., Fanidi, A. and Evan, G.I., 1994. c-Myc-induced apoptosis in fibroblasts is inhibited by specific cytokines. *EMBO Journal*, 13, 3286–3295.

43. Davey Smith, George, Gunnell, David and Holly, Jeff, 2000. Cancer and insulin-like growth factor-I. *BMJ*, 321, 847–8.

3. THE THIRD STRAWBERRY

1. Forbes, Alec, 1984. *The Bristol Diet*. Century.
2. http://www.nci.nih.gov/cancerinfo/wyntk/prostate
3. Trichopoulos, Dimitrios, Li, Frederick, P. and Hunter, David J., 1996. What Causes Cancer? *Scientific American*, Special Issue, What you need to know about Cancer. September, 275, 3, 80–85.
4. Boots the Chemist, 1998. *Breast Awareness – an essential guide*, Be enlightened, not frightened. Published in association with the charity Breast Cancer Care.
5. Waxman, Jonathan, 2001. *The Prostate Cancer Book*. London: Vermillion.
6. Holland, J.C., 1996. Cancer's Psychological Challenges. *Scientific American*, Special Issue, What you need to know about Cancer, September, 275, 3, 158–161.
7. http://www.who.int/nut/malnutrition-worldwide.htm
8. *Cancer Incidence in Five Continents*, 1997. Vol. V11, published by the IARC (International Agency for Research on Cancer).
9. Medical Report: Prostate Cancer. *ICON*, 2002, 1(5), 8–10.
10. Parkin, D.M., Whelan, S.L., Ferlay, J., Raymond, L., Young, J. *Cancer in five Continents vol. VII*. Lyon: IARCPress, 1997.
11. http://www.rense.com/general/dair.htm
12. America Cancer Society, 2006. Cancer facts and figures 2006. Atlanta.
13. http://www.cancer.med.umich.edu/prostcan/
14. Waxman, Jonathan, 2001. *The Prostate Cancer Book*. London: Vermillion; http://www.cancer.med.umich.edu/prostcan/
15. Medical Report: Prostate Cancer. *ICON*, 2002, 1(5), 8–10.
16. http://www.cancer.med.umich.edu/prostcan/
17. Oishi, K., Yoshida, O. and Schroeder, F.H., 1995. The geography of prostate cancer and its teatment in Japan. *Cancer Surveys*, 23, 267–280.
18. *Proceedings of the European Cancer Conference*, September 23, 2003, quoted in *The Times (Public Agenda)*, 30 September 2003.
19. Mayor, Susan, 2003. UK improves cancer control. *BMJ*, 326, 72.
20. *The Atlas of Cancer Mortality in the People's Republic of China*.
21. Pike, M.C., Kolonel, L.N., Henderson, B.E., Wilkens, L.R., Hankin, J.H., Feigelson, H.S., Wan, P.C., Stram, D.O. and Nomura, A.M., 2002. Breast cancer in a multiethnic cohort in Hawaii and Los Angeles: risk factor-adjusted incidence in Japanese equals that in Hawaiians exceeds that in whites. *Cancer Epidemiology Biomarkers and Prevention*, 11(9), 795–800.
22. http://www.hawaii.edu/crch/ProfileKolonel.htm
23. World Cancer Research Fund, 1997. *Food, nutrition and the prevention of cancer: a global perspective*. Washington, DC: American Institute of Cancer Research; Gunnell, D.L. and 10 others, 2003. Are diet – prostate-cancer associations mediated by the IGF axis? A cross-sectional analysis of diet, IGF-I

and IGFBP-3 in healthy middle-aged men. *British Journal of Cancer*, 88, 1682–1686.

24. America Cancer Society, 2006. Cancer facts and figures 2006. Atlanta.
25. www.cancerresearchuk.org
26. Minino, A.M., Arias, E., Kochanek, K.D., Murphy, S.L. and Smith, B.L., 2002. *Deaths: Final Data for 2000. National vital statistics reports.* Hyattsville, Maryland: National Center for Health Statistics.
27. www-dep.iarc.fr/GLOBOCAN
28. http://www.prostatepointers.org/cmyers/pf0696.html
29. http://www.prostatepointers.org/cmyers/pf0696.html
30. Plant, Jane and Tidey, Gill, 2003. *Understanding, Preventing and Overcoming Osteoporosis.* Virgin Books.
31. Campbell, T.C. and Junshi, C., 1994. Diet and chronic degenerative disease perspectives from China. *American Journal of Clinical Nutrition*, 59 (Suppl.), 11,535–11,615.
32. Remer, T. and Manz, F., 1995. Potential renal acid load of foods and its influence on urine pH. *Journal of the American Dietetic Association*, 95, No. 7, 791–797.
33. Lark, Susan and Richards, James A., 2000. *The Chemistry of Success.* San Fransisco: Bay Books, 55.
34. *Statistical Abstracts of the US*, 1994 edition.
35. Anon, 2007. Healthy products breed healthy sales for Danone. www.foodnavigator.com
36. Campbell, T.C., quoted in http://www:milksucks.com/osteo.html; Robbins, John, 1987. *A Diet for a New America.* Stillpoint Publishing; McDougall, John, 2000. *The McDougall Program for Women.*
37. Plant, Jane and Tidey, Gill, 2003. *Understanding, Preventing and Overcoming Osteoporosis.* Virgin Books.
38. Frassetto, L.A., Todd, K.M., Morris, R.C., Jr and Sebastian, A., 2000. Worldwide incidence of hip fracture in elderly women: relation to consumption of animal and vegetable foods. *J Geront: Med Sci*, 55A, 10, M585–M592.
39. Forbes, Alec, 1984. *The Bristol Diet.* Century.
40. Cramer, D.W. and others, 1989. Galactose consumption and metabolism in relation to the risk of ovarian cancer. *Lancet*, 2, 66–71.
41. Newcomb, P.A. and Egan, K.M., 2006. Dairy food and ovarian cancer risk. *The Lancet*, March 2006, 797–799.

4. MILK IS A FOUR-LETTER WORD

1. Pringle, H., 1998. Neolithic agriculture: reading the signs of ancient animal domestication. *Science*. 282, 1448.
2. Latham, M.C., 1997. Human nutrition in the developing world, Rome, 1997. FAO Food and Nutrition Series No 29, Cornell University, Ithaca, NY.
3. Cox, Peter and Brusseau, Peggy, 1995. *LifePoints For Kids.* Bloomsbury.
4. Butler, J., 2006. *White lies.* Vegetarian and Vegan Foundation.
5. AbuGhazaleh, A.A. and others, 2004. CLA increases in milk when cows fed fish meal and extruded soybeans for an extended period of time. *Journal of Dairy Science*, 87 (6), 1758–1766.

6. Petit, H.V., 2002. Digestion, milk production, milk composition, and blood composition of dairy cows fed whole flax seed. *Journal of Dairy Science*, 85 (6), 1482–1490.

7. Wahle, K.W. and others, 2004. CLAs: are they beneficial or detrimental to health? *Progress in Lipid Research*, 43 (6), 553–587.

8. The Royal Society, 2000. Endocrine-disrupting chemicals. *Document* 06/00. The Royal Society.

9. Butler, J., 2006. *White lies*. Vegetarian and Vegan Foundation.

10. Qin, L.Q. and others, 2004. Estrogen: one of the risk factors in milk for prostate cancer. *Medical Hypotheses*, 62 (1), 133–142.

11. Hartman, S. and others, 1998. Natural occurrence of steroid hormones in food. *Food Chemistry*, 62, 7–20.

12. Butler, J., 2006. *White lies*. Vegetarian and Vegan Foundation.

13. Ganmaa, D. and Sato, A., 2005. Possible role of female sex hormones in milk from pregnant cows in the development of breast, ovarian and corpus uteri cancers. *Medical Hypotheses*, 65 (6), 1028–1037.

14. DEFRA, 2005. *Agriculture in the UK*, 2004. Norwich, UK: HMSO.

15. *Statistical Abstracts of the US*, 1994 edition.

16. Campbell, T.C. and Junshi, C., 1994. Diet and chronic degenerative disease perspectives from China. *Am J Clin Nutr*, 59, Suppl., 11,535–11,615.

17. Charatan, Fred, 2003. Book Review: Fat Land: How Americans Became the Fattest People in the World, by Greg Critser. *BMJ*, 326, 229.

18. Charatan, Fred, 2003. Book Review: Fat Land: How Americans Became the Fattest People in the World, by Greg Critser. *BMJ*, 326, 229.

19. Charatan, Fred, 2003. Book Review: Fat Land: How Americans Became the Fattest People in the World, by Greg Critser. *BMJ*, 326, 229.

20. Grosvenor, C.E. and others, 1992. Hormones and growth factors in milk. *Endocrine Reviews*, 14 (6), 710–728.

21. http://www.dhn.csiro.au/crctissue.html

22. http://www.13.waisays.com/cancer2.htm

23. le Huerou-Luron, I. and others, 1998. Source of dietary protein influences kinetics of plasma gut regulatory peptide concentration to feeding in preruminant calves. *Comparative Biochemistry and Physiology: A – Molecular and Integrative Physiology*, 119 (3), 817–824.

24. Koldovski, O. and others, 1995. Milk-borne hormones: possible tools of communication between mother and suckling. *Physiological Research*, 1995, 44 (6), 349–351; Koldovsky, O. and others, 1994. Hormonally active peptides in human milk. *Acta Paediatrica* Suppl., 402, 89–93; Lehy,T. and others, 1990. Promoting effect of bombesin on the cell proliferation in the rat endocrine pancreas during the early post natal period. *RegulatoryPeptides*, 27 (1), 87–96; Pollack, P.F., 1989. Effects of enterally- and parenterally-administrated bombesin on intestinal luminal tryptic activity and protein in the suckling rat. *Experienta*, 45 (4), 385–388; Lazarus, L.H. and others, 1986. An immunoreactive peptide in milk contains bombesin-like bioactivity. *Experienta*, 42 (7), 822–823; Jahnke, G.D. and others, 1984. A bombesin immunoreactive peptide in milk. *Proc Natl Acad Sci USA.*, 81 (2), 578–582.

25. Berseth, C.I. and others, 1990. Postpartum changes in pattern of gastrointestinal regulatory peptides in human milk. *Am J Clin Nutr*, 51 (6), 985–990.

26. Markwalder, R. and others, 1999. Gastrin-releasing peptide receptors in the human prostate: relation to neoplastic transformation. *Cancer Research*, 59 (5), 1152–1159; Festuccia, C. and others, 1998. In vitro regulation of pericellular proteolysis in prostatic tumor cells treated with bombesin. *Int. J. Cancer*, 75 (3), 418–431; Krongrad, A. and others, 1997. Endopeptidase 24.11 activity in the human prostate cancer cell lines LNCaP and PPC-1. *Urological Research*, 25 (2), 113–116; Jungwirth, A. and others, 1997. LHRH antagonist Cetrolix (SB-75) and bombesin-antagonist RC-3940-II inhibit the growth of androgen-independent PC-3 prostate cancer in nude mice. *Prostate*, 32 (3), 164–172; Larran, J. and others, 1996. In vitro characterization of bombesin and calcitonin on the proliferation of PC3, DK145 and LNCaP cancer prostatic cell lines. International Journal of Developmental Biology, 1996 (Suppl. 1), 275S–276S; Aprickian, A.G. and others, 1996. Bombesin specifically induces intracellular calcium mobilization via gastrin-releasing peptide receptors in human prostatic cancer cells. *Journal of Molecular Endocrinology*, 16 (3), 297–306; Bologna, M. and others, 1989. Bombesin stimulates growth of human prostatic cancer cells in vitro. *Cancer*, 63 (9), 1714–1720; Wasilenko, W.J. and others, 1996. Effects of the calcium influx inhibitor carboxyamido-triazole on the proliferation and invasiveness of human prostate tumor cell lines. *Int J Cancer*, 68 (2), 259–264.

27. Burns, D.M. and others, 1999. Breast cancer cell-associated endopeptidase EC24.11 modulates proliferative response to bombesin. *British Journal of Cancer*, 79 (2), 214–220; Bold, R.J. and others, 1998. Bombesin stimulates in vitro growth of human breast cancer independent of estrogen receptor status. *Anticancer Research*, 18 (16A), 4051–4056; Miyazaki, M. and others, 1998. Inhibition of growth of MDA-MB-231 human breast cancer xenografts in nude mice by bombesin/gastrin-releasing peptide (GRP) antagonists RC-3940-II and RC-3095. *European Journal of Cancer*, 34 (5), 710–717; Nelson, J. and others, 1991. Bombesin stimulates proliferation of human breast cancer cells in culture. *Br. J. Cancer*, 63 (6), 933–936; Giacchetti, S. and others, 1990. Characterization, in some human breast cancer cell lines, of gastrin-releasing peptide-like receptors which are absent in normal breast epithelial cells. *Int J Cancer*, 46 (2), 293–298; Weber, C.J. and others, 1989. Gastrin-releasing peptide, calcitonin gene-related peptide, and calcitonin-like immuno-reactivity in human breast cyst fluid and gastrin-releasing peptide-like immunoreactivity in human breast carcinoma cell lines. *Surgery*, (6), 1134–1139 (disc.1139–1140).

28. Takeyama, M. and others, 1989. Enzyme immunoassay of gastrin-releasing peptide (GRP)-like immunoreactivity in milk. *Int J Pept Protein Res*, 34 (1), 70–74.

29. Ducroc, R. and others, 1995. Immunoreactive substance P and calcitonin-gene-related peptide (CGRP) in rat milk and in human milk and infant formula's. *Am J Clin Nutr*, 62 (3), 554–558.

30. Lembeck, F. and others, 1979. Substance P as neurogenic mediator of antidromic vasodilation and neurogenic plasma extravasation. *Arch Pharmacol*, 310 (2), 175–183.

31. Khare, V.K. and others, 1998. The neuropeptide/mast cell secretagogue substance P is expressed in cutaneous melanocyticlesions. *Journal of Cutaneous Pathology*, 25 (1), 2–10.

32. Ducroc, R. and others, 1995. Immunoreactive substance P and calcitonin-gene-related peptide (CGRP) in rat milk and in human milk and infant formula's. *Am J Clin Nutr*, 62 (3), 554–558.
33. Faulkner, A., 1998. Insuline-like growth factor 1 concentrations in milk and plasma after growth hormone treatment. *Biochemical Society Transactions*, 26 (4), 386; Silanikove, N. and others, 1998. Metabolic and productive response of dairy cows to increased ion supplementation at early lactation in warm weather. *Journal of Dairy Research*, 65 (4), 529–543; Ginjala, V. and others, 1998. Determination of transforming growth factor-beta 1 (TGF-beta 1) and insulin-like growth factor-1 (IGF-1) in bovine colostreum samples. *Journal of Immunoassay*, 19 (2–3), 195–207; Schober, D.A. and others, 1990. Perinatal expression of type 1 IGF receptors in porcine small intestine. *Endocrinology*, 126 (2), 1125–1132.
34. Rao, R.K. and others, 1998. Luminal stability of insulin-like growth factor-1 and -2 in developing rat gastrointestinal tract. *Journal of Pediatric Gastroenterology and Nutrition*, 26 (2), 179–185.
35. Untergasser, G. and others, 1999. Proliferative disorders of the aging human prostate: involvement of protein hormones and their receptors. *Experimental Gerontology*, 34 (2), 275–287; Xu, Z.D., 1999. Hammerhead ribozyme-mediated cleavage of the human insulin-like growth factor-2 ribonucleic acid in vitro and in prostate cancer cells. *Endocrinology*, 140 (5), 2134–2144; Marelli, M.M. and others, 1999. Luteinizing hormone-releasing hormone agonists interfere with the antagonic activity of the insulin-like growth factor system in androgen-dependent prostate cancer cells. *Endocrinology*, 140 (1), 329–334; Lamharzi, N. and others, 1998. Growth hormone-releasing hormone antagonist MZ-5-156 inhibits growth of DY-145 human androgen-independent prostate carcinoma in nude mice and suppresses the levels and mRNA expression of insulin-like growth factor-2 in tumors. *Proc Natl Acad Sci USA*, 95 (15), 8864–8868; Wang, Y.Z. and others, 1998. Sex hormone-induced prostatic carcinogenesis in the noble rat: the role of insulin-like growth factor-1 (IGF-1) and vascular endothelial growth factor (VEGF) in the development of cancer. *Prostate*, 35 (3), 165–177.
36. Parisot, J.P. and others, 1999. Altered expression of the insulin-like growth factor-1 receptor in a tamoxifen-resistant human breast cancer cell line. *Br J Cancer*, 79 (5–6), 693–700; Sciacca, L. and others, 1999. Insulin receptor activation by insulin-like growth factor-2 in breast cancers: evidence for a new autocrine/paracrine mechanism. *Oncogene*, 18 (15), 2471–2479; Grothey, A. and others, 1999. The role of insuline-like growth factor and its receptor in cell growth transformation, apoptosis, and chemoresistance in solid tumors. *Journal of Cancer Research and Clinical Oncology*, 125 (3–4), 166–173; Perks, C.M. and others, 1999. Activation of integrin and ceramide signalling pathways can inhibit the mitogenic effect of insulin-like growth factor-1 (IGF-1) in human breast cancer cell lines. *Br J Cancer*, 79 (5–6), 701–706; de Cupis, A. and others, 1998. Responsiveness to hormone, growth factor and drug treatment of a human breast cancer cell line: comparison between early and late cultures. *In Vitro Cellular and Developmental Biology – Animal*, 34 (10), 836–843; Kobari, M. and others, 1998. The inhibitory effect of an epidermal growth factor receptor specific tyrokinase inhibitor on

pancreatic cancer cell lines was more potent than inhibitory antibodies against the receptors for EGF and IGF-1. *International Journal of Pancreatology*, 24 (2), 85–95; Gooch, J.L. and others, 1998. Interleukin 4 inhibits growth and induces apoptosis in human breast cancer cells. *Cancer Res*, 58 (18), 4199–4205; Choki, I. and others, 1998. Osteoblast-derived growth factors enhance adriamycin-cytostasis of MCF-7 human breast cancer cells. *Anticancer Res*, 18 (16A), 4213–4224; Jackson, J.G. and others, 1998. Insulin receptor substrate-1 is the predominant signaling molecule activated by insulin-like growth factor-1, insulin, and interleukin-4 in estrogen receptor-positive human breast cancer cells. *Journal of Biological Chemistry*, 273 (16), 9994–10003; Westley, B.R. and others, 1998. Interactions between the oestrogen and IGF signalling pathways in the control of breast epithelial cell proliferation. *Biochemical Society Symposium*, 63, 35–44; Surmacz, E. and others, 1995. Overexpression of insulin receptor substrate 1 (IRS-1) in the human breast cancer cell line MCF-7 induces loss of estrogen requirements for growth and transformation. *Clinical Cancer Research*, 1 (11), 1429–1436.

37. He, Y., 1999. Comment on the Association between Insulin-Like Growth Factor-I (IGF-I) and Bone Mineral Density: Further Evidence Linking IGF-I to Breast Cancer Risk. *Journal of Cellular Endocrinology and Metabolism*, 84, 1760.

38. Perks, C. M. and Holly, J.M.P., 2000. Insulin-Like Growth Factor Binding Proteins (IGFBPs) in Breast Cancer. *Journal of Mammary Gland Biology and Neoplasia*, 5, 75–84.

39. Murphy, M.S. and others, 1998. Growth factors and the gastrointestinal tract. *Nutrition*, 14 (10), 771–774; Buts, J.P., 1998. Bioactive factors in milk. (in French.) *Archives de Pediatrie*, 5 (3), 298–306.

40. Shen, W.H. and others, 1998. Stability and distribution of orally administered epidermal growth factor in neonatal pigs. *Life Sciences*, 63 (10), 809–820; Rao, R.K. and others, 1998. Bovine milk inhibits proteolytic degradation of epidermal growth factor in human gastric and duodenal lumen. *Peptides*, 19 (3), 495–504; McCuskey, R.S. and others, 1997. Effect of milk-borne epidermal growth factor on the hepatic microcirculation and Kupfer cell function in suckling rats. *Biology of the Neonate*, 7 (3), 202–206; Oguchi, S. and others, 1997. Growth factors in breast milk and their effect on gastrointestinal development. *Chang Hua Min Kuo Hsiao Erh Ko I Hsuek Tsa Chih*, 38 (5), 332–337.

41. Zhau, H.J. and others, 1996. Androgen-depressed phenotype in human prostate cancer. *Proc. Natl. Acad. Sci. U.S.A.*, 93 (26), 15152–15157.

42. Salomon, D.S. and others, 1999. Cripto: a novel epidermal growth factor (EGF)-related peptide in mammary gland development and neoplasia. *Bioessays*, 21 (1), 61–70; Chou, Y.C. and others, 1999. Induction of mammary carcinomas by N-methyl-N-nitrosurea in ovariectomized rats treated with epidermal growth factor. *Carcinogenesis*, 20 (4), 677–684; Kurtz, A. and others, 1998. Local control of mammary gland differentation: mammary-derived growth inhibitor and pleiotrophin. *Biochemical Society Symposium*, 63, 51–69. , Taylor, M.R. and others, 1997. Lactadherin (formerly BA46); a membrane-associated gycoprotein expressed in human

milk and breast carcinomas, promotes Arg-Gly-Asp (RGD)-dependent cell adhesion. *DNA and Cell Biology*, 16 (7), 861–869.

43. Thornburg, W. and others, 1984. Gastrointestinal absorption of epidermal growth factor in suckling rats. *American Journal of Physiology*, 246, G80–G85.

44. www.prostatepointers.org/cmyers/pf0696.html

45. Gaull, G.E. and others, 1985. Significance of growth modulators in human milk. *Pediatrics*, 75 (2), 142–145.

46. Ganmaa, D. and Sato, A., 2005. Possible role of female sex hormones in milk from pregnant cows in the development of breast, ovarian and corpus uteri cancers. *Medical Hypotheses*, 65 (6), 1028–1037.

47. Hartman, S. and others, 1998. Natural occurrence of steroid hormones in food. *Food Chemistry*, 62, 7–20.

48. Delgrange, E. and others, 1997. Sex related differences in the growth of prolactinomas : a clinical and proliferation marker study. *Journal of Clinical Endocrinology and Metabolism*, 82 (7), 2102–2107.

49. Leav, I. and others, 1999. Prolactin receptor expression in the developing human prostate and in hyperplastic, dysplastic, and neoplastic lesions. *American Journal of Pathology*, 154 (3), 863–870; Horti, J. and others, 1998. A phase 2 study of bromocriptine in patients with androgen-independent prostate cancer. *Oncology Reports*, 5 (4), 893–896; Franklin, R.B. and others, 1997. Prolactin regulation of mitochondrial aspartate aminotransferase and proteinkinase C *Molecular and Cellular Endocrinology*, 127 (1), 19–25; Janssen, T. and others, 1996. In vitro characterization of prolactin-induced effects on proliferation in the neoplastic LNCaP, DU145, and PC3 models of the human prostate. *Cancer*, 77 (1), 144–149; Janssen, T. and others, 1995. Organ culture of human tissue as study model of hormonal and pharmacological regulation of benign prostatic hyperplasia and of prostatic cancer. (frans) *Acta Urol Belg*, 63 (1), 7–14; Oliver, R.T. and others, 1995. New directions with hormone therapy in prostate cancer: possible benefit from blocking prolactin and use of hormone treatment intermittently in combination with immunotherapy. *Eur J Cancer*, 31A (6), 859–860; Rana, A. and others, 1995. A case for synchronous reduction of testicular androgen, adrenal androgen and prolactin for the treatment of advanced carcinoma of the prostate. *Eur J Cancer*, 31A (6), 871–875.

50. Vonderhaar, B.K., 1998, Prolactin: The forgotten hormone of human breast cancer. *Pharmacology and Therapeutics*, 79 (2), 169–178; Das, R. and others, 1996. Involvement of SHC, GRB2, SOS and RAS in prolactin signal transduction in mammary epithelial cells. *Oncogene*, 13 (6), 1139–1145; Mershon, J. and others, 1995. Prolactin is a local growth factor in rat mammary tumors. *Endocrinology*, 136 (8), 3619–3623; Ginsberg, E. and others, 1995. Prolactin secretion by human breast cancer cells. *Cancer Res*, 55 (12), 2591–2595; Fuh, G. and others, 1995. Prolactin receptor antagonists that inhibit the growth of breast cancer cell lines. *J Biol Chem*, 270 (22), 13133–13137.

51. Hinuma, S. and others, 1998. A prolactin-releasing peptide in the brain. *Nature*, 393 (6682), 272–276.

52. Smith, S.S. and others, 1986. Presence of luteinising hormone-releasing hormone (LHRH) in milk. Endocrinol Exp., 20 (2–3), 147–153; Koldovsky,

O., 1989. Search for the role of milk borne biologically active peptides for the suckling. *J. Nutr.*, 119 (11), 1543–1551; Nair, R.M. and others, 1987. Studies on LHRH and physiological fluid amino acids in human colostreum and milk. *Endocrinolologia Experimentalis*, 21 (1), 23–30.

53. White, M.E. and others, 1986. Milk progesterone concentrations following simultaneous administration of buserelin and cloprostenol in cattle with normal corporal lutea. *Canadian Journal of Veterinary Research*, 50 (2), 285–286; Dinsmore, R.P. and others, 1989. Effect of gonadotropin-releasing hormone on clinical response and fertility in cows with cystyic ovaries, as related to milk progesterone concentration and days after partarition. *Journal of the American Veterinary Medical Association*, 195 (3), 327–330.

54. Hartman, S. and others, 1998. Natural occurrence of steroid hormones in food. *Food Chemistry*, 62, 7–20.

55. Berseth, C.I. and others, 1990. Postpartum changes in pattern of gastrointestinal regulatory peptides in human milk. *Am J Clin Nutr*, 51 (6), 985–990.

56. Berseth, C.I. and others, 1990. Postpartum changes in pattern of gastrointestinal regulatory peptides in human milk. *Am J Clin Nutr*, 51 (6), 985–990.

57. Flood, J.F. and others, 1991. Increased food intake by neuropeptide Y is due to an increased motivation to eat. *Peptides*, 12 (6), 1329–1332.

58. Amarant, T. and others, 1982. Luteinising hormone-releasing hormone and thyrotropin-releasing hormone in human and bovine milk. *European Journal of Biochemistry*, 127 (3), 647–650; Baram, T. and others, 1977. Gonadotropin-releasing hormone in milk. *Science*, 198 (4314), 300–302.

59. Koike, K. and others, 1997. The pituitary folliculo-stellate cell line TtT/GF augments basal and TRH-induced prolactin secretion by GH3 cells. *Life Sci*, 61 (25), 2491–2497; Tyson, J.E. and others, 1975. The influence of prolactine secretion on human lactation. *J Clin Endocrinol Metab*, 40 (5), 764–773.

60. Grochowska, R. and others, 1999. Stimulated growth hormone (GH) release in Friesian cattle with respect to GH genotypes. *Reproduction Nutrition Development*, 39 (2), 171–180; Bourne, R.A. and others, 1977. Serum growth hormone concentrations after growth hormone or thyroid-releasing hormone in cows. *Journal of Dairy Science*, 60 (10), 1629–1635.

61. Chomczinsky, P. and others, 1993. Stimulatory effect of thyroid hormone on growth hormone gene expression in a human pituitary cell line. *J Clin Endocrinol Metab*, 77 (1), 281–285; Reynolds, A.M., 1991. The effects of chronic exposure to supraphysiological concentrations of 3,5,3/triiodo-L-thyronine (T3) on cultured GC cells. *Journal of Cellular. Physiology*, 149 (3), 544–547.

62. Tenore, A. and others, 1980. Thyroidal response to peroral TSH in suckling and weaned rats. *American Journal of Physiology*, 238 (5), E428–430.

63. Slebodzinski, A.B. and others, 1998. Triiodothyronine (T3), insulin and characteristics of 5/-monodiodinase (5/-MD) in mare's milk from partarition to 21 days post-partum. *Reproduction Nutrition Development*, 38 (3), 235–244.

64. Fujimoto, N. and others, 1997. Upregulation of the estrogen receptor by triiodothyronine in rat pituitary cell lines. *Journal of Steroid Biochemistry and Molecular Biology*, 61 (1–2), 79–85.

65. Koldovsky, O., 1989. Search for the role of milk borne biologically active peptides for the suckling. *J Nutr*, 119 (11), 1543–1551; Buts, J.P., 1998. Bioactive factors in milk. (in French.) *Arch Pediatr*, 5 (3), 298–306.

66. Faulkner, A., 1998. Insulin-like growth factor concentrations in milk and plasma after growth hormone treatment. *Biochemical Society Transactions*, 26 (4), S386; Baldini, E. and others, 1994. In vivo cytokinetic effects of recombinant human growth hormone (rhGH) in patients with advanced breast carcinoma. *Journal of Biological Regulators and Homeostatic Agents*, 8 (4), 113–116; Scheven, B.A. and others, 1991. Effects of recombinant human insulin-like growth factor-1 and -2 (IGF) and growth hormone (GH) on the growth of normal adult human osteoblast-like cells and human osteogenic sarcoma cells. *Growth Regulation*, 1 (4), 160–167; Hodate, K. and others, 1990. Plasma growth hormone, insuline-like growth factor-1, and milk production response to exogenous human growth hormone-releasing factor analogs in dairy cows. *Endocrinologia Japonica*, 37 (2), 261–273.

67. Koldovsky, O., 1989. Search for the role of milk borne biologically active peptides for the suckling. *J Nutr*, 119 (11), 1543–1551; Buts, J.P., 1998. Bioactive factors in milk. (in French.) *Arch Pediatr*, 5 (3), 298–306.

68. Westrom, B.R. and others, 1987. Levels of immunoreactive insulin, neurotensin, and bombesin in porcine colostreum and milk. *J Pediatr Gastroenterol Nutr*, 6 (3), 460–465; Ehman, R. and others, 1985. Bombesin, neurotensin and pro-gamma-melanotropin in immunoreactants in human milk. *Regulatory Peptides*, 10 (2–3), 99–105.

69. Shutt, D.A. and others, 1985. Comparison of total and free cortisol in bovine serum and milk colostreum. *J Dairy Sci*, 68 (7), 1832–1834.

70. Vaarala, O. and others, 1998. Cow milk feeding induces antibodies to insulin in children – a link between cow milk and insulin-dependent diabetes mellitus? *Scandinavian Journal of Immunology* 47 (2), 131–135; Slebodzinsky, A.B. and others, 1998. Triiodothyronine (T3), insulin and characteristics of 5/-monodiodinase (5/-MD) in mare's milk from partarition to 21 days post-partum. *Reprod Nutr Dev*, 38 (3), 235–244; Westrom, B.R. and others, 1987. Levels of immunoreactive insulin, neurotensin, and bombesin in porcine colostreum and milk. *J Pediatr Gastroenterol Nutr*, 6 (3), 460–465.

71. Ferrando, T. and others, 1990. Beta-endorphin-like and alpha-MSH-like immunoreactivities in human milk. *Life Sci*, 47 (7), 633–635.

72. http://www.13.waisays.com/cancer2.htm; Newcomb, P.A. and Egan, K.M., 2006. Dairy food and ovarian cancer risk. *The Lancet*, March 2006, 797–799; Stang, A. and others, 2006. Adolescent milk fat and galactose consumption and testicular germ cell cancer. *Cancer Epidemiology and Biomarkers Prevention*, 15, 2189–2195.

73. Reiter, E. and others, 1999. Effects of pituitary hormones on the prostate. *Prostate*, 38 (2), 159–165; Lamharzi, N. and others, 1998. Luteinising hormone-releasing hormone (LH-RH) antagonist Cetrorelix inhibits growth of DU-145 human androgen-independent prostate carcinoma in nude mice and suppresses the levels and mRNA expression of IGF-2 in tumors. *Regulatory Peptides.*, 77 (1–3), 185–192; Jungwirth, A. and others, 1997.

Luteinising hormone-releasing hormone (LH-RH) antagonist Cetrorelix (SB-75) and bombesin antagonist RC-3940-2 inhibit the growth of androgen-independent PC-3 prostate cancer in nude mice. *Prostate*, 32 (3), 164–172; Maezawa, H. and others, 1997. Potentiating effect of buserelin acetate, an LHRH agonist, on the proliferation of ventral prostatic epithelial cells in testosterone-treated castrated rats. *Int J Urol*, 4 (4), 411–416; Hsing, A.W. and others, 1993. Serological precursers of cancer serum hormones and risk of subsequent prostate cancer. *Cancer Epidemiol Biomarkers Prev*, 2 (1), 27–32; Garde, S. and others, 1993. Effect of prostatic inhibiting peptide on prostate cancer cell growth in vitro and in vivo. *Prostate*, 7 (2), 183–194.

74. Maruuchi, T. and others, 1998. Effects of gonadotropin-releasing hormone agonist on rat ovarian adenocarcinoma cell lines in vitro and in vivo. *Japanese Journal of Cancer Research*, 89 (9), 977–983; Kuroda, H. and others, 1998. Human chorionic gonadotrophin (hCG) inhibits cisplatin-induced apoptosis in ovarian cancer cells: possibe role of up-regulation of IGF-1 by hCG. *Int J Cancer*, 76 (4), 571–578; Kurbacher, C.M. and others, 1995. Influence of luteinising hormone on cell growth and CA 125 secretion of primary epithelial ovarian carcinomas in vitro. *Tumour Biology*, 16 (6), 374–384; Manetta, A. and others, 1995. Inhibition of growth of human ovarian cancer in nude mice by luteinising hormone-releasing hormone antagonist Cetrorelix (SB-75). *Fertility and Sterility*, 63 (2), 282–287.

75. Bosland, M.C., 1996. Hormonal factors in carcinogenesis of the prostate and testis in humans and in animal models. *Progress in Clinical and Biological Research*, 394, 309–352.

76. Chapman, S. and others, 1992. Changes in adult cigarette consumption per head in 128 countries, 1986–1990. *Tobacco Control*, 1, 281–284.

77. http://www.who.int

78. Chapman, S. and others, 1992. Changes in adult cigarette consumption per head in 128 countries, 1986–1990. *Tobacco Control*, 1, 281–284.

79. http://www.who.int

80. http://www.13.waisays.com/cancer2.htm

81. Underwood, L.E., D'Ercole, J.A. and Van Wyk, J.J., 1980. Somatomedin-C and the assessment of growth. *Ped Clin N Amer*, 27, 4, 771–782, and Perdue, J.F., 1984. Chemistry, structure and function of insulin-like growth factors and their receptors: a review. *Can J Biochem Cell Bio*, 62, 1237–1245.

82. Evidence for a zinc uptake transporter in human prostate cancer cells which is regulated by prolactin and testosterone. *J Biol Chem*, 274, 17499–504.

83. Medical Report: Prostate Cancer. *ICON*, 2002, 1(5), 8–10.

84. http://vvv.com/healthnews/milk.html

85. Pollack, Michael, 2003. Cancer, aging and IGF physiology. Meeting of the Royal Society of Medicine in London in October 2003, entitled 'Biology of IGF-I: its interaction with insulin in health and malignant states'.

86. Lonning, Per Eystein, 2003. IGF-I and breast cancer. Meeting of the Royal Society of Medicine in London in October 2003, entitled 'Biology of IGF-I: its interaction with insulin in health and malignant states'.

87. Yee, Doug, 2003. Targeting the IGF system for anti-tumour therapy. Meeting of the Royal Society of Medicine in London in October 2003,

entitled 'Biology of IGF-I: its interaction with insulin in health and malignant states'.

88. Rudman and others, 1990. *N Eng J Med*, 323.

89. Chan, J.M., Stampfer, M.J., Giovannucci, E., Gann, P.H., Ma, J., Wilkinson, P. and others, 1998. Plasma insulin-like growth factor-I and prostate cancer risk: a prospective study. *Science*, 279, 563–566; Hankinson, S.E., Willett, W.C., Colditz, G.A., Hunter, D.J., Michaud, D.S., Deroo, B. and others, 1998. Circulating concentrations of insulin-like growth factor-I and risk of breast cancer. *Lancet*, 1998, 351, 1393–1396; Ma, P., Pollak, M.N., Giovannucci, E., Chan, J.M., Tao, Y., Hennekens, C.H. and others, 1999. Prospective study of colorectal cancer risk in men and plasma levels of insulin-like growth factor (IGF)-I and IGF-binding protein-3. *J Natl Cancer Inst*, 91, 620–625.

90. Chan, J.M., Stampfer, M.J., Giovannucci, E., Gann, P.H., Ma, J., Wilkinson, P. and others, 1998. Plasma insulin-like growth factor-I and prostate cancer risk: a prospective study. *Science*, 279, 563–566; Hankinson, S.E., Willett, W.C., Colditz, G.A., Hunter, D.J., Michaud, D.S., Deroo, B. and others, 1998. Circulating concentrations of insulin-like growth factor-I and risk of breast cancer. *Lancet*, 1998, 351, 1393–1396; Ma, P., Pollak, M.N., Giovannucci, E., Chan, J.M., Tao, Y., Hennekens, C.H. and others, 1999. Prospective study of colorectal cancer risk in men and plasma levels of insulin-like growth factor (IGF)-I and IGF-binding protein-3. *J Natl Cancer Inst*, 91, 620–625.

91. Holly, J.M.P., Gunnell, D.J. and Davey Smith, G., 1999. Growth hormone, IGF-I and cancer. Less intervention to avoid cancer? More intervention to prevent cancer? *J Endocrinol*, 162, 321–330.

92. Chan, J.M., Stampfer, M.J., Giovannucci, E., Gann, P.H., Ma, J., Wilkinson, P. and others, 1998. Plasma insulin-like growth factor-I and prostate cancer risk: a prospective study. *Science*, 279, 563–566.

93. Pollack, M.N. and others, 1998. IGF-1 Risk Factor for Prostate Cancer. *Science*, 279.

94. Pollack, Michael, 2003. Cancer, aging and IGF physiology. Meeting of the Royal Society of Medicine in London in October 2003, entitled 'Biology of IGF-I: its interaction with insulin in health and malignant states'.

95. Holly, Jeff, 1998. Insulin-like growth factor-1 and new opportunities for cancer prevention. *Lancet*, 351, 9113, 9 May, 1373–1375.

96. Chan, J.M., Stampfer, M.J., Giovannucci, E. and others, 1998. Plasma insulin-like growth factor-I and prostate cancer risk: a prospective study. *Science*, 279, 563–566; Harman, S.M., Metter, E.J., Blackman, M.R., Landis, P.K. and Carter, H.B., 2000. Serum levels of insulin-type growth factor 1 (IGF-I), IGF II, IGF-binding protein-3, and prostate-specific antigen as predictors of clinical prostate cancer. *J Clin Endocrinol Metab*, 85, 4258–4265; Stattin, P and nine others, 2000. Plasma insulin-like growth factor-I insulin-like growth-binding proteins, and prostate cancer risk: a prospective study. *J Natl Cancer Inst*, 92, 1910–1917; Chokkalingam, A.P. and 12 others, 2001. Insulin-like growth factors and prostate cancer: a population-based case-control study in China. *Cancer Epidemiol Biomarkers Prev*, 10, 421–427; Chan, J.M., Stampfer, M.J., Ma, J. and others, 2002.

Insulin-like growth factor-I (IGF-I) and IGF binding protein-3 as predictors of advanced-stage prostate cancer. *J Natl Cancer Inst*, 94, 1099–1106; Mantzoros, C.S., Tzonou, A., Signorello, L.B. and others, 1997. Insulin-like growth factor 1 in relation to prostate cancer and benign prostatic hyperplasia. *British Journal of Cancer*, 76, 1115–1118; Wolk, A., Mantzoros, C.S., Andersson, S.O. and others, 1998. Insulin-like growth factor 1 and prostate cancer risk: a population-based, case-control study. *J Natl Cancer Inst*, 90, 911–915.

97. Holly, J.M.P., Gunnell, D.J. and Davey Smith, G., 1999. Growth hormone, IGF-I and cancer. Less intervention. Less intervention to avoid cancer? More intervention to prevent cancer. *J Endocrinol*, 162, 321–330.

98. Yu, H. and others, 1999. Plasma levels of IGF-I and lung cancer risk. *Journal of the National Cancer Institute*, 91, 151–156.

99. Ma, J. and others, 2001. Milk intake, circulating levels of IGF-I and risk of colorectal cancer in men. *Journal of the National Cancer Institute*, 93 (17), 1330–1336.

100. LeRoith, D. and others, 1995. The role of the IGF-I receptor in cancer. *Annals of the New York Academy of Sciences*, 766, 402–408; Butler, J., 2006. *White lies*. Vegetarian and Vegan Foundation.

101. Campbell, T.C. and Campbell, T.M., 2006. *The China Study*.

102. Robbins, John, 1987. *A Diet for a New America*. Stillpoint Publishing.

103. Xian, C., 1995. Degradation of IGF-1 in the Adult Rat Gastrointestinal Tract is limited by a Specific Antiserum of the Dietary Protein Casein. *Journal of Endocrinology*, 146, 2, 1 August, 215; Thornburg, W. and others, 1984. Gastrointestinal absorption of epidermal growth factor in suckling rats. *American Journal of Physiology*, 246, G80–G85.

104. The European Commission. Health and Consumer Protection. Scientific Committee on Veterinary Measures relating to Public Health – Outcome of discussions. http://europa.eu.int/comm/dg24/health/sc/scv/out19_en.html

105. Allen, N.E., and others, 2000. Hormones and Diet: Low Insulin-like Growth Factor-1 but Normal Bioavailable Androgens in Vegan Men. *Brit J Canc*, 83 (1), 95–97.

106. Norat and others, 2007. Diet, serum IGF-1 and IGF-BP3 in European women. *European Journal of Clinical Nutrition*, 61, 91–98.

107. Miller, M.A., Hildebrand, J.R., White, T.C., Hammond, B.G., Madson, K.S. and Collier, R.J., 1989. Determination of insulin-like growth factor-1 (IGF-1) concentrations in raw pasteurised and heat treated milk. *Journal of Dairy Science*, 72, Supplement 1, 186–187.

108. Outwater, J.L., Nicholson, A. and Barnard, N., 1997. Dairy products and breast cancer; the IGF-1 estrogen, and bGH hypothesis. *Medical Hypotheses*, 48, 453–461.

109. The European Commission. Health and Consumer Protection. Scientific Committee on Veterinary Measures relating to Public Health – Outcome of discussions. http://europa.eu.int/comm/dg24/health/sc/scv/out19_en.html

110. Heaney, R.P. and others, 1999. Dietary changes favourably affect bone remodelling in older adults, *Journal of the American Dietetic Association*, 99 (10), 1228–1233.

111. http://www.cancernetwork.com/journals/oncnews/n0007hh.htm

112. Chan, J.M., Stampfer, M.J., Ma, J., Gann, P.H., Gaziano, J.M. and Giovannucci, E.L., 2001. *American Journal of Clinical Nutrition*, 74, 549–554.

113. Hansen, C.M., Binderup, L., Hamberg, K.J. and Carlberg, C., 2001. Vitamin D and cancer: effects of 1,25 $(OH)_2D_3$ and its analogs on growth control and tumorigenesis. *Frontiers in Bioscience*, 6, d820–848.

114. Neal D. Barnard, 2002. Milk Consumption and Prostate Cancer, http://www.pcrm.org/health/Dairy_and_Prostate_Cancer/d_p_article.html

115. Giovannucci, E, 1999. *Advances in Experimental Medicine and Biology*, 472, 29–42.

116. Giovannucci, E, 1998. *Cancer Causes Control*, 9 (6), 567–582.

117. Medical Report: Prostate Cancer. *ICON*, 2002, 1 (5), 8–10.

118. Morimoto, L.M. and others, 2005. Variation in plasma IGF-I and IGFBP-3: personal and lifestyle factors (US). *Cancer Causes Control*, 16 (8), 917–927.

119. Hoppe, C. and others, 2004. Animal protein intake, serum IGF-1 and growth in healthy 2.5-year-old Danish Children. *American Journal of Clinical Nutrition*, 80 (2), 447–452.

120. Outwater, J.L., Nicholson, A. and Barnard, N., 1997. Dairy products and breast cancer: the IGF-1, estrogen, and bGH hypothesis. *Medical Hypotheses*, 48, 453–461.

121. Leonard, Rodney E., 1995. Codex at the Crossroads: Conflict on Trade Health. *Nutrition Week*, Vol. 25, No 26, 14 July, 4–5. *Nutrition Week* is published by the Community Nutrition Institute, 910 17th Street, N.W., Suite 413, Washington DC 20006; The European Commission. Health and Consumer Protection. Scientific Committee on Veterinary Measures relating to Public Health – Outcome of discussions. http://europa.eu.int/comm/dg24/health/sc/scv/out19-en.html

122. Heaney, R.P. and seven others, 1999. Dietary changes favorably affect bone remodelling in older adults. *J Am Diet Assoc*, 99, 1228–1233.

123. Chan, J.M. and Giovannucci, E.L., 2001. Dairy products, calcium and vitamin D and risk of prostate cancer. *Epidemiol Rev*, 23, 87–92.

124. Bradford Hill, A., 1965. The environment and disease: association or causation? *Proceedings of the Royal Society of Medicine*, 58, 295–300.

125. Holly, J.M.P., Gunnell, D.J. and Davey Smith, G., 1999. Growth hormone, IGF-I and cancer. Less intervention. Less intervention to avoid cancer? More intervention to prevent cancer. *J Endocrinol*, 162, 321–330.

126. Ornish, D. and others, 2005. Intensive lifestyle changes may affect the progression of prostate cancer. *Journal of Urology*, 174(3).

127. World Cancer Research Fund, 1997. *Food, nutrition and the prevention of cancer: a global perspective*. Washington, DC: American Institute of Cancer Research.

128. Gunnell, D.L. and 10 others, 2003. Are diet – prostate-cancer associations mediated by the IGF axis? A cross-sectional analysis of diet, IGF-I and IGFBP-3 in healthy middle-aged men. *British Journal of Cancer*, 88, 1682–1686.

129. Allen, N.E., Appleby, P.N., Davey, G.K. and Key, T.J., 2000. Hormones and diet: low insulin-like growth factor-I but normal bioavailable androgens in vegan men. *Br J Cancer*, 83, 95–97.

130. Mucci, L.A. and six others, 2001. Are dietary influences on the risk of prostate cancer mediated through the insulin-like growth factor system. *BJU Int*, 87, 814–820.

131. Yaker, S. and others, 2005. The role of the growth hormone/IGF axis in tumour growth and progression: lessons from animal models. *Cytokine and Growth Factor Reviews*, 16 (4–5), 407–420; Butler, J., 2006. *White lies*. Vegetarian and Vegan Foundation.

132. Schuurman, A.G. and others, 1999. Animal products, calcium and protein and prostate cancer risk in The Netherlands Cohort Study. *Br J Cancer*, 80 (7), 1107–1113; Giovannucci, E., 1999. Nutritional factors in human cancers. *Advances in Experimental Medicine and Biology*, 472, 29–42; Giovanucci, E., 1998. Dietary influences of 1,25(OH)2 vitamin D in relation to prostate cancer: a hypothesis. *Cancer Causes and Control*, 9 (6), 567–582; Willet, W.C., 1997. Nutrition and Cancer. *Salud Publica de Mexico*, 39 (4), 298–309; De Stefani, E. and others, 1995. Tobacco, alcohol, diet and risk of prostate cancer. *Tumori*, 81 (5), 315–320; Le Marchand, L. and others, 1994. Animal fat consumption and prostate cancer: a prospective study in Hawaii. *Epidemiology*, 5 (3), 276–282; Talamini, R. and others, 1992. Diet and prostate cancer: a case control study in northern Italy. *Nutrition and Cancer*, 18 (3), 277–286; La Vecchia, C. and others, 1991. Dairy products and the risk of prostatic cancer. *Oncology*, 48 (5), 406–410; Mettlin, C. and others, 1989. Beta-carotene and animal fats and their relationship to prostate cancer risk. A case control study. *Cancer*, 64 (3), 605–612; Snowdon, D.A., 1988. Animal product consumption and mortality because of all causes combined, coronary heart disease, stroke, diabetes, and cancer in Seventh-day Adventists. *Am J Clin Nutr*, 48 (3 Suppl.), 739–748; Talamini, R. and others, 1986. Nutrition, social factors, and prostate cancer in a northern Italian population. *Br J Cancer*, 53 (6), 817–821; Rose, D.P. and others, 1986. International comparisons of mortality rates for cancer of the breast, ovary, prostate, and colon, and per capita food consumption. *Cancer*, 58 (11), 2263–2271.

133. Mannisto, S. and others, 1999. Diet and the risk of breast cancer in a case control study: does the threat of disease have an influence on recall bias? *Journal of Clinical Epidemiology*, 52 (5), 429–439; Outwater, J.L. and others, 1997. Dairy products and breast cancer: the IGF-1, estrogen and bGH hypothesis. *Medical Hypotheses*, 48 (6), 453–461; Gaard, M. and others, 1995. Dietary fat and the risk of breast cancer: a prospective study of 25,892 Norwegian women. *Int J Cancer*, 63 (1), 13–17; Decarli, A. and others, 1986. Environmental factors and cancer mortality in Italy: correlational exercise. *Oncology*, 43 (2), 116–126; Rose, D.P. and others, 1986. International comparisons of mortality rates for cancer of the breast, ovary, prostate, and colon, and per capita food consumption. *Cancer*, 58 (11), 2363–2371; Shimada, A. and others, Ecological approach to the eating habits and the cancer mortality of Brazilian people. (in het japans.) *Gan No Rinsho*, 32 (6), 631–640; La Vecchia, C. and others, 1986. Age at first birth, dietary practises and breast cancer mortality in various Italian regions. *Oncology*, 43 (1), 1–6; Talamini, R. and others, 1984. Social factors, diet and breast cancer in a northern Italian population. *Br J Cancer*, 49 (6), 723–729.

134. Mepham, T.B. and others, 1994. Safety of Milk from Cows Treated with Bovine Somatotropin. *Lancet*, 334, November 19, 1445–1446; Mepham, T.B. and Schonfield, P.N., 1995. *Health Aspects of BST Milk*, prepared for the International Dairy Federation Nutrition Week conference in Paris, France, June 1995.

135. Plant, Jane, 2003. *Your Life in Your Hands*. Second edition. Virgin Books.

136. Butler, J., 2006. *White lies*. Vegetarian and Vegan Foundation.

137. Butler, J., 2006. *White lies*. Vegetarian and Vegan Foundation.

138. Outwater, J.L., Nicholson, A. and Barnard, N., 1997. Dairy products and breast cancer; the IGF-1 estrogen, and bGH hypothesis. *Medical Hypotheses*, 48, 453–461.

139. Lawrence R., 1994 *Breastfeeding – A Guide to the Medical Profession*, Fourth edition, Mossby, USA.

140. http://www.shef.ac.uk/uni/academic/a-c/csi/1997/pir2.html

141. Clevenger, C.V., Chang, W.P., Ngo, W., Pasha, T.L., Montone, K.T. and Tomaszewski, J.E., 1995. Expression of prolactin and prolactin receptor in human breast carcinoma. Evidence for an autocrine/paracrine loop. *Am J Pathol*, 146, 695–705.

142. Struman, I., Bentzien, F., Lee, H., Mainfroid, V., D'Angelo, G., Goffin, V., Weiner, R.I. and Martial, J.A., 1999. Opposing actions of intact and N-terminal fragments of the human prolactin/growth hormone family members on angiogenesis: an efficient mechanism for the regulation of angiogenesis. *Proc Natl Acad Sci USA*, 96, 1246–1251.

143. Lawrence R., 1994 *Breastfeeding – A Guide to the Medical Profession*, Fourth edition, Mossby, USA.

144. e.g. http://www.inter-medico.com/prolactn.html

145. Holly, J.M.P., Gunnell, D.J. and Davey Smith, G., 1999. Growth hormone, IGF-I and cancer. Less intervention to avoid cancer? More intervention to prevent cancer? *J Endocrinol*, 162, 321–330.

146. Clark, P.A. and Rogol, A.D., 1996 Growth hormones and sex steroid interactions at puberty. *Endocrinology and Metabolism Clinics of North America*, 25, 665–681.

147. Chan, J.M., Stampfer, M.J., Giovannucci, E., Gann, P.H., Ma, J., Wilkinson, P., Hennekens, C.H. and Pollak, M., 1998. Plasma insulin-like growth factor-I and prostate cancer risk: a prospective study. *Science*, 279, 563–566.

148. De Mellow, J.S.M., Handelsman, D.J. and Baxter, R.C., 1987 Short-term exposure to insulin-like growth factors stimulates testosterone production by testicular interstitial cells. *Acta Endocrinologica*, 115, 483–489.

149. Giudice, L.A., 1992. Insulin-like growth factors and ovarian follicular development. *Endocrine Reviews*, 13, 641–669.

150. Westley, B.R. and May, F.E.B., 1994. Role of insulin-like growth factors in steroid modulated proliferation. *Journal of Steroid Biochemistry and Molecular Biology*, 51, 1–9; Marcelli, M., Haidacher, S.J., Plymate, S.R. and Birnbaum, R.S., 1995. Altered growth and insulin-like growth factor-binding protein-3 production in PC-3 prostate carcinoma cells stably transfected with a constitutively active androgen receptor complementary deoxyribonucleic acid. *Endocrinology*, 136, 1040–1048.

151. Culig, Z., Hobisch, A., Cronauer, M.V., Radmayr, C., Trapman, J., Hittmair, A., Bartsch, G. and Klocker, H., 1994. Androgen receptor activation in prostate tumor cell lines by insulin-like growth factor-I, keratinocyte growth factor, and epidermal growth factor. *Cancer Research*, 54, 5474–5478.

152. Holly, J.M.P., Gunnell, D.J. and Davey Smith, G., 1999. Growth hormone, IGF-I and cancer. Less intervention to avoid cancer? More intervention to prevent cancer? *J Endocrinol*, 162, 321–330.

153. Outwater, J.L., Nicholson, A. and Barnard, N., 1997. Dairy products and breast cancer: the IGF-1, estrogen, and bGH hypothesis. *Medical Hypotheses*, 48, 453–461.

154. The European Commission. Health and Consumer Protection. Scientific Committee on Veterinary Measures relating to Public Health – Outcome of discussions. 1999. Report on Public Health Aspects of the Use of Bovine Somatotropin. http://europa.eu.int/comm/dg24/health/sc/scv/out19-en.html

155. Kradjian, R.D., 1994. *Save Yourself from Breast Cancer*, Berkley Books, New York.

156. http://www.afpafitness.com/milkdoc.htm

157. Plant, Jane and Tidey, Gill, 2005. *Eating for Better Health*. London: Virgin Books.

158. Anyon, C.P. and Clarkson, K.G., 1971. A cause of iron-deficiency anaemia in infants. *N Z Med J*, 74, 24–25.

159. American Academy of Pediatrics Committee on Nutrition (1992). The use of whole cows' milk in infancy. *Pediatrics*, 89, 1105–1109.

160. Anon, 2003. UK supports exclusive breast feeding for six months. *BMJ*, 326, 1052.

161. Clyne, P.S. and Kulczycki, A. 1991. Human breast milk contains bovine IgG. Relationship to infant colic? *Pediatrics*, 87 (4), 439–444.

162. Wilson, J.F., Lahey, M.E. and Heiner, D.C., 1974. Studies on iron metabolism. V. Further observations on cow's milk-induced gastrointestinal bleeding in infants with iron-deficiency anaemia. *J Pediatr*, 84, 335–344.

163. Bahna, S.L., 1987. Milk allergy in infancy. *Ann Allergy*, 59, 131.

164. Dunea, G., 1982. Beyond the Etheric. *BMJ*, 285, 428–429.

165. Kretchmer, N., 1981. The Significance of lactose intolerance. In: Paige, D.M. and Bayless, T.M., Editors., *Lactose Digestion: Clinical and nutritional implications*. Johns Hopkins University Press.

166. http://www.fda.gov/fdac/features/2001/401_food.html

167. http://www.ifst.org/hottop19.htm

168. Taylor, S L, 1992. Chemistry and detection of food allergens. *Food Technology*, 46 (5), 146–152.

169. Saarinen, K.N. and others, 2005. Clinical course and prognosis of cow's milk allergy are dependent on milk-specific IgE status. *Journal of Allergy and Clinical Immunology*, 116 (4), 869–875.

170. http://www.ifst.org/hottop19.htm

171. Martin, Peter, 2002. Milk: Nectar or poison? *Sunday Times Magazine*, July 21, 2002.

172. Scott, F.W., 1990. Cow milk and insulin-dependent diabetes mellitus: is there a relationship? *Am J Clin Nutr*, 51, 489–491.

173. Thorsdottir, I. and Ramel, A., 2003. Dietary intake of 10- to 16-year-old children and adolescents in Central and Northern Europe and association with the incidence of type-1 diabetes. *Annals of Nutrition and Metabolism*, 47 (6), 267–275.

174. Chiodini, R.J. and Hermon-Taylor, J., 1993. The thermal resistance of Mycobacterium paratuberculosis in raw milk under conditions simulating pasteurisation. *J Vet Diagn Invest*, 5, 629–631; Grant, I.R., Ball, H.J., and Rowe, M.T., 1996. Inactivation of Mycobacterium paratuberculosis in cows' milk at pasteurisation temperatures. *Appl and Env Microbiology*, 62, 631–636.

175. The Institute of Food Science & Technology Position Statement, 1998. Food Science & Technology Today, 12 (4), 223–228, September. http://www.ifst.org/hottop23.html

176. Financial Times for the weekend 20–21 November 1999.

177. Bull, T.J. and others, 2003. Detection and verification of *Mycobacterium avium* subsp. *paratuberculosis* in fresh ileocolonic mucosal biopsy specimens from individuals with and without Crohn's disease. *Journal of Clinical Microbiology*, 41 (7), 2915–2923.

178. Millar, D. and others, 1996. IS900 PCR to detect *Mycobacterium paratuberculosis* in retail supplies of whole pasteurized cows' milk in England and Wales. *Applied and Environmental Microbiology*, 62 (9), 3446–3452.

179. Pickup, R.W. and others, 2005. MAP in the catchment area and water of the River Taff in South Wales, UK and its potential relationship to clustering of Crohn's disease cases in the city of Cardiff. *Applied and Environmental Microbiology*, 71 (4), 2130–2139.

180. FSA/SE, 2001. Task force on E.coli 0157. www.food.gov.uk/multimedia/pdfs/ecolitaskfinreport.pdf

181. The Institute of Food Science & Technology Position Statement http://www.ifst.org/hottop2.html. Hard copies available from IFST, 5 Cambridge Court, 210 Shepherds Bush Road, London, W6 7NJ.

182. Butler, J., 2006. *White lies*. Vegetarian and Vegan Foundation.

183. EU Directive 70/524 February 1999.

184. US FDA websites: http://vm.cfsan.fda.gov/'ear/m190-11.html; http://vm.cfsan.fda.gov/'ear/

185. Ingersoll, Bruce, 1990. Technology and Health: FDA Detects Drugs in Milk but Fails to Confirm Results. *Wall Street Journal*, 6 February pB6; Ingersoll, Bruce, 1990. Politics and Policy: GAO Says FDA Can't Substantiate Claims About Milk. *Wall Street Journal*, 21 November pA16; and Ingersoll, Bruce, 1990. Technology & Health: FDA Plans a Nationwide Test of Milk for Antibiotics, Other Drug Residues. *Wall Street Journal*, 28 December p10.

186. European Commission, Scientific Committee on Veterinary Measures relating to Public Health, 1999. *Report on Public Health Aspects of the Use of Bovine Somatotropin*, 15–16 March.

187. Plant, Jane and Tidey, Gill, 2003. *Understanding, Preventing and Overcoming Osteoporosis*. London: Virgin Books.

188. Robbins, John, 1987. *A Diet for a New America*. Stillpoint Publishing.

189. Hegsted D.M. 1986. Calcium and Osteoporosis. *J. Nutr.*, 116, 2316–2319.

190. Campbell, T.C. and Campbell, T.M. 2006. *The China Study*. BenBella Books.

191. Ademamowo, C.A. and others, 2005. High-school dietary dairy intake and teenage acne. *Journal of the American Academy of Dermatology*, 52 (2), 207–214.

192. Butler, J., 2006. *White lies*. Vegetarian and Vegan Foundation.

193. Toohey, M.L. and others, 1998. Cardiovascular disease risk factors are lower in African-American vegans compared to lacto-ovo-vegetarians. *Journal of the American College of Nutrition*, 17 (5), 425–434.

194. Park, M. and others, 2005. Consumption of milk and calcium in mid-life and the future risk of Parkinson disease. *Neurology*, 64, 1047–1051.

5. THE FOOD FACTORS

1. World Cancer Research Fund and American Institute for Cancer Research. 1997. *Food, Nutrition and the Prevention of Cancer: a Global Perspective*. Washington DC: American Institute for Cancer Research. (http://www.aicr.org/report2.htm)

2. http://www.pcrm.org/health/Dairy_and_Prostate_Cancer/d_p_article.html

3. Plant, Jane, 2003. *Your Life in Your Hands*. Second edition. Virgin Books; Plant, Jane and Tidey, Gill, 2002. *The Plant Programme*. Paperback edition. Virgin Books; Plant, Jane and Tidey, Gill, 2005. *Eating for Better Health*. Virgin Books.

4. Smith-Warner, S.A. and Giovannucci, E., 1999. Fruit and vegetable intake and cancer. In: Heber, D., Blackburn, G.L. and Go, V.L.W., editors. *Nutritional oncology*. San Diego: Academic Press. 153–183.

5. American Institute for Cancer Research, 2000. Press Release (August 31, 2000) from the AICR Annual Research Conference 2000: New Methods in Clinical Trials Lending New Insights on Diet-cancer Connection, Expert Says.

6. Greenwald, Peter, 2002. Cancer chemoprevention. *BMJ*, 324, 714–718.

7. National Cattlemen's Beef Association, 1999. Conjugated Linoleic Acid and Dietary Beef – An Update. *Beef Facts: Nutrition*, Series No. FS/N 016.

8. Ip, C., Scimeca, J.A. and Thompson, H.J, 1994. Conjugated linoleic acid. A powerful anticarcinogen from animal fat sources. *Cancer*, 74, 1050–1054.

9. Steinhart, Carol, 1996. Conjugated Linoleic Acid: The Good News about Animal Fat. *Journal of Chemical Education*, 73, A302. (http://jchemed.chem.wisc.edu/Journal/Issues/1996/Dec/absA302.html)

10. Campbell, T.C. and Junshi, C., 1994. Diet and chronic degenerative disease perspectives from China. *American Journal of Clinical Nutrition*, 59 (Suppl.), 11,535–11,615.

11. Campbell, T.C. and Junshi, C., 1994. Diet and chronic degenerative disease perspectives from China. *American Journal of Clinical Nutrition*, 59 (Suppl.), 11,535–11,615.

12. Waxman, Jonathan, 2001. *The Prostate Cancer Book*. London: Vermillion.

13. Waxman, Jonathan, 2001. *The Prostate Cancer Book*. London: Vermillion.

14. Campbell, T. Colin, Campbell, Thomas M. II, 2006. *The China Study*. BenBella Books.

15. Ornish, D and others, 2005. Intensive lifestyle changes may affect the progression of prostate cancer. *Journal of Urology*, 174 (3), 1065–1069.

16. Waxman, Jonathan, 2001. *The Prostate Cancer Book*. London: Vermillion.

17. Campbell, T. Colin, Campbell, Thomas M. II, Robbins, John and Lyman Howard, 2006. *The China Study: The Most Comprehensive Study of Nutrition Ever Conducted and the Startling Implications for Diet, Weight Loss and Long-term Health*. BenBella Books.

18. Plant, Jane and Tidey, Gill, 2005. *Eating for Better Health*. Virgin Books. See also, Campbell, T. Colin, Campbell, Thomas M. II, Robbins, John and Lyman Howard, 2006. *The China Study: The Most Comprehensive Study of Nutrition Ever Conducted and the Startling Implications for Diet, Weight Loss and Long-term Health*. BenBella Books; Robbins, John, 1987. *A Diet for a New America*. Stillpoint Publishing.

19. Newby, J.A. and Howard, C.V., 2006. Environmental influences in cancer aetiology. *Journal of Nutritional and Environmental Medicine*, 2006, 1–59.

20. Campbell, T.C. and Junshi, C., 1994. Diet and chronic degenerative disease perspectives from China. *American Journal of Clinical Nutrition*, 59 (Suppl.), 11,535–11,615.

21. *Food Chemical News*, April 29, 1996.

22. Medical Report: Prostate Cancer. *ICON*, 2002, 1 (5), 8–10.

23. Pritchard, K.I. and others, 1996. Increased thromboembolic complications with concurrent tamoxifen and chemotherapy in a randomized trial of adjuvant therapy for women with breast cancer. *Journal of Clinical Oncology*, 14 (10), 2731–2738.

24. Gooderham, M.J., Adlercreutz, H., Sirpa, T.O., Wahala, K. and Holub, B.J., 1996. A Soy Protein Isolate Rich in Genistein and Daidzein and its Effects on Plasma Isoflavone Concentrations, Platelet Aggregation, Blood Lipids and Fatty Acid Composition of Plasma Phospholipid in Normal Men. *J Nutr*, 126, 2000–2006.

25. Greenwald, Peter, 1996. Chemoprevention of Cancer. *Scientific American*, Special Issue, What you need to know about Cancer, September, 275, 3, 96–99.

26. Setchell, K.D.R., 1998. Phyto-oestrogens: the biochemistry, physiology and implications for human health of soy isoflavones. *Nutrition*, 68, 1333S–1346S.

27. Kurzer, M.S. and Xu, X., 1999. Dietary Phytoestrogens. *Annual Reviews of Nutrition*, 17, 353–381.

28. Conil, Christopher and Conil, Jean. *New Tofu Recipes*.

29. Shurtleff, William and Aoyagi, Akiko, 1975. *The Book of Tofu*. Autumn Press Inc.

30. Conil, Christopher and Conil, Jean. *New Tofu Recipes*.

31. Kurzer, M.S. and Xu, X., 1999. Dietary Phytoestrogens. *Annual Reviews of Nutrition*, 17, 353–381.

32. Glenville, Marilyn, 2003. *The New Natural Alternatives to HRT*. Second edition. Kyle Cathie.

33. Campbell, T. Colin, Campbell, Thomas M. II, Robbins, John and Lyman Howard, 2006. *The China Study: The Most Comprehensive Study of Nutrition Ever Conducted and the Startling Implications for Diet, Weight Loss and Long-term Health*. BenBella Books.

34. Glenville, Marilyn, 2003. *The New Natural Alternatives to HRT*. Second edition. Kyle Cathie.

35. Adlercreutz, H., 1995. Phyto-oestrogens: Epidemiology and a Possible Role in Cancer Protection. *Environmental Health Perspectives*, 103 (Supppl 7), 103–112; Adlercreutz, H., Mazur, W., Bartels, P., Elomaa, V.-V., Watanabe, S., Wähälä, K., Landström, M., Lundin, E., Bergh, A., Damber, J.-E., Åman, P., Widmark, A., Johansson, A., Zhang, J.-X. and Hallmans, G., 2000. Phyto-oestrogens and Prostate Disease. *J Nutr*, 130, 658S–659S.
36. http://www.ifst.org/hottop34.htm
37. Adlercreutz, H., Mazur, W., Bartels, P., Elomaa, V.-V., Watanabe, S., Wähälä, K., Landström, M., Lundin, E., Bergh, A., Damber, J.-E., Åman, P., Widmark, A., Johansson, A., Zhang, J.-X. and Hallmans, G., 2000. Phyto-oestrogens and Prostate Disease. *J Nutr*, 130, 658S–659S.
38. Zhou, J.-R., Gugger, E.T., Tanaka, T., Guo, Y., Blackburn, G.L. and Clinton, S.K., 1999. Soy-bean phytochemicals inhibit the growth of transplantable human prostate carcinoma and tumor angiogenesis in mice. *J Nutr*, 129, 1628–1635; Davis, J.N., Singh, B., Bhuiyan, M. and Sarkar, F.H., 1998. Genistein-induced upregulation of p21WAF1, downregulation of cyclin B, and induction of apoptosis in prostate cancer cells. *Nutr Cancer*, 32, 123–131; The Royal Society, 2000. Endocrine-disrupting chemicals. *Document 06/00*. The Royal Society; Setchell, K.D.R., 1998. Phyto-oestrogens: the biochemistry, physiology and implications for human health of soy isoflavones. *Nutrition*, 68, 1333S–1346S.
39. Robbins, John, 1987. *A Diet for a New America*. Stillpoint Publishing; Kradjian, R.M., 1994. *Save Yourself from Breast Cancer*. New York: Berkley Books; McDougall, John, 2000. *The McDougall Program for Women*; Lee, John R., 1999. *Natural Progesterone*. Second revised edition. Jon Carpenter; Plant, Jane and Tidey, Gill, 2003. *Understanding, Preventing and Overcoming Oteoporosis*. Virgin Books; Fox, Douglas, 2001. Hard cheese. *New Scientist*, 15 December 2001, 42–45.
40. http://wayne.unl.edu/00aprilcolumn.htm
41. Martin, Peter, 2002. Milk: Nectar or Poison? *Sunday Times Magazine*, July 21, 2002, 46–54.
42. Website of the American Cancer Society, http://www.cancer.org/docroot/eto/content/eto_5_3x_soybean.asp?sitearea = &viewmode = print
43. Gottlieb, Scott, 2003. Men should eat nine servings of fruit and vegetables a day. *BMJ*, 326, 1003.
44. UK Ministry of Agriculture, Fisheries and Food advice as reported in the *Sunday Times*, 1999.
45. Willet, W.C., 1994. Micronutrients and cancer risk. *Am J Clin Nutr*, 59, (suppl), 1162S–5S. See also: Willett, Walter C., Colditz, Graham A. and Mueller, Nancy A., 1996. Strategies for Minimising Cancer Risk. *Scientific American*, Special Issue, What you need to know about Cancer, September, 275, 3, 88–95.
46. Greenwald, Peter, 1996. Chemoprevention of Cancer. *Scientific American*, Special Issue, What you need to know about Cancer, September, 275, 3, 96–99.
47. Huang, M.-T., Asawa T., Ho C.-T., Rosen R.T., eds, 1994. *Food phytochemicals for cancer prevention I – fruits and vegetables*. Washington, DC: American Chemical Society; Ho, C.-T., Osawa, T., Huang, M.-T.

and Rosen, R.T., eds, 1994. *Food phytochemicals for cancer prevention II – teas, spices, herbs*. Washington, DC: American Chemical Society; American Institute for Cancer Research, ed., 1996. *Dietary phytochemicals in cancer prevention and treatment*. New York: Plenum Press; Liu, R.H. and Espinosa, A., 2000. Bio-active Compounds from Fruits and Vegetables in the Prevention of Cancer. In: *Agriculture in the New Century: Managing Bio-Resources and Bio-Diversity*, National Taiwan University, Taipei, Taiwan, 53–59.

48. Greenwald, Peter, 2002. Cancer chemoprevention. *BMJ*, 324, 714–718.

49. Alpha-Tocopherol Beta-Carotene Cancer Prevention Study Group, Heinonen, O.P., Huttunen, J.K. and Albanes, D., 1994. The effect of vitamin E and beta-carotene on the incidence of lung cancer and other cancers in male smokers. *N Engl J Med*, 330, 1029–35; Omenn, G.S., Goodman, G.E., Thornquist, M.D., Balmes, J., Cullen, M.R. and Glass, A., 1996. Effects of a combination of beta carotene and vitamin A on lung cancer and cardiovascular disease. *N Engl J Med*, 334, 1150–1155.

50. Ursell, Amanda, 2007. Eat a rainbow to stay healthy. *The Times* (T2), 6 February 2007.

51. Medical Report: Prostate Cancer. *ICON*, 2002, 1 (5), 8–10.

52. Levy, J., Bosin, E., Feldman, B., Giat, Y., Miinster, Danilenko, M. and Sharoni, Y., 1995. Lycopene is more potent inhibitor of human cancer cell proliferation than either A-carotene or B-carotene. *Nutr Cancer*, 24, 257–266.

53. Gunnell, D.L. and 10 others, 2003. Are diet – prostate-cancer associations mediated by the IGF axis? A cross-sectional analysis of diet, IGF-I and IGFBP-3 in healthy middle-aged men. *British Journal of Cancer*, 88, 1682–1686.

54. Mucci, L.A. and six others, 2001. Are dietary influences on the risk of prostate cancer mediated through the insulin-like growth factor system. *BJU Int*, 87, 814–820.

55. Giovannucci, E, 1999. Tomatoes: tomato-based products, lycopene and cancer: review of the epidemiological literature. *J Nat Cancer Inst*, 91, 317–331.

56. Willett, Walter C., Colditz, Graham A. and Mueller, Nancy A., 1996. Strategies for Minimising Cancer Risk. *Scientific American*, Special Issue, What you need to know about Cancer, September, 275, 3, 88–95.

57. Ortega, R.M. and others, 1996. Functional and Psychic Deterioration in Elderly People may be aggravated by folate deficiency. *J Nutr*, 126, 1992–1999.

58. http://www.flax.com.fda

59. Greenwald, Peter, 1996. Chemoprevention of Cancer. *Scientific American*, Special Issue, What you need to know about Cancer, September, 275, 3, 96–99.

60. Coghlan, Andy, 1999. Crunch Time for Cancer. *New Scientist*, 13 November, 264, 2212.

61. Pinto, J.T., Qiao, C.H., Xing, J., Rivlin, R.S., Protomastro, M.L., Weissler, M.L. and Heston, W.D.W., 1999. Effects of garlic thioallylic derivatives on growth, glutathione concentration, and polyamine formation of human prostate carcinoma cells in culture. *Am J Clin Nutr*. See also: Li, G., Qiao,

C.H., Lin, R.I., Pinto,J., Osborne, M.P. and Tiwari, R.K., 1995. Antiproliferative effects of garlic constituents in cultured human breast cancer cells. *Oncology Rpts*, 2, 787–791.

62. http://www.3mistral.co.uk/garlic/cancer.htm; see also: http://www.mskcc.org/rande/pharmacology/189.html

63. Inside Story. *Which?* April 2002, 4.

64. Lu, C. and others, 2006. Organic diets significantly lower children's dietary exposure to organophosphous pesticides. *Environmental Health Perspectives*, 114 (2), 260–263.

65. Doll, R. and Peto, R., 1981. *The causes of cancer: quantitative estimates of avoidable risks of cancer in the United States today*. New York: Oxford University Press.

66. Boseley, Sarah, 2006. Expert revered for painstaking work that proved link between smoking and cancer. *Guardian*, 8 December, 2006.

67. Lang, T. and Clutterbuck, C., 1991. *P is for Pesticides*, Ebury Press, Random Century Group, 256p.

68. Colborn, T.T., 1993. Developmental effects of endocrine-disrupting chemicals in wildlife and humans. *Environmental Health Perspectives*, 101 (5), 378–384.

69. McKinlay, R. and others, 2007. Endocrine-disrupting pesticides: implications for risk assessment.

70. Royal Commission on Environmental Pollution, 2005. *Special report, crop spraying and health of residents and bystanders*.

71. Mittelstaedt, Martin, 2002. Data point to breast-cancer risk. *Globe and Mail*, 22 November 2002, A5.

72. McMichael, A.J., 1993. *Planetary Overload – Global Environmental Change and the Health of the Species*. Cambridge University Press.

73. Royal Commission on Environmental Pollution, 2002. *A Short Report on the Environmental Effects of Civil Aircraft in Flight*. Royal Commission on Environmental Pollution.

74. Bristow, Amanda, 2002. *Which?*, April 2002, 22–23.

75. Campbell, T. Colin, Campbell, Thomas M. II, 2006. *The China Study*. BenBella Books; McDougall, J. and others, 1995. Rapid reduction of serum cholesterol and blood pressure by a twelve-day, very low fat, strictly vegetarian diet. J. Am. Coll. Nutr. 14, 491–496.

76. *ICON*, September 2002.

77. http://www.eurocbc.org/page641.html; http://www.ciwf.co.uk/Trust/FF/farm_facts_fish_farming.htm

78. Cho, E. and others, 2006. Red meat intake and risk of breast cancer among premenopausal women. *Archives of International Medicine*, 166, 2253–2259.

79. Simpson and others. Effect of exogenous estradiol on plasma concentrations of somatotropin, insulin-like growth factor 1, insulin-like growth factor-binding protein activity, and metabolites in ovariectomised Angus and Brahman cows. http://www.nal.usda.gov/ttic/tektran/glimpse/data/000007/75/0000077539.html

80. The Globe and Mail, 31 July 1999.

81. Hendler, S.S., 1990. The Doctors' Vitamin and Mineral Encyclopaedia, Simon and Schuster, New York.

82. Hetzel, B.S. and Maberly, G.F., 1986. Iodine, In: *Trace Elements in Human and Animal Nutrition*, Fifth Edition, Mertz, W., Ed. Academic Press, Inc, London.

83. http://www.prostatepointers.org/cmyers/pf0696.html

84. http://www.prostatepointers.org/cmyers/pf0696.html

85. http://www.prostatepointers.org/cmyers/pf0696.html; *American Heart Association Cookbook*, fifth edition, 1995. New York: Times Books, Random House; Pritikin, Nathan, 1979. *The Pritikin Program for Diet and Exercise*. New York: Bantam Books; Ornish, D., 1990. *Dr Dean Ornish's Program for Reversing Heart Disease*. New York: Ballantyne Books.

86. Van de Weyer, Courtney, 2005. Changing diets, changing minds. Sustain.

87. www.annieappleseedproject.org/nutgenprotin.html

88. TV ban on adverts for cheese, the latest 'junk food'. www.dailymail.co.uk, 3 January 2007

89. Kohlmeier, L. and others, 1997. Adipose tissue trans fatty acids and breast cancer in the European Community Multicenter Study on Antioxidants, Myocardial Infarction, and Breast Cancer. *Cancer Epidemiol Biomarkers Prev*, 6, 9, 705–710.

90. Koletzko, B., 1992. Trans fatty acids may impair biosynthesis of long-chain polyunsaturates and growth in man. *Acta Paediatr*, 81, 302–306.

91. Dupont, J., White, P.J., Johnston, K.M. and others, 1989. Food safety and health effects of canola oil. *J Am Coll Nutr*, 8, 360–375.

92. Simopoulos, A.P., 1991. Omega-3 fatty acids in health and disease and in growth and development. *Am J Clin Nutr*, 54, 438–463.

93. Quoted in Small, Meredith F., 2002. The happy fat. *New Scientist*, Aug 2002, 34–37.

94. Small, M.F., 2002. The happy fat. *New Scientist*, 24 August 2002.

95. Small, Meredith F., 2002. The happy fat. *New Scientist*, Aug 2002, 34–37.

96. Ingram, A.J. and others, 1995. Effects of a Flaxseed and Flax Oil Diet in a Rat – 5/6 Renal Ablation Model. *American Journal of Kidney Disease*, February 25, 2, 320–329.

97. Obermeyer, W.R., Musser, S.M., Betz, J.M., Casey, R.E., Pohland, A.E. and Page, S.W., 1995. Chemical studies of phytoestrogens and related compounds in dietary supplements – flax and chaparral. *Proceedings of the Society for Experimental Biology and Medicine*. See also Obermeyer, W.R., Warner, C., Casey, R.E. and Musser, S., 1993. Flaxseed lignans isolation metabolism and biological effects. *Fed Am Soc Exp Biol J*, A863.

98. Van de Weyer, Courtney, 2005. Changing diets, changing minds. Sustain.

99. Trichopoulos, Dimitrios, Li, Frederick P. and Hunter, David J., 1996. What Causes Cancer? *Scientific American*, Special Issue, What you need to know about Cancer, September, 275, 3, 80–85.

100. Djamgoz, M.B.A. and Isbilen, B., 2006. Dietary compounds as anti-cancer agents: a preliminary evaluation of ion channels and membrane excitability as possible target mechanisms. *The Lancet*.

101. http://www.findarticles.com/cf_0/m0FKA/5_62/62702338/p1/article.jhtml?term=turmeric%2C+Liz+Brown

102. Steinmetz, K.A. and Potter, J.D, 1991. Vegetables, fruit, and cancer, II. Mechanisms. *Cancer Causes Control*, 2, 427–442; Lam, L.K.T., Zhang, J.,

Hasegawa, S. and others, 1994. Inhibition of chemically induced carcinogenesis by citrus liminoids. In: Huang, M-T., Asawa, T., Ho, C-T. and Rosen, R.T., eds. *Food phytochemicals for cancer prevention, I – fruits and vegetables*. Washington, DC: American Chemical Society, pp. 209–219; Zheng, G,Q., Zhang, J., Kenney, P.M. and Lam, L.K.T., 1994 Stimulation of glutathione S-transferase and inhibition of carcinogenesis in mice by celery seed oil constituents. In: Huang, M.-T., Asawa, T., Ho, C.-T. and Rosen, R.T., eds. *Food phytochemicals for cancer prevention, I – fruits and vegetables*. Washington, DC: American Chemical Society, pp.230–238.

103. Nakatani, N, 1994. Chemistry of antioxidants from Labiatae herbs. In: Ho, C.-T., Osawa, T., Huang, M.-T. and Rosen, R.T., eds. *Food phytochemicals for cancer prevention, II – teas, spices, herbs*. Washington, DC: American Chemical Society, pp. 144–153.

104. Ho, C.-T., Ferraro, T., Chen, Q and others, 1994. Phytochemicals in teas and rosemary and their cancer-preventive properties. In: Ho, C.-T., Osawa, T., Huang, M.-T. and Rosen, R.T., eds. *Food phytochemicals for cancer prevention, II – teas, spices, herbs*. Washington, DC: American Chemical Society, pp. 2–19.

105. Kikuzaki, H. and Nakatani, N, 1993. Antioxidant effects of some ginger constituents. *Journal of Food Science*, 58, 1407–1410.

106. Zheng, G.Q., Kenney, P.M. and Lam, L.K.T., 1993. Potential anticarcinogenic natural products isolated from lemongrass oil and galanga root oil. *Journal of Agricultural and Food Chemistry*, 41, 153–156; Zheng, G.Q., Kenney, P.M. and Lam, L.K.T., 1992. Anethofuran, carvone, and limonene: potential cancer chemopreventive agents from dill weed oil and caraway oil. *Planta Medica*, 58, 338–341; Zheng, G.Q., Kenney, P.M., Zhang, J. and others, 1993. Chemoprevention of benzo[a]pyrene-induced forestomach cancer in mice by natural phthalides from celery seed oil. *Nutr Cancer*, 19, 77–86; Zheng, G.Q., Kenney, P.M. and Lam, L.K.T., 1992. Sesquiterpenes from clove (Eugenia caryophyllata) as potential anticarcinogenic agents. *Journal of Natural Products*, 55, 999–1003; Zheng, G.Q., Kenney, P.M. and Lam, L.K.T., 1992. Myristicin: a potential cancer chemopreventive agent from parsley leaf oil. *J Agric Food Chem*, 40, 107–110.

107. http://www.pcrm.org/health/Dairy_and_Prostate_Cancer/d_p_article.html; World Cancer Research Fund and American Institute for Cancer Reseach. 1997. *Food, Nutrition and the Prevention of Cancer: a global perspective*. Washington DC: American Institute for Cancer Research. (http:// www.aicr.org/report2.htm)

108. *Journal of the American Diabetic Association*, May 2001; http:// www.wadsworth.com/nutrition_d/special_features/news/nutu1201.html.

109. Thompson, L.U., 1994. Antioxidants and hormone-mediated health benefits of whole grains. *Critical Reviews in Food Science and Nutrition*, 34, 473–497.

110. Thompson, L.U., 1992. Potential health benefits of whole grains and their components. *Contemp Nutr*, 17 (6), 1–2.

111. Elson, C.E. and Yu, S.G., 1994. The chemoprevention of cancer by mevalonate-derived constituents of fruits and vegetables. *J Nutr*, 124, 607–614.

112. Elson, C.E. and Yu, S.G., 1994. The chemoprevention of cancer by mevalonate-derived constituents of fruits and vegetables. *J Nutr*, 124, 607–614.
113. Fox, Douglas, 2002. Bread to blame for plague of pimples. *New Scientist*, 7 December 2002.
114. Forbes, Alec, 1984. The Bristol Diet, Century.
115. Forbes, Alec, 1984. The Bristol Diet, Century.
116. Ingram, A.J., Parbtani, A., Clark, W.F, Spanner, E., Huff, M.W., Philbrick, D.J. and Holub, B.J., 1995. Effects of flaxseed and flax oil diets in a rat-5/6 renal ablation model. *Am J Kidney Dis*, February, 25, 2, 320–329.
117. http://www.dorway.com/badnews.html
118. http://www.stevia.net; http://www.holisticmed.com/sweet/
119. Lee, S. and others, 1999. Monitoring of Drinking Water in terms of Natural Organic Matter and Disinfection By-products. Proc 2nd Intern. Symp. On Advanced Env. Monitoring, Kwangju, Korea.
120. Pesticide residues found in Indian bottled water. 2003. *BMJ*, 326, 352.
121. Herrick, D., 1996. Cryptosporidium and Giardia: Should you be concerned? *Water Well Journal*, 50, 4, 49, 44–46.
122. Jankun, Jerzy, Selman, Steven H., Swiercz, Rafal and Skrzypczak-Jankun, Ewa, 1997. Why drinking green tea could prevent cancer. *Nature*, 387, 15 June, p. 561; see also: Greenwald, Peter, 1996. Chemoprevention of Cancer. *Scientific American*, Special Issue, What you need to know about Cancer, September, 275, 3, 96–99.
123. Jankun, Jerzy, Selman, Steven H., Swiercz, Rafal and Skrzypczak-Jankun, Ewa, 1997. Why drinking green tea could prevent cancer. *Nature*, 387, 15 June, p. 561.
124. Meiers and others, 2001. The Anthocyanidins Cyanidin and Delphinidin are potent inhibitors of the epidermal growth-factor receptor. *J Agric Food Chem*, 49, 958–962.
125. http://www.annieappleseedproject.org/nutgenprotin.html, reporting on a conference on nutritional genomics and proteomics in cancer prevention in September 2002, at the USNIH, Bethesda.
126. Campion, K., 1986. Vegetarian Encyclopaedia, Century Hutchinson Ltd, London.
127. Jankun, Jerzy, Selman, Steven H., Swiercz, Rafal and Skrzypczak-Jankun, Ewa, 1997. Why drinking green tea could prevent cancer. *Nature*, 387, 15 June, p. 561.
128. Why tea is not so good for you after all. *The Times*, 9 January 2007.
129. Oliver, S.E., Gunnell, D.G., Donovan, J. and others, 2004. Screen-detected prostate cancer and the insulin-like growth factor axis: Results of a population-based case-control study. *International Journal of Cancer*, 108, 887–892.
130. http://research.kib.ki.se/e-uven/public/51419.html
131. ENDS Report.
132. http://www.vegansociety.com/html/info/info28.html
133. http://www.vegansociety.com
134. Royal College of Physicians, 2002. Nutrition and patients: a doctor's responsibility.
135. http://www.pcrm.org/health/Dairy_and_Prostate_Cancer/d_p_article.html

6. THE LIFESTYLE FACTORS

1. Berger, Abi, 2002. Science commentary: What does zinc do? *BMJ*, 325, 1062–1063.
2. Hambridge, K. M., Casey, C. E. and Krebs, N. F., 1986. Zinc, In: *Trace Elements in Human and Animal Nutrition*, Fifth Edition, Mertz, W., Ed. Academic Press, Inc, London.
3. Medical Report: Prostate Cancer. *ICON*, 2002, 1 (5), 8–10.
4. McCusker, R.H., 1998. Controlling Insulin-Like Growth Factor Activity and the Modulation of Insulin-Like Growth Factor Binding Protein and Receptor Binding. *J Dairy Sci*, 81, 1790–1800.
5. Josefson, Deborah, 2002. Popping a multivitamin daily can keep disease at bay. *BMJ*, 324, 1544.
6. Van de Weyer, C., 2005. *Changing diets, changing minds*. Sustain.
7. Van de Weyer, C., 2005. *Changing diets, changing minds*. Sustain.
8. Johnson, C., 1999, Environmental controls in iodine deficiency disorders (IDD), *Earthworks*, 9 November, p. 3, British Geological Survey.
9. Greenwald, Peter, 1996. Chemoprevention of cancer. *Scientific American*, September 1996, 96–99.
10. Olivotto, Ivo, Hoffer, Abram and Lesperance, Mary, 2002. In *Breast Cancer Research and Treatment*, http://www.nlm.nih.gov/medlineplus/news/fullstory_10706.html
11. Bender, David A., 2002. Daily doses of multivitamin tablets. *BMJ*, 325, 173–174.
12. *Annals of Internal Medicine*, July 1, 2003; http://www.nlm.nih.gov/medlineplus/news/fullstory_13210.html
13. Kmietowicz, Zosia, 2003. Food watchdog warns against high doses of vitamins and minerals. *BMJ*, 326, 1001.
14. http://www.nlm.nih.gov/medlineplus/news/fullstory_13219.html
15. Oakley, Godfrey P., 2002. Delaying folic acid fortification of flour. *BMJ*, 324, 1348–1349.
16. Reynolds, Edward, 2002. Fortification of flour with folic acid. BMJ, 324, 918.
17. Campbell, T.C. and Campbell, T.M., 2006. *The China Study*. BenBella Books.
18. Feldman, David, 2002. Pathways of Vitamin D Action to Inhibit Prostate Cancer Cell Growth. www.annieappleseedproject.org/nutgenprotin.html
19. Seol, J.G. and five others, 1998. Telomerase activity in acute myelogenous leukemia: clinical and biological implications. *Br J Haematology*, 100, 156–165; Savoysky, E. and seven others, 1996. Down-regulation of telomerase activity is an early event in the differentiation in HL-60 cells. *Biochem Biophys Res Commun*, 226, 329–334; Albanell, J. and five others, 1996. Telomerase activity is repressed during differentiation of maturation-sensitive but not resistant human tumor cell lines. *Cancer Res*, 56, 1503–1508.
20. Gross, C. Stamey, T.A. Hancock, S. and Feldman, D., 1998. Treatment of early recurrent prostate cancer with 1,25-Dihydroxyvitamin D_3 (Calcitriol). *J Urol*, 159, 2035–2040.

21. http://bioscience.igh.cnrs.fr/2001/v6/d/hansen/2.asp
22. Neal D. Barnard, 2002. Milk Consumption and Prostate Cancer, http://www.pcrm.org/health/Dairy_and_Prostate_Cancer/d_p_article.html
23. http://www.rense.com/general/dair.htm
24. Medical Report: Prostate Cancer. *ICON*, 2002, 1(5), 8–10.
25. Barretto, A.M., Schwartz, G.G., Woofruff, R. and Cramer, S.C., 2000. 5-hydroxyvitamin D-3, the prohormone of 1,25-dihydroxyvitamin D-3, inhibits the proliferation of primary prostatic epithelial cells. *Cancer Epidemiology Biomarkers & Prevention*, 9, 3, 265–270.
26. Spallholz, J.E., Stewart, J.R., 1989. Advances in the role of minerals in immunobiology. Center for Food and Nutrition, Texas Tech University, Lubbock 79409. *Biol Trace Elem Res Mar*, 19 (3) pp. 129–151.
27. Redbook, April, 1989, v172, n6, p. 96 (5).
28. Niki, E., Noguchi, N, Tsuchihashi, H. and others, 1995. Interaction among vitamin C, vitamin E and beta-carotene. *Am J Clin Nutr*, 62 (Suppl), 1322S–1326S.
29. Craig, Winston J., 2002. Phytochemicals: Guardians of Our Health, http://www.andrews.edu/NUFS/phyto.html, 03/12/02.
30. *New Scientist*, August 2006.
31. Monographs on the Evaluation of the Carcinogenic Risk of Chemicals to Man, 1982. Geneva: World Health Organization, International Agency for Research on Cancer, 1972-present. (Multivolume work). V29 p. 282.
32. Anon, 2003. Growing problems: Endocrine disruptors under the spotlight. *ENDS Report*, 336, 20–23.
33. Vikse, R. and others, 1999. Heterocyclic amines in cooked meat. *Tidsskr Nor Laegeforen*, 119 (1), 45–49.
34. Skog, K. and others, 1997. Polar and non-polar heterocyclic amines in cooked fish and meat products and their corresponding pan residues. *Food Chemical Toxicology*, 35 (6), 555–565.
35. *BMJ*, 325, 1250.
36. http://www.who.int/inf/en/pr-2002-51.html
37. JIFSTAN/NCFST Acrylamide in Food Workshop, 1989. White paper for Working Group 5: Risk Communication. National Research Council, National Academy of Sciences (NRC-NAS). *Improving Risk Communication*. National Academy Press, Washington DC.
38. Fleck, Fiona, 2002. Experts launch action on staple foods. *BMJ*, 325, 120.
39. Anon, 2002. Acrylamide clues found in Asparagine. *ICON*, 1 (6), 24.
40. Anon, 1997. Acrylamide. Toxic Air Contaminant Identification. List Summaries – ARB/SSD/SES. September 1997.
41. website of the US Environmental Protection Agency, http://www.epa.gov/ttn/atw/hlthef/acrylami.html
42. website of the US Environmental Protection Agency, http://www.epa.gov/ttn/atw/hlthef/acrylami.html
43. http://ntp-server.niehs.nih.gov/htdocs/Chem_H&S/NTP_Chem7/Radian79-06-1.html
44. http://www.nsc.org/library/chemical/Acrylami.htm
45. Anon, 1997. Acrylamide. Toxic Air Contaminant Identification. List Summaries – ARB/SSD/SES. September 1997.

46. Advisory Committee on Hazardous Substances. *Sixth Annual Report* (2001–2002). Department for Environment, Food and Rural Affairs; The Royal Commission on Environmental Pollution, 2003. Chemicals in products: safeguarding the environment and human health. *Report* 24.
47. website of the US Environmental Protection Agency, http://www.epa.gov/ttn/atw/hlthef/acrylami.html
48. http://ntp-server.niehs.nih.gov/htdocs/Chem_H&S/NTP_Chem7/Radian79-06-1.html
49. http://www.foodstandards.gov.uk/multimedia/webpage/acrylamide_study_faq
50. Waxman, Jonathan, 2001. *The Prostate Cancer Book*. London: Vermillion.
51. White, Craig A. and Macleod, Una, 2002. ABC of psychological medicine: Cancer. *BMJ*, 325, 377–380.
52. Walsh, Kiri, King, Michael, Jones, Louise, Tookman, Adrian and Blizzard, Robert, 2002. Spiritual beliefs may affect outcome of bereavement: prospective study. *BMJ*, 324, 1551–1554.
53. White, Craig A. and Macleod, Una, 2002. ABC of psychological medicine: Cancer. *BMJ*, 325, 377–380.
54. White, Craig A. and Macleod, Una, 2002. ABC of psychological medicine: Cancer. *BMJ*, 325, 377–380.
55. White, Craig A. and Macleod, Una, 2002. ABC of psychological medicine: Cancer. *BMJ*, 325, 377–380.
56. Petticrew, Mark, Bell, Ruth and Hunter, Duncan, 2002. Influence of psychological coping on survival and recurrence in people with cancer: systematic review. *BMJ*, 325, 1066–1069.
57. Beales, D., 2004. Beyond mind-body dualism: implications for patient care. *Journal of Holistic Healthcare*, 1 (3).
58. Ernst, Edzard (ed.), 2001. *The desktop guide to complementary and alternative medicine*. Mosby.
59. http://www.nccn.org/patient_gls/_english/_prostate/
60. King, Michael and five others, 2002. Effectiveness of teaching general practitioners skills in brief cognitive behaviour therapy to treat patients with depression: randomised controlled trial. BMJ, 324, 947.
61. *European Journal of Cancer*, 2003, 39, 1562–1567; quoted in *BMJ*, 327, 402.
62. Plant, Jane and Stephenson, Janet, in preparation. *Breakthrough Anxiety and Depression*.
63. Based on Holland, J.C., 1996. Cancer's Psychological Challenges. *Scientific American*, Special Issue, What you need to know about Cancer, September, 275, 3, 158–161.
64. Plant, Jane and Stephenson, Janet, in preparation. *Breakthrough Anxiety and Depression*.
65. Bartram, Thomas, 1998. *Bartram's Encyclopedia of Herbal Medicine*. London: Robinson.
66. *Cancer Epidemiology, Biomarkers and Prevention*, July 2003; http://www.nlm.nih.gov/medlineplus/news/fullstory_13352.html
67. Oliver, S.E., Gunnell, D.G., Donovan, J. and others, 2004. Screen-detected prostate cancer and the insulin-like growth factor axis: Results of a

population-based case-control study. *International Journal of Cancer*, 108, 887–892.

68. Signorello, L.B., Kuper, H., Lagiou, P. and others, 2000. Lifestyle factors and insulin-like growth factor 1 levels among elderly men. *European Journal of Cancer Prevention*, 9, 173–178.

69. Chan, J.M., Stampfer, M.J., Giovannucci, E., 1998. Plasma insulin-like growth factor-I and prostate cancer risk: a prospective study. *Science*, 279, 563–566; Stattin, P., Bylund, A., Rinaldi, S. and others, 2000. Plasma insulin-like growth factor-I, insulin-like growth factor-binding proteins, and prostate cancer risk: a prospective study. *J Natl Cancer Inst*, 92, 1910–1917.

70. *Cancer Epidemiology, Biomarkers and Prevention*, July 2003; http://www.nlm.nih.gov/medlineplus/news/fullstory_13352.html

71. Plant, Jane and Tidey, Gill, 2003. *Understanding, Preventing and Overcoming Osteoporosis*. Virgin Books.

72. Goodman-Gruen, D. and Barrett-Connor, E., 1997. Epidemiology of insulin-like growth factor-I in elderly men and women. The Rancho Bernardo Study. *American Journal of Epidemiology*, 145, 970–976; Kaklamani, V.G., Linos, A., Kaklamani, E., Markaki, I. and Mantzoros, C., 1999. Age, sex, and smoking are predictors of circulating insulin-like growth factor 1 and insulin-like growth factor-binding protein 3. *Journal of Clinical Oncology*, 17, 813–817.

73. Levy, Len, 1998, Biomed II: Exposure to low-level benzene, p. 76. In: Institute for Environment and Health, Annual Report, 100pp.

74. Pearson, J.K., 2000. The Air Quality Challenge, American Society of Automotive Engineers and HMSO.

75. North Atlantic Treaty Organisation, 1988. International Toxicity Equivalency Factor (I-TEF) method of risk assessment for complex mixtures of dioxins and related compounds. Pilot study on international information exchange on dioxins and related compounds. *CCMS Report* Number 176, Environmental Protection Agency, Washington DC, USA.

76. EPA Dioxin Reassessment Summary, 1994, 4//94 – Vol. 1, CER/ORD Publication Centre, USEPA.

77. MAFF, 1997. Dioxins and PCBs in retail cows' milk in England. *Food Surveillance* No. 136, December, Ministry of Agriculture, Fisheries and Food, London.

78. Tanabe, S., 1988. PCB Problems in the Future: Foresight from Current Knowledge. *Environmental Pollution*, 50, 5–28.

79. Department of the Environment, 1989. Dioxins in the Environment. *Pollution Paper*, No. 27, HMSO, London.

80. MAFF, 1997. Dioxins and Polychlorinated Biphenyls in Fish Oil Dietary Supplements and Licensed Medicines. *Food Surveillance Information Sheet*, No 106, Ministry of Agriculture, Fisheries and Food, London.

81. MAFF, 1996. Dioxins in Human Milk. *Food Surveillance Information Sheet*, No 88, Ministry of Agriculture, Fisheries and Food, London.

82. MAFF, 1996. Polychlorinated Biphenyls in Food – UK Dietary Intakes. *Food Surveillance Information Sheet*, No 89, Ministry of Agriculture, Fisheries and Food, London.

83. The Environment Agency, March 2000. *Endocrine-disrupting substances in the environment: The Environment Agency's Strategy*, The Environment Agency, Bristol, UK.

84. Miller, W.R. and Sharpe, R.M., 1998. Environmental oestrogens and human reproductive cancers. *Endocrine-Related Cancer*, 5, 69–96; Plant, J.A. and Davis, D.L., 2003. Breast and prostate cancer: sources and pathways of endocrine-disrupting chemicals (EDCs). In *Geology and Health*. Skinner, H.C.W. and Berger, A.R. (editors). OUP. 95–99.

85. McKinlay, R. and others, 2007. Endocrine disrupting pesticides: implications for risk assessment.

86. Toppari, J., Larsen, J.C., Christiansen, P., Giwercman, A., Grandjean, P., Guillette, L.J., Jr, Jégou, B., Jensen, T.K., Jouannet, P., Keiding, N., Leffers, H., McLachlan, J.A., Meyer, O., Müller, J., Rajpert-De Meyts, E., Scheike, T., Sharpe, R.M., Sumpter, J.S. and Skakkebaek, N. E., 1996. Male reproductive health and environmental xenoestrogens. *Environmental Health Perspectives*, 104, 741–803.

87. Soto, A.M., 1994. Pesticides and estrogenic effects on human estrogen-sensitive cells. *Environmental Health Perspectives*, 2004, 105(4), 380–383.

88. The Royal Commission on Environmental Pollution, 2003. Chemicals in products: safeguarding the environment and human health. *Report* 24; Annual Reports of the (UK) Chemical Stakeholders Forum, 2002, and The Advisory Committee on Hazardous Substances, 2002; Miller, W.R. and Sharpe, R.M., 1998. Environmental oestrogens and human reproductive cancers. *Endocrine-Related Cancer*, 5, 69–96.

89. Charlier, C.C.J., 2002. Determination of organochlorine pesticide residues in the blood of healthy individuals. *Clinical Chemistry and Laboratory Medicine*, 44, 361–364; WWF, 2003. *UK national biomonitoring survey*. WWF.

90. MDuffie, H.H., 2005. Host factors and genetic susceptibility: a paradigm of the conundrum of pesticide exposure and cancer associations. *Reviews on Environmental Health*, 20 (2), 77–101.

91. Mathur, V., 2002. Breast cancer incidence and exposure to pesticides among women originating from Jaipur. *Environment International*, 28 (5), 331–336; Starek, A., 2003. Estrogen and organochlorine xenoestrogens and breast cancer risk. *International Journal of Occupational Medicine and Environmental Health*, 16 (2), 113–124.

92. Frigo, D.E., 2004. Mechanism of AP-1-mediated gene expression by select organochlorines through the p38 MAPK pathway. *Carcinogenesis*, 25 (Feb), 249–261; Lewis, J.S. and others, 2005. Differential effects of 16-hydroxyestrone and 2-methoxyestradiol on cyclin D1 involving the transcription factor ATF-2 in MCF-7 breast cancer cells. *Journal of Molecular Endocinology*, 34, 91–105; Tessier, D.D., 2001. Increased ErbB-2 tyrosine kinase activity, MAPK phosporylation, and cell proliferation in the prostate cancer cell line LNCaP following treatment by select pesticides. *Toxicological Sciences*, 60 (1), 38–43.

93. Kawauchi, H., 2002. Identification of growth hormone in the sea lamprey, an extant representative of a group of the most ancient vertebrates. *Endocrinology*, 143 (12), 4916–4921; Park, J.I., 2005 Conservation of the heterodimeric glycoprotein hormone subunit family proteins and the LGR

signaling system from nematodes to humans. *Endocrine Journal*, 26 (3), 267–276.

94. *Environmental Endocrine Disruptors: A Handbook of Property Data*, John Wiley and Sons.

95. Edwards, T.T., 2006. Reproductive dysgenesis in wildlife: a comparative view. *International Journal of Andrology*, 29 (1), 109–121; Guillette, L.L., 1999. Plasma steroid concentrations and male phallus size in juvenile alligators from seven Florida lakes. *General and Comparative Endocrinology*, 116 (3), 356–372.

96. Colborn, T., Dumanoski, D. and Myers, J.P., 1996. *Our Stolen Futures*, Dutton, Penguin Books, USA.

97. Clapp, R.W., Howe, K.H. and Jacobs, M.M., 2005. Environmental and occupational causes of cancer. www.sustainableproduction.org

98. Webb, S.F., 2000. Risk assessment approaches for Pharmaceuticals. In: International Seminar: Pharmaceuticals in the Environment, Technological Institute, Section on Environmental Technology, Brussels, 2000.

99. Kolpin, D.A., Furlong, E.T., Meyer, M.T., Thurman, E.M., Zaugg, S.D., Barber, L.B. and Buxton, H.T., 2002. Pharmaceuticals, Hormones, and Other Organic Wastewater Contaminants in US Streams, 1999–2000: A National Reconnaissance. *Environmental Science & Technology*, 36, 1202–1211.

100. McQuillan, D., Mullany, J., Parker, J., Mills, D., Sherrell, K. and Chapman, T.H., 2000. Drug Residues in Ambient Water: Initial Surveillance in New Mexico, USA. December 2000 Progress Report, http://www.nmenv.state.nm.us/gwb/drugs.html; Morelli, J., 2000. Are Our Medicines Tainting the Environment? http://webmd.lycos.com/content/article/25/1728_58159?

101. McQuillan, D., Mullany, J., Parker, J., Mills, D., Sherrell, K. and Chapman, T.H., 2000. Drug Residues in Ambient Water: Initial Surveillance in New Mexico, USA. December 2000 Progress Report, http://www.nmenv.state.nm.us/gwb/drugs.html

102. The Royal Commission on Environmental Pollution, 2003. Chemicals in products: safeguarding the environment and human health. *Report* 24.

103. Hamburger Umwelt Institute, 1997. Poor Design Practices – gaseous emissions form complex products.

104. Brown, S.K. and Cheng, M., 2000. Volatile Organic Compounds (VOCs) in New Car Interiors. Presented at the 15th International Clean Air & Environment Conference Sydney, 26–30 November 2000.

105. http://www.le.ac.uk/ieh

106. Dyson, T., 1999. Prospects for feeding the world. *BMJ*, 319, 988–991.

107. McMichael, A.J., 1993. *Planetary Overload*. Cambridge University Press.

108. Park, J.I., 2005. Conservation of the heterodimeric glycoprotein hormone subunit family proteins and the LGR signaling system from nematodes to humans. *Endocrine Journal*, 26 (3), 267–276.

109. Reuters, 8 October 1998.

110. McMurry, Laura M., Oethinger, Margaret, Levy, Stuart B., 1998. Triclosan targets lipid synthesis. *Nature*, 394, 6693, 531–532.

111. Trichopoulos, Dimitrios, Li, Frederick, P. and Hunter, David J, 1996. What Causes Cancer? *Scientific American*, Special Issue, What you need to know about Cancer, September, 275, 3, 80–85.

112. Kross, B.B.C., 1996. Proportionate mortality study of golf-course superintendents. *American Journal of Industrial Medicine*, 29(5), 501–506.
113. www.cancersupportinternational.com
114. Waxman, Jonathan, 2001. *The Prostate Cancer Book*. London: Vermillion.
115. www.ananova.com/news/story/sm_800400.html.

7. WHY ARE OUR LIVES IN OUR OWN HANDS? TEN SIMPLE GUIDELINES

1. Kannel W.B. and others, 1961. Factors of risk in the development of coronary heart disease – six year follow up experience. *Anna. Internal medi.*, 55.
2. Campbell, T.C. and Campbell, T.M., 2006. *The China Study*. BenBella Books.
3. Campbell, T.C. and Junshi, C., 1994. Diet and chronic degenerative disease perspectives from China. *Am. J Clin. Nutr*, 59, Suppl., 11,535–11,615.
4. Plant, Jane, 2000 and 2003. *Your Life in Your Hands*. Virgin Books; Plant, Jane and Tidey, Gill, 2001. *The Plant Programme*. Virgin Books; Plant, Jane and Tidey, Gill, 2003. *Understanding, Preventing and Overcoming Osteoporosis*. Virgin Books; Plant, Jane and Tidey, Gill, 2005. *Eating for Better Health*. Virgin Books.
5. Marwick, Charles, 2003. Food industry obfuscates healthy eating message. *BMJ*, 327, 121.
6. Campbell, T.C. and Campbell, T.M., 2006. *The China Study*. BenBella Books.
7. Schlosser, E., 2002. *Fast Food Nation*. Penguin.
8. Martin, Peter, 2002. Milk: Nectar or Poison? *Sunday Times Magazine*, 21 July 2002, 46–54.
9. Mercer, Chris, 2007. EU unveils milk shake-up plans. www.foodnavigator.com
10. http://www.cafod.org.uk
11. Spock, B. *Baby and Child Care*.
12. Anon, 2003. UK supports exclusive breast feeding for six months. *BMJ*, 326, 1052.
13. Laurens, Claire, 2003. Baby milk company fined for advertising direct to consumers. *BMJ*, 327, 307.
14. Butler, J., 2006. *White Lies*. Vegetarian and Vegan Foundation.
15. Atkins, P.J., 2005. Fattening children or fattening farmers. School milk in Britain, 1921–1941. *Economic History Review*, 58(1), 57–78.
16. http://www.nationaldairycouncil.org
17. Plant, Jane, 2000 and 2003. *Your Life in Your Hands*. Virgin Books.
18. Kradjian, R.M., 1994. *Save Yourself from Breast Cancer*. Berkley Books, New York.
19. Martin, Peter, 2002. Milk: Nectar or Poison? *Sunday Times Magazine*, 21 July 2002, 46–54.
20. Outwater, J.L. and others, 1997. Dairy Products and Breast Cancer: the IGF-1, estrogen and bGH hypothesis. *Med Hypotheses*, 48, 453–461.
21. European Commission, Scientific Committee on Vetinerary Measures relating to Public Health. 1999. Report on Public Health Aspects of the Use of Bovine Somatotropin, 15–16 March.
22. Yu, H. and Rohan, T., 2002. Role of the insulin-like growth factor family in cancer development and progression. *J Natl Cancer Inst*, 92, 1472–1489.

23. http://www.milksucks.com/osteo.html
24. New, S.A. and Francis, R.M., 2003. *Science in Parliament*, 60 (4), 21.
25. Plant, Jane and Tidey, Gill, 2004. *Science in Parliament*, 61 (1), 28.
26. Kradjian, R.M., 1994. *Save Yourself from Breast Cancer*. Berkley Books, New York.
27. New, S.A. and Francis, R.M., 2004. *Science in Parliament*, 61 (3), 21.
28. Robbins, John, 1987. *Diet for a New America*. Stillpoint.
29. www.food-navigator.com
30. Parry, Vivienne, 2007. It's udder confusion. *The Times (Body and Soul)*, 20 January, 2007.
31. Butler, Justine, 2007. Second opinion. *The Times (Body and Soul)*, 27 January, 2007.
32. *ICON*, 2006, issue 4.
33. Martin, Peter, 2002. Milk: Nectar or Poison? *Sunday Times Magazine*, 21 July 2002, 46–54.
34. Bristow, A., 2002. Organic processed food. *Which?* April 2002, 22–23.
35. Bristow, A., 2002. Organic processed food. *Which?* April 2002, 22–23.
36. Inside Story. *Which?* April 2002, 4.
37. Clapp, R.W., Howe, K.H. and Jacobs, M.M., 2005. Environmental and occupational causes of cancer. www.sustainableproduction.org
38. Plant, J.A., Turner, K.T. and Highley, D.E., 1998. Minerals and the environment. Proceedings of Minerals '98 Conference, June 1998; Republished in the *Mineralogical Society Bulletin*, No.119, July 1998, 3–11; *Mineral Planning* 77, December 1998, 3–8; *IM&M Journal*, December 1998, 1, 12, 331–336.
39. Getz, Linn, Sigurdsson, Johann A. and Hetlevik, Irene, 2003. Is opportunistic disease prevention in the consultation ethically justifiable? *BMJ*, 327, 498.
40. Waxman, Jonathan, 2001. *The Prostate Cancer Book*. London: Vermillion.
41. Kushi L. H. and others, 2007. Lifestyle Factors and Survival in Women with Breast Cancer. *The Journal of Nutrition. Special supplement; Intern. Research conf. on Food, Nutrition and Cancer*, 236S–242S
42. Research muddled by political pressures. *The Times (Public Agenda)*, 19 August 2003.
43. Chaturvedi, P., 2003. Medical community may be partly responsible for cancer misery. *BMJ*, 326, 1146.
44. Kmietowicz, Zosia, 2002. Research spending on cancers doesn't match their death rates. *BMJ*, 325, 920.
45. Smith, Richard, 2003. Do patients need to read research? *BMJ*, 326, 1307.
46. Smith, Richard, 2003. Do patients need to read research? *BMJ*, 326. 1307.
47. Corrie, Pippa, Shaw, Justin and Harris, Roy, 2003. Rate limiting factors in recruitment of patients to clinical trials in cancer research: descriptive study. *BMJ*, 327, 320–321.
48. Wald, Nicholas J. and Morris, Joan K., 2003. Teleoanalysis: combining data from different types of study. *BMJ*, 327, 616–618.
49. Smith, Richard, 2003. Editor's choice: The screening industry. *BMJ*, 326, 26 April 2003.
50. Gottlieb, Scott, 2003. US drug sales continue to rise. *BMJ*, 326, 518.
51. Gottlieb, Scott, 2002. Drug companies maintain 'astounding' profits. *BMJ*, 324, 1054.

52. Kjaergard, Lise L. and Als-Nielsen, Bodil, 2002. Association between competing interests and authors' conclusions: epidemiological study of randomised clinical trials published in the *BMJ*. *BMJ*, 325, 249–252.
53. Eaton, Lynn, 2003. Readers want transparency in link between doctors and drug firms. *BMJ*, 326, 1352.
54. Mayor, Susan, 2002. Researchers claim clinical trials are reported with misleading statistics. *BMJ*, 324, 1353.
55. *JAMA*, 2003, 389, 454–465, quoted by Hopkins Tanne, Janice, 2003. Industry is deeply involved in funding US research. *BMJ*, 326, 179.
56. Tonks, Alison, 2002. Authors of guidelines have strong links with drugs industry. *BMJ*, 324, 383.
57. Spurgeon, David, 2002. Doctors accept $50 a time to listen to drug representatives. BMJ, 324, 1113.
58. Gottlieb, Scott, 2003. A fifth of Americans contact their doctor as a result of direct to consumer drug advertising. *BMJ*, 325, 854.
59. *BMJ*, 2003. Drug companies want to inform patients. *BMJ*, 326, 1286.
60. Watson, Rory, 2003. EU health ministers reject proposal for limited direct to consumer advertising. *BMJ*, 326, 1284.
61. Mayor, Susan, 2002. GMC issues new guidance on clinical research. *BMJ*, 324, 384.
62. Marwick, Charles, 2002. US tackles drug company gifts to doctors. *BMJ*, 325, 795.
63. Mosconi, Paola, 2003. Declaration of competing interests is rare in Italian breast cancer associations. *BMJ*, 327, 344.
64. Herxheimer, A., 2003. Relationships between the pharmaceutical industry and patients' organisations. *BMJ*, 326, 1208–1210.
65. Hirst, J., 2003. Charities and patient groups should declare interests. *BMJ*, 326, 1211.
66. Clark, Jocalyn, 2003. A hot flush for Big Pharma. *BMJ*, 327, 400.
67. Writing Group for the Women's Health Initiative Investigators, 2002. Risks and benefits of estrogen plus progestin in healthy postmenopausal women. *JAMA*, 288, 321–333.
68. Moynihan, Ray, 2003. US seniors group attacks pharmaceutical industry 'fronts'. *BMJ*, 326, 351.
69. Cho, E. and others, 2006. Red meat intake and risk of breast cancer among premenopausal women. *Archives of International Medicine*, 166, 2253–2259.
70. Lenzer, Jeanne, The operation was a success (but the patient died). *BMJ*, 325, 664.
71. Walsh, P.C., 2002. Surgery and the Reduction of Mortality from Prostate Cancer. *N Engl J Med*, 347, 781–789.
72. Lenzer, Jeanne, 2002. The operation was a success (but the patient died). *BMJ*, 325, 664
73. Moynihan, Ray, 2003. Blurring the boundaries. *BMJ*, 326, 1094.
74. The selling of a wonder drug. *The Guardian*, 29 March 2006.
75. http://en.wikipedia.org/wiki/Trastuzumab.
76. Bartlett, Christopher, Sterne, Jonathan and Egger, Matthias, 2002. What is newsworthy? Longitudinal study of the reporting of medical research in two British newspapers. *BMJ*, 325, 81.

77. Several versions of the poem, of which this is an extract, may be found on the internet; for example, http://www.madnessmansion.com/~jimkc/txt/ambulanc.txt; http://www.public.asu.edu/~tadams2/Quotes/Ambulance

78. McMichael, A.J. and Powles, J.W., 1999. Human numbers, environment, sustainability and health. *BMJ*, 319, 977–980.

INDEX